Brain Sciences in Psychiatry

Brain Sciences in Psychiatry

David M. Shaw, MB BS, FRCP, PhD, FRCPsych
Clinical Tutor, Department of Psychological Medicine, Whitchurch Hospital, Cardiff

A.M.P. Kellam, MD, MRCPsych, MB BS, MRCS, LRCP, DPM
Consultant Psychiatrist, South Glamorgan Area Health Authority
Clinical Teacher, Department of Psychological Medicine, Welsh National School of Medicine, Cardiff

R.F. Mottram, MB BS, BSc, PhD, LMSSA
Senior Lecturer, Department of Physiology, University College, Cardiff

Butterworth Scientific
London   Boston   Durban   Singapore   Sydney   Toronto   Wellington

First published 1982

© Butterworth & Co (Publishers) Ltd, 1982

British Library Cataloguing in Publication Data

Shaw, David
    Brain sciences in psychiatry.
    1. Neurology
    I. Title   II. Kellam, A.M.P.
    III. Mottram, R.F.
    616.8   RC346

    ISBN 0–407–00236–7
    ISBN 0–407–00237–5 Pbk

Typeset by Scribe Design, Gillingham, Kent
Printed and bound by Page Bros (Norwich) Ltd

Preface

The book starts with a review of neuroanatomy, neurochemistry and physiology. The chapter on biochemistry was felt to be of particular importance, because it has been found essential to refresh and to update a subject most students have not considered for 5–10 years. The chapter on pharmacology is directed towards its application to psychiatry and towards the light it throws on underlying brain processes in health and disease. There are chapters on central and peripheral mechanisms, which may accompany or underlie some psychiatric illnesses and emotional states.

The authors are only too aware of the gaps between these basic issues and the treatment of individual psychiatric patients. However, they feel certain that any psychiatrist who is going to be able to assess new therapies and to modify his practice over the years accordingly, must have this basic scientific training. This book is not by any means a complete account of the subjects discussed, and students must expect to undertake further reading while studying for MRCPsych and hopefully they will develop this into a lifelong habit. Even if the psychiatrist does not undertake applied research himself, he will need his knowledge to be updated continuously in order to follow debate and criticize articles in the professional journals and to assess for himself claimed advances in the understanding of disease processes and new therapies.

We would like to acknowledge the help and advice of a number of colleagues. These have included Dr Keith Collard, Dr Stephen Barasi, Dr Graham Riley and Dr Frank Vingoe.

We are indebted to Professor F. Gibbons for his useful criticism. We thank Mrs Gerrie Ballard, Mrs Jean Clark and Mrs Tina Harris for their secretarial assistance and Mr Malcolm Jenkins for the illustrations.

The postgraduate students attending the MRCPsych Part I course have been of great assistance in deciding on content, etc.

Contents

vii

Chapter 1

Neuroanatomy

The complexity of the relationships between brain functions and behaviour are a source of wonder even to people who spend their whole lives studying the brain. The brain is remarkable for many different features. One is the sheer size of the memory stores, the number of factors in the internal and external environment which are controlled simultaneously, and the precision of that control is remarkable. Other facts underline the unique nature of the brain. At a rough estimate there are 10 000 000 000 nerve cells in the human brain, and each cell receives between 5000 and 20 000 contacts from other cells. This amounts to something like 10^{14} contacts, each with the function of a graded switch—or potentiometer—transferring or not transferring information, and doing so strongly or weakly. As this description of function is reasonably similar to the function of a transistor, computers are a suitable comparison. A large modern computer contains something like 10^{10} gates, or switches; these are often not graded but are simply ON or OFF. This means that the human brain is many times more than 10 000 times more complex than a very powerful modern computer. There also seems to be some principle concerning the way in which the brain handles data which is beyond the current understanding of its activities. When this knowledge is available, it may be that the brain is more powerful than even these calculations imply. Perhaps the variety and complexity of the input–output relationships of the brain are less difficult to comprehend with these figures, but the internal organization of the brain has assumed a greater importance.

Major divisions of the central nervous system

Nerve cell bodies are found in the grey areas of the central nervous system (CNS), and the axons of these cells (i.e. fibres) are found in the white parts. The differences in colour are due mostly to the layers of lipid which surround the axons and impart a white colour on dissection. In the brain some grey areas overlie fibre tracts, but in the spinal cord they lie inside the enclosing white matter. The central grey of the spinal cord projects up into the centre of the brain, giving the basic structure of midline masses of cells (nuclei) separated from the outer grey (cortex) by white fibre tracts.

1

Conventionally the CNS is divided into four parts by planes which pass roughly at right angles to the neuraxis. These parts are forebrain, midbrain, hindbrain and spinal cord. Their approximate positions are shown in *Figure 1.1*, and not too much attention should be given to the precise location of the borders between them. These terms are useful in practical dealings with the brain, and will often be found in current research literature: the phrase 'electrical stimulation of hindbrain raphe nuclei' excludes those nuclei of the raphe group which fall in the midbrain; the statement 'The whole forebrain was rapidly removed and frozen for analysis' means that cortex—deep nuclei, fibre tracts, and all—was collected but the cerebellum

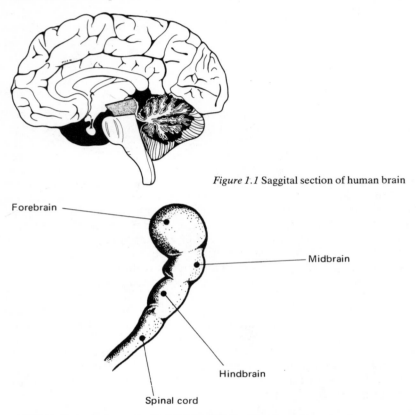

Figure 1.1 Saggital section of human brain

Forebrain

Midbrain

Hindbrain

Spinal cord

Figure 1.2 The anterior end of the CNS in the 4th week of gestation, showing the division into the four major parts

and much else was not. It is also remarkable that psychophysiologists can discuss brain–behaviour relationships in terms of subdivisions. Complex behaviours of many sorts can often be ascribed to the forebrain, while the integration of these behaviours occurs in the midbrain and the hindbrain. Complex reflexes—e.g. balance and respiration—also depend upon the hindbrain or even more anterior structures, but simple reflexes are spinal. Incidentally, it is a mistake to ascribe precision to rough rules like the ones just outlined. There are several exceptions to the general principle. 'Learning', for example, is usually thought of as a complex behaviour, but also it can be shown to occur at the level of the spinal cord.

The four major divisions of the CNS are most obvious during embryological development. *Figure 1.2* shows that at the fourth week of gestation, forebrain, midbrain and hindbrain are clearly differentiated and roughly equal in size. The forebrain then divides into two; the most anterior enlargement becomes the cerebral hemispheres and the part behind it becomes the thalamus.

The major structures visible on the brain surface

The lateral view of the mature brain (*Figure 1.3*) consists mostly of cerebral cortex, with part of the cerebellum, medulla and spinal cord. The deep fissures running through the cortex are called *sulci*, and the folds of cortex between them are called *gyri*. The most important are named in *Figure 1.3*: gyri to the left and sulci to the right. The cerebral cortex is subdivided into the lobes shown in *Figure 1.4*.

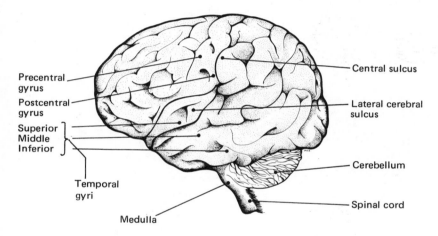

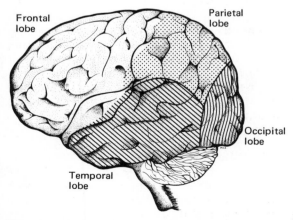

Figure 1.4 Surface anatomy of the brain, II (lateral view)

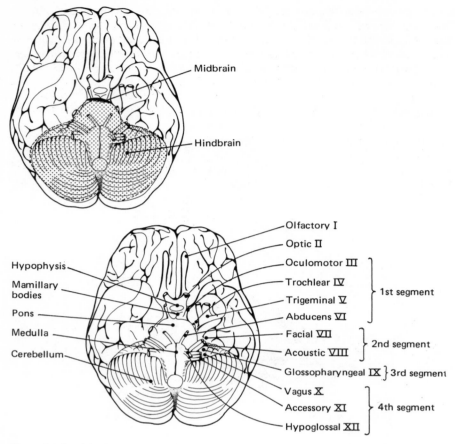

Figure 1.6 Cranial nerves

The ventral view of the human brain presents a more complex picture of forebrain, midbrain and hindbrain (*Figure 1.5*). The hindbrain is represented by the medulla, the pons and the cerebellum; the midbrain is barely visible below the oculomotor nerve. All other structures form parts of the forebrain. During development the brain shows the segmented arrangement which the spinal cord still displays at maturity. As the brain develops, however, the segmentation is no longer obvious but four of the original segmental nerves—fifth, seventh, ninth and tenth—can still be identified (*Figure 1.6*). The hypophysis, or pituitary gland, lies just posterior to the optic chiasma and just anterior to the mamillary bodies.

The major structures visible on cutting into the brain

Perhaps the simplest dissection revealing the internal structures of the brain is the sagittal section. This view of the brain in *Figures 1.7* and *1.8* includes the hindbrain structures—medulla, pons and cerebellum—which can be seen to surround an enlargement of the central canal of the spinal cord. This enlargement is the fourth ventricle of the brain and is connected by a canal, the cerebral aqueduct, to the third ventricle. The position of this ventricle and the two lateral ventricles is not clear from *Figure 1.7* but is clarified in *Figure 1.9*. All the ventricles connect with one another and the central canal of the spinal cord. They contain cerebrospinal fluid (CSF), which is produced by active secretion from the epithelial cells of the choroid plexuses, which are found mainly on the floors of the lateral ventricles. The fluid is absorbed by the arachnoid villi which project into the venous sinuses. The hydrostatic pressure in the CSF is between 5 and 10 mmHg, and the ventricles form a type of internal skeleton to support the brain tissue.

The production of CSF by the choroid plexuses and absorption by the arachnoid villi leads to a circulation of the CSF throughout the ventricles. As absorption is also occurring along the length of the spinal cord, the fluid here is *to a degree* representative of the fluid within the brain. This fluid is in close contact with several

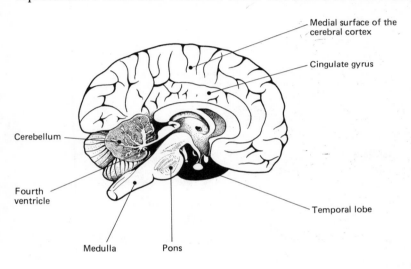

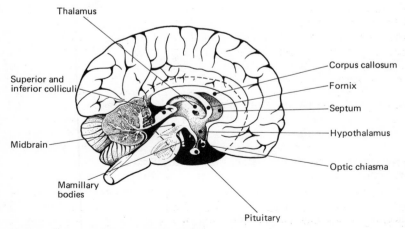

Figure 1.8 Sagittal section of the brain, II

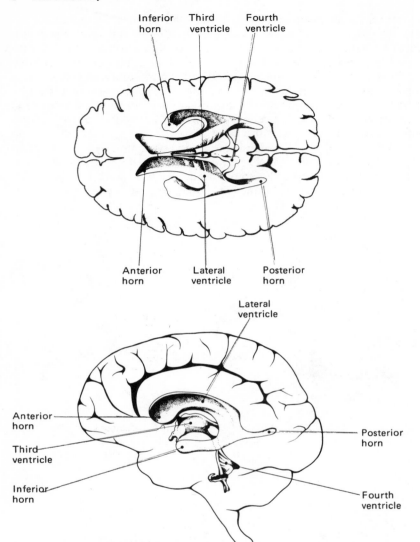

Figure 1.9 The ventricular system

internal structures which are not normally accessible for study and yet, as we shall see later, are of great interest to the psychiatrist and the psychologist. In the 1950s and 1960s Feldberg conducted a series of laboratory experiments on cats in which he perfused fluid past the hippocampus, the caudate nucleus and the hypothalamus. He was able to show that some substances added to these fluids penetrated the brain and also that the fluid contained substances which had come from the brain. For a time these techniques became an important tool for the investigation of the biochemistry of some parts of the brain. Clinically, CSF may be obtained by lumbar puncture. Analysis of the fluids obtained from patients may contribute to the knowledge of the nature of any biochemical disturbances which exist.

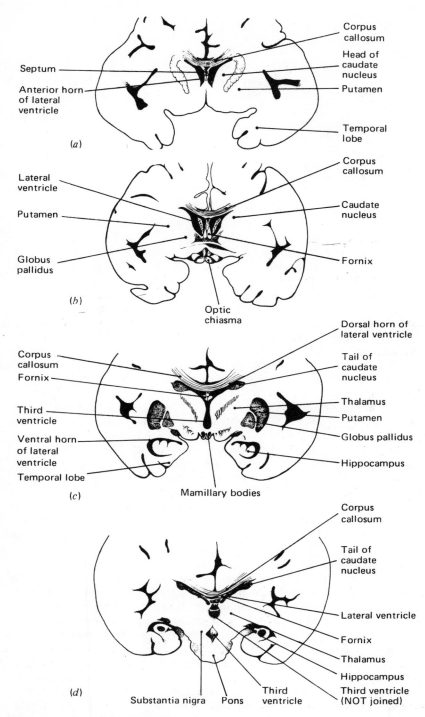

Figure 1.10 Coronal sections of the brain

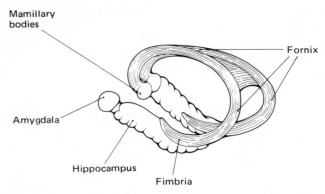

Mamillary
bodies

Fornix

Amygdala

Hippocampus

Fimbria

Figure 1.11 The 'Papez circuit'

To return to the sagittal section of the brain, *Figure 1.8* gives an enlarged view of the central part of *Figure 1.7*. The thalamus forms the lateral wall of the third ventricle and the septum separates the two lateral ventricles. A tongue of the third ventricle projects down into the hypothalamus, which lies just above the optic chiasma. The stalk of the pituitary (hypophysis) projects from the hypothalamus. The midbrain surrounds the cerebral aqueduct, which is the channel joining the third and fourth ventricles. Above the aqueduct lies the corpora quadrigemina (the superior and inferior colliculi). The corpus callosum lies above the lateral ventricles, and its position is best understood from *Figure 1.10*. The fornix passes through the corpus callosum and curls along the posterior margin of the septum, and passes through the hypothalamus to end in the mamillary bodies. These lie on the ventral surface of the brain just on the posterior surface of the hypothalamus. Directly above the thalamus the fornix diverges from the midline, and its path cannot be seen in *Figure 1.9*. However, it can be reconstructed from the four coronal sections in *Figure 1.10* and by reference to *Figure 1.11*. The fornix is a fibre tract containing axons from the hippocampus which flow towards the mamillary bodies. The close connection thus existing between the hippocampus and the hypothalamus is of considerable interest to behaviourists, owing to the probable importance of these structures in the elaboration of emotive behaviour (*see* below).

The curved path of the fornix seems to be repeated by the curling path of the caudate nucleus. This can be seen also in the sections of the brain shown in *Figure 1.10* and the reconstruction of *Figure 1.12*. The massive interconnection between the lenticular nucleus and the caudate nucleus (together forming the corpus striatum) suggests a close correlation of function of these nuclei. The tail of the caudate nucleus curls around the ventral and lateral surfaces of the ventricles to join the amygdala. As *Figure 1.11* shows, the amygdala has many connections with the hippocampus, and thus with the hypothalamus. These circular pathways have been referred to by Papez as the limbic lobe of emotion.

The section given in *Figure 1.10* reveals that the corpus callosum spans the roofs of the lateral ventricles joining the two hemispheres together. This is a physiological role, as fibre tracts run transversely in the callosum, and these fibres radiate from most parts of the cerebral cortex of one hemisphere across to the cortex of the other side. Two other commissures also have this function: the anterior commissure, which lies at the anterior edge of the hypothalamus just below the septum, and the posterior commissure, which is just anterior to the corpora quadrigemina.

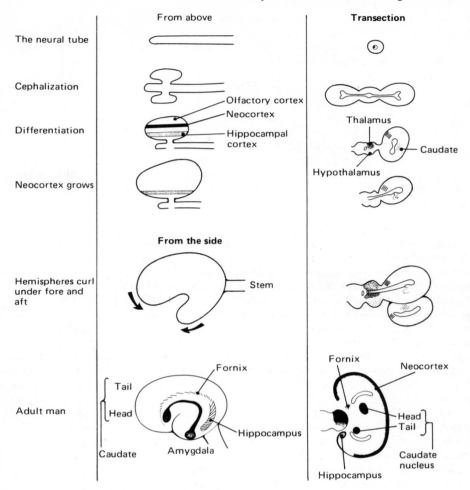

Figure 1.12 Brain development

Before we leave this brief survey of gross anatomy, it may be useful to suggest how these curling paths followed by the fornix and tail of the caudate nucleus probably reflect the development of the brain. At a primitive stage the CNS consists of a tube without visible differentiation along its axis. The lumen of the tube becomes the ventricular system of the brain in the course of further development. The process of cephalization was presumably associated phylogenetically with the animal moving through its environment 'one end first'. As that end was encountering the novel environment, the anterior part of the neural tube developed many receptors. The resultant swelling took the form shown in *Figure 1.12*. Lateral enlargements, containing the evaginated lumen of the tube, look like, and are, early representations of the cerebral hemispheres. The development of midbrain and hindbrain have been referred to earlier and are omitted from the very schematic diagram. Further development and differentiation of types of cortex have been deduced from comparative anatomical and embryological studies. The primitive cortex was sensory, with dense connections with olfactory organs, and had a simpler structure than the newer cortex or neocortex, which developed from the dorsolateral position shown in *Figure 1.12*. The large growth and development of the neocortex caused the primitive olfactory cortex (paleocortex) to be pushed to the ventral surface of the hemispheres, where a primitive cortex with a largely olfactory function is found in man. The portion of old cortex medial to the neocortex was pushed medial and towards the fusion of the hemispheres. This cortex (archecortex) is also simpler in structure than the neocortex and gives rise during embryological development to the hippocampus. The continued growth of the neocortex is associated with a 'curling inwards' of the anterior and the posterior lobes of the hemispheres. The internal structures follow this curling, and, as indicated by the highly simplified diagrams to the right of *Figure 1.12*, some insight into the structure of the adult brain can be gained by a study of this possible phylogenetic development.

The meninges and the blood vessels of the CNS

The CNS is completely enclosed by three membranes, or meninges. From the outside, these are the dura mater, the arachnoid and the pia mater. The dura mater is thick and tough. Within the skull it incorporates the periosteum and lies in close contact with the inner surface of the cranium. A major fold of the dura mater lies between the cerebral hemispheres (the falx cerebri) and another between the cerebrum and the cerebellum (the tentorium cerebelli). Within the dura mater are large venous sinuses (*Figure 1.13*). Below the dura mater and between the arachnoid and the pia mater are spaces filled with CSF. Arachnoid trabeculae traverse the subarachnoid space, and these support the blood vessels which run over the surface of the cortex. Arachnoid villi penetrate the dura mater and project into the venous sinuses. These are the sites where CSF is returned to the circulation.

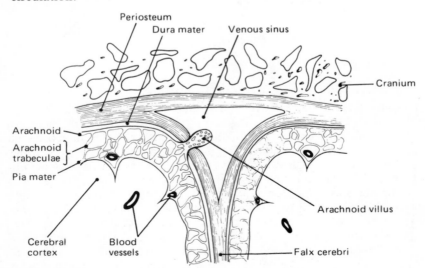

Figure 1.13 Membranes; arachnoid villi, etc.

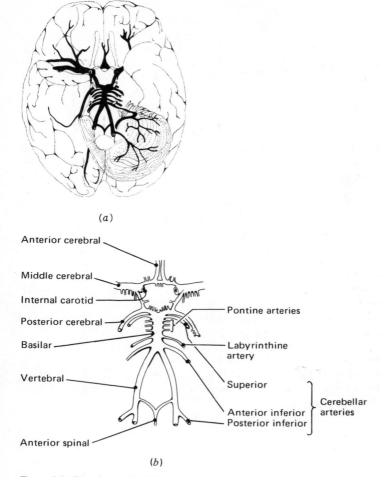

Anterior cerebral

Middle cerebral

Internal carotid

Posterior cerebral

Basilar

Vertebral

Anterior spinal

Pontine arteries

Labyrinthine artery

Superior

Anterior inferior
Posterior inferior

Cerebellar arteries

(b)

Figure 1.14 Blood vessels of the brain

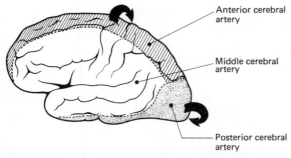

Anterior cerebral artery

Middle cerebral artery

Posterior cerebral artery

Figure 1.15 Areas supplied by cerebral arteries. (The student should attempt to name the areas supplied by the various arteries)

Figure 1.14 is a diagram of the arterial blood supply to the brain. The circle of Willis is formed by anastomoses between the anterior, middle and posterior cerebral arteries. Blood enters the circle from right and left internal carotid arteries and also from the two vertebral arteries via the basilar artery. Occlusion of one of these major supplies does not necessarily prevent adequate perfusion of any part of the brain. Occlusion of any of the branches from the circle of Willis or basilar arteries will lead to a relatively localized ischaemia, however. Each cerebral artery supplies a specific cortical area (*Figure 1.15*). Comparison of *Figure 1.15* with diagrams of cortical function which appear later will give some idea of the broad type of neurological deficit which may result from an arterial occlusion or haemorrhage. The middle cerebral artery, for example, supplies the three cortical areas especially concerned with language, the auditory receptive area and the greater part of the motor and somataesthetic areas. The many small arteries illustrated in *Figure 1.14* which come directly from the circle of Willis ramify within the midbrain; those from the anterior cerebral arteries supply the hypothalamus and those from the middle cerebral artery supply the corpus striatum, the internal capsule and the thalamus. These latter vessels are particularly susceptible to thrombosis or haemorrhage, which give rise to serious disabilities.

Blood from the brain drains through veins which lie on the pia mater into the large venous sinuses of the dura mater.

The brain forms only 2 per cent of the total body weight, and yet receives about 30 per cent of the blood leaving the left ventricle and accounts for about 40 per cent of the body's metabolic activity. A cubic millimetre of grey matter may contain capillaries totalling over a metre in length and having a surface area of $20–30\,mm^2$ for exchange with the tissues. These facts underline the importance of an adequate supply of blood to nervous tissue. Consciousness is lost within six or seven seconds following occlusion of the blood supply to the head, and there is irreversible tissue damage within a few minutes. It is easy to see that many diseases of the CNS may be due to localized disturbances of circulation, although this is very difficult to prove. Such diseases would not be precisely replicated from case to case, owing to variability in the position of the disturbance. However, much of our knowledge of gross localization of function in the cortex is obtained by studying precisely which region is affected by arterial disease and what disturbance of function or behaviour results.

Chapter 2

Neurochemistry

Introduction

The purpose of this chapter is to provide the basic information required to understand the chemistry of brain function. Within the space available, attention to each topic is brief but the treatment includes most of the terms used frequently in biochemical texts. In this way the chapter is intended to provide a bridge to more comprehensive accounts of neurochemistry. There may be topics that appear in both this chapter and Chapter 3, on neuronal physiology. The repetition of such material is deliberate, since it is in context in both places.

General biochemistry

Charged atomic or molecular particles (ions) have important metabolic roles. However, in neurons ions have a central function. Movements of sodium and potassium ions are involved in depolarization of the axon membrane (see Chapter 3). These ions carry a single positive charge formed when sodium and potassium atoms lose a negative charged electron. Non-metal atoms are able to acquire electrons to form negative ions. This means that a solution of sodium chloride is a mixture of positive sodium and negative chloride ions, with electrical neutrality overall. Positive ions are known as cations and negative ions as anions.

In aqueous solution ionic particles are independent of one another and move freely in the solvent. This mobility gives an ionic solution the property of being able to conduct electricity. For this reason water-soluble ions are classified as electrolytes. Despite ions of a salt being independent in solution, in the solid state positive and negative ions form a highly ordered crystal structure. In order to do so, the cations are repelled by one another but are attracted to the anions. The attraction is strong enough to form a stable bond between charged particles and leads to the formation of intermolecular ionic bonds.

In ionic bonds electrons are donated by one atom and received by another, and the resultant charge difference creates an attractive force between the ions. This bond, therefore, is formed by a reallocation of available electrons. Covalent bonding, which is a feature of most organic chemistry, also occurs as a result of electron relocation. However, in this case, instead of electrons being donated by one atom and incorporated into the other, the electrons available for donation are shared between the two atoms. This leads to a bond between the atoms. The simplest example of a covalent bond is seen in the hydrogen molecule (*Figure 2.1*). Hydrogen atoms have a single electron which is available for sharing with another atom. Two hydrogen atoms can form the hydrogen molecule (H_2), in which the two electrons are shared equally between the two nuclei. This is a stable arrangement and is the form found in hydrogen gas.

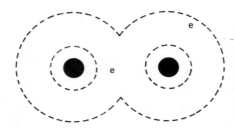

Figure 2.1 The hydrogen molecule. The nucleus of a hydrogen atom consists of one proton. An electron travels at very high speed around the nucleus but is confined within an orbital which has the form of a hollow sphere. In the hydrogen molecule the orbitals of two atoms overlap and the nuclei share both electrons. This figure represents a section through the hydrogen molecule. The orbital boundaries, indicated by dotted lines, retain two electons (**e**)

Bonds formed between identical atoms share electrons equally. However, when different atoms are combined, one of them may have a greater than equal share of the electrons. As a result, this atom has a small negative charge and is described as electronegative. When electronegative atoms are involved in covalent bonds, they have a partial ionic character. This is responsible for the reactivity of many compounds, as the inequality of electron sharing can be accentuated by changes in the chemical environment.

The oxygen atom is electronegative, and this has a major effect on the chemical properties of the water molecule. Whereas the two O–H bonds of water are basically covalent in nature, the oxygen atom attracts a greater share of the electrons. This weakens the covalent bonds and they have a tendency to break. The result is two ions, OH^- and H^+, formed by the donation of a hydrogen electron to the O–H.

This reaction is reversible:

$$H_2O \rightleftharpoons H^+ + OH^-$$

A sample of pure water contains certain proportions of these three species. Equilibrium is reached when the amount of water dissociating is equal to the recombination of H^+ and OH^-. The concentrations of these three molecular species at this point form a constant ratio at a stated temperature:

$$\text{constant} = K = \frac{[H^+] \times [OH^-]}{[H_2O]} \tag{2.1}$$

The square brackets are a conventional symbol denoting the molar concentration* of the reacting ion or molecule.

---

*If $[H^+]$ is 1 molar (abbreviated 1 M), then the solution contains a gram-ion of hydrogen ions per litre of the stated solvent. Since the atomic (or ionic weight) of hydrogen is 1.0, then this is 1 g H^+ per litre. In the case of water 1 litre weighs 1 kilogram and the molecular weight of water is 18. Therefore, there are 55.5 mol water per litre—i.e. 55.5 M.

It has been found that the amount of dissociation of water is small. Therefore, the change in $[H_2O]$ is negligible, and for practical purposes remains constant. Equation (2.1) therefore reduces to

$$K_w = [H^+] \times [HO^-] \tag{2.2}$$

where K_w is the product of the original K in equation (2.1) and the constant $[H_2O]$. Estimations of K_w have produced a value of about 1×10^{-14} M.

pH

pH is defined as a negative logarithm of the concentration of hydrogen ions in aqueous solutions—i.e. $- \log_{10} [H^+]$. In pure water $[H^+] = [OH^-]$; therefore, from equation (2.2) $[H^+] = 1 \times 10^{-7}$ M, so that the pH of pure water is $-\log_{10}[10^{-7}] =$ pH 7.

Acids are solutes which increase the concentration of hydrogen ions. Hydrochloric acid is a strong acid which, in solution, is completely dissociated into ions, H^+ and Cl^-. A 0.1 M solution of hydrochloric acid contains 0.1 M$[H^+]$ and 0.1 M$[Cl^-]$. However, the K_w constant must be satisfied, so that if $[H^+] = 1 \times 10^{-1}$ M, then $[OH^-]$ must equal 1×10^{-13} M. Taking negative logs, we find that the pH of the solution is 1.0. Similarly, an alkali increases the concentration of OH^- and reduces the concentration of H^+. Hence, the pH scale is used to describe the acidity or alkalinity of an aqueous solution.

Buffer solutions

Hydrochloric acid is a strong acid, because in solution it dissociates completely into ions. The majority of acids, particularly organic acids, are weak acids, because they are only partially ionized.

Buffer solutions are usually mixtures of a weak acid and its salt. Such solutions have the ability to maintain a constant pH when acids or alkalis are added. Biological fluids are well buffered to maintain a constant pH. This is usually in the region of 7.4 but may vary from tissue to tissue. A constant pH is important, since enzyme activities are sensitive to changes.

The relationship between the acid and salt concentrations and pH is derived from a form of equation (2.1):

$$K_a = \frac{[H^+] \times [A^-]}{[HA]} \tag{2.3}$$

where A^- is the acid anion, HA is the undissociated acid, and K_a is the acid dissociation constant. Rearranging,

$$[H^+] = \frac{K_a \times [HA]}{[A^-]} \tag{2.4}$$

Taking logarithms,

$$\log_{10}[H^+] = \log K_a + \log \frac{[HA]}{[A^-]} \tag{2.5}$$

Multiplying by −1 gives

$$pH = pK_a - \log \frac{[HA]}{[A^-]} \qquad (2.6)$$

where pK_a is defined in a manner analogous to pH—i.e. $pK_a = \log_{10}K_a$. [HA] corresponds to the concentration of acid, and $[A^-]$ to that of salt. Equation (2.6) then becomes the Henderson–Hasselbalch equation:

$$pH = pK_a + \log \frac{[salt]}{[acid]} \qquad (2.7)$$

As an example of the buffer effect, consider a pH 5.0 0.1 M acetate buffer prepared from acetic acid and sodium acetate. When 100 ml of this buffer is mixed with 10 ml of 0.1 M hydrochloric acid, the calculated pH is about 4.9, a change of only 0.1 pH units. However, 10 ml of the same acid diluted with 100 ml of water would have a pH of about 2.0. Since the pH scale is logarithmic, this represents a thousand-fold difference in acidity of the two solutions.

Equilibrium reactions

Many chemical reactions, particularly inorganic ones, continue until one or other of the starting reactants has been completely used up. A simple example is the formation of sodium chloride by neutralizing hydrochloric acid with sodium hydroxide. In contrast, many chemical and biochemical reactions are completed with some of the original reactants remaining in the mixture. This is because the products formed react together to re-form the starting material. When no further change in the concentration of all reacting substances is observed, the reaction is said to be at equilibrium. A common reaction type in organic chemistry is the formation of esters, which is analogous to salt formation in inorganic chemistry. Esters are produced by the reaction of acids and alcohols, and are typically equilibrium reactions:

$$CH_3 COOH + C_2H_5OH \rightleftharpoons CH_3 COOC_2H_5 + H_2O$$

acetic	ethyl	ethyl
acid	alcohol	acetate

Reactions of this type tend to be slow compared with acid–alkali reactions, and a completed reaction contains an equilibrium mixture of the acid, the alcohol, the ester and water. At equilibrium the concentrations of reactants can be specified in terms of a constant:

$$K = \frac{[ester] \times [water]}{[acid] \times [alcohol]}$$

where K is the equilibrium constant and for a particular reaction is dependent on temperature. The dissociation of water and weak acids described above is an equilibrium reaction, so that both K_w and K_a are special forms of the general constant.

Oxidation and reduction

Cellular energetics centre on oxidation and reduction (redox) reactions. For example, sugars are oxidized to carbon dioxide and water, yielding energy in the process. This energy is used by the cell to perform its functions:

$$C_6H_{12}O_6 + 6O_2 \longrightarrow 6CO_2 + 6H_2O + energy$$
glucose

In this reaction glucose is oxidized by oxygen to carbon dioxide and water. At the same time, oxygen is *reduced* by glucose; thus, oxidation and reduction are simultaneous reactions. The term applied to a particular reaction depends on the reactant which is under consideration. Whereas oxidation reactions consuming oxygen are readily identified, in biochemical reactions molecular oxygen is a reactant in only a few of the cases.

Reduction can be viewed as an addition of hydrogen and oxidation as its removal. This is a biochemically more useful concept, since hydrogen transfer reactions occur very frequently. In the glucose oxidation equation above, the glucose is oxidized to carbon dioxide and in the process loses hydrogen, whereas oxygen which is reduced gains hydrogen to form water.

Most redox reactions in the cell are controlled by enzymes, often known as dehydrogenases. This name illustrates the importance of hydrogen transfer in the reaction. Perhaps the most intensively studied of these is alcohol dehydrogenase. The non-enzymic reaction is

$$C_2H_5-OH + \tfrac{1}{2}O_2 \longrightarrow CH_3-CHO + H_2O$$
ethyl   acetaldehyde
alcohol

Here the hydrogen atoms of the ethyl alcohol are transferred to oxygen. The enzymic reaction utilizes a hydrogen carrier, which is nicotinamide adenine dinucleotide (NAD). This coenzyme was formerly known as DPN or coenzyme 1. The biological reaction is

$$C_2H_5OH + NAD \rightleftharpoons CH_3-CHO + NADH_2$$

The utilization of a hydrogen carrier by the cell has an important consequence. This is that NAD/NADH$_2$ can link different redox reactions together:

where A and B represent the oxidized forms of substances whose reactions are linked by the hydrogen carrier.

General metabolism

Although living cells have complex metabolic patterns, they are based on a relatively small number of molecules, behaving as chemical 'bricks' from which the complex structures are produced. The human diet contains these metabolic building blocks, which fall into three broad classes. These are lipids (fats), carbohydrates and amino acids. The bulk of the latter are ingested as proteins but during digestion they are hydrolysed to amino acids (*Figure 2.2*).

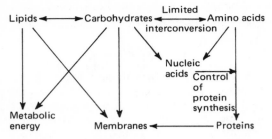

Figure 2.2 Inter-relationships of the major metabolites. The interconversion of lipid via acetyl coenzyme A to carbohydrate allows stored fats to be made available to the cell in a more convenient form. Similarly, excess dietary carbohydrate may be stored as lipid. Some amino acids may be converted to carbohydrates by a single step. Alanine on transamination becomes pyruvic acid

Lipids

Extraction of animal tissues with organic solvents yields a mixture of fats. Some of them may be converted by hydrolysis to soaps (saponification). The group of saponifiable fats contains the glycerides, the phospholipids and the cholestrol esters. These have two major roles. One is to provide an essential part of cell membrane structure and the other is to act as a reserve store of metabolic fuel. The group of non-saponifiable fats contains a number of hormones, particularly steroids.

Fatty acids

The fatty acids obtained from animal tissues are unbranched chains of carbon atoms. Each chain is terminated by a carboxylic acid group (–COOH). Animal fatty acids have even numbers of carbon atoms, because they are synthesized by progressive addition of the two-carbon molecule acetic acid. This produces saturated acids with the general formula $C_nH_{(2n + 1)}COOH$. The most abundant of these are palmitic acid (*Figure 2.3*) and stearic acid ($C_{17}H_{35}COOH$).

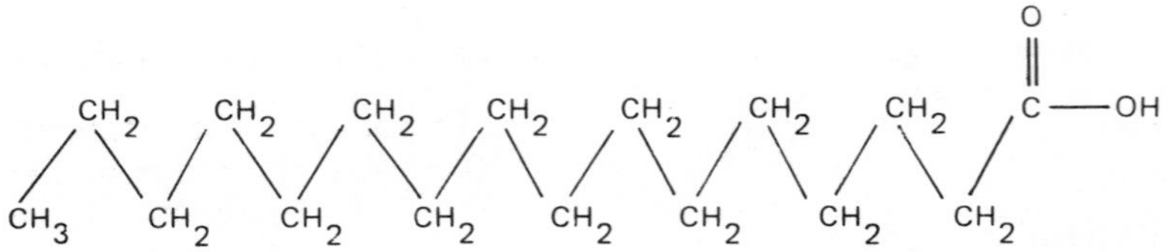

Figure 2.3 Palmitic acid ($C_{15}H_{31}COOH$)

Chemically, fatty acids are saturated when carbon–carbon double bonds are absent. Unsaturated fatty acids with double bonds are also found in mixtures of the saponified fats. Some of the unsaturated fatty acids provide the starting material for the synthesis of prostaglandins. Apart from this, the detailed specific functions of the saturated, compared with the unsaturated, fatty acids is not clear. However, lipids containing unsaturated fatty acids are liquid at lower temperatures, whereas saturated fats tend to be solid. The fluidity of membranes may well be controlled by a balance of the two groups of fatty acids.

Glycerides

The glycerides are esters of glycerol and fatty acids. Glycerol has three alcohol hydroxyl groups which can be substituted to give monoglycerides, diglycerides or

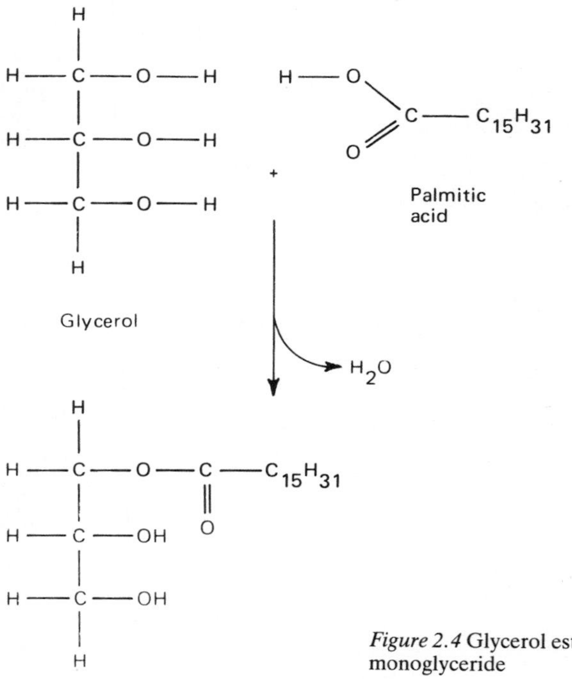

Figure 2.4 Glycerol esterified to palmitic acid to form a monoglyceride

triglycerides (*Figure 2.4*). In most animal tissues the fully esterified triglycerides predominate.

Phospholipids

Phospholipids (*Figure 2.5*) are diglycerides with the third hydroxyl group esterified to inorganic phosphoric acid instead of an organic fatty acid. In addition, the phosphoric acid is further esterified to an amino alcohol. This is usually one of either choline, serine or ethanolamine.

Cholesterol

Cholesterol (*Figure 2.6*) is a steroid of major importance. It has a role in the structure of cell membranes, both in its free form and when esterified to a fatty acid. A second metabolic function is as the starting point for synthesis of the many steroid hormones.

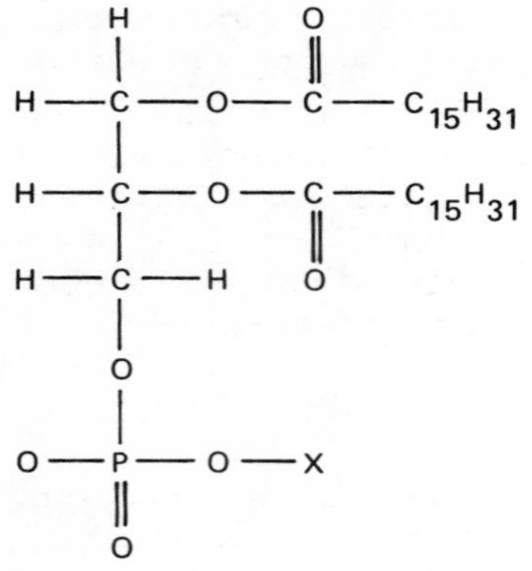

$$
\begin{array}{ccc}
\text{H} & & \text{O} \\
| & & \| \\
\text{H}-\text{C}-\text{O}-\text{C}-\text{C}_{15}\text{H}_{31} \\
| \\
\text{H}-\text{C}-\text{O}-\text{C}-\text{C}_{15}\text{H}_{31} \\
| & & \| \\
\text{H}-\text{C}-\text{H} & & \text{O} \\
| \\
\text{O} \\
| \\
\text{O}-\text{P}-\text{O}-\text{X} \\
\| \\
\text{O}
\end{array}
$$

Where X is from one of the three organic bases (HO—X):

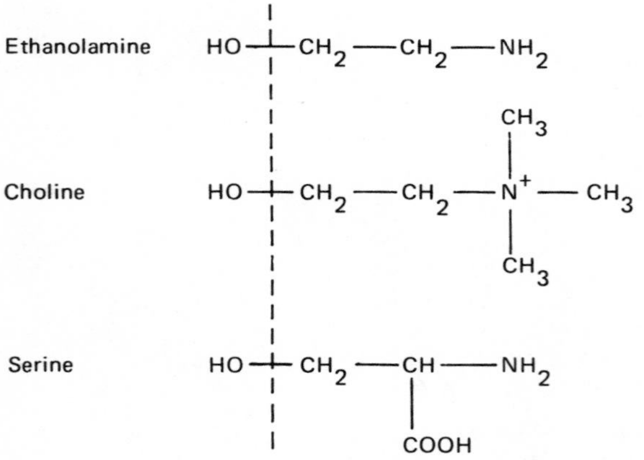

Ethanolamine $\text{HO}-\text{CH}_2-\text{CH}_2-\text{NH}_2$

Choline $\text{HO}-\text{CH}_2-\text{CH}_2-\overset{+}{\text{N}}(\text{CH}_3)_3$

$$
\begin{array}{c}
\text{CH}_3 \\
| \\
\text{HO}-\text{CH}_2-\text{CH}_2-\overset{+}{\text{N}}-\text{CH}_3 \\
| \\
\text{CH}_3
\end{array}
$$

Serine
$$
\begin{array}{c}
\text{HO}-\text{CH}_2-\text{CH}-\text{NH}_2 \\
| \\
\text{COOH}
\end{array}
$$

Figure 2.5 General structure of the phosphoglycerides

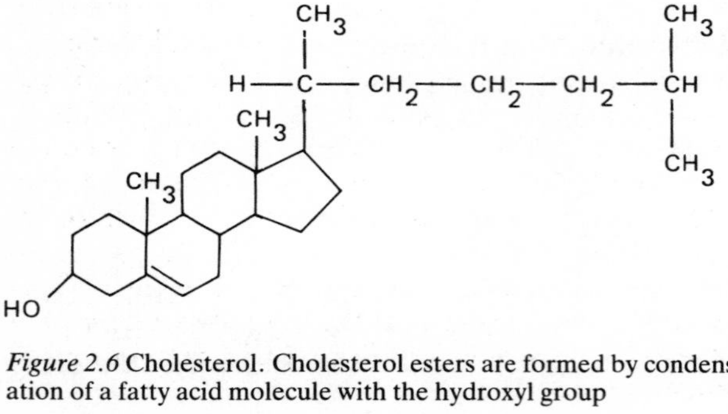

$$
\begin{array}{c}
\text{CH}_3 \qquad\qquad\qquad \text{CH}_3 \\
| \qquad\qquad\qquad\qquad | \\
\text{H}-\text{C}-\text{CH}_2-\text{CH}_2-\text{CH}_2-\text{CH} \\
| \qquad\qquad\qquad\qquad | \\
\text{CH}_3 \qquad\qquad\qquad \text{CH}_3
\end{array}
$$

Figure 2.6 Cholesterol. Cholesterol esters are formed by condensation of a fatty acid molecule with the hydroxyl group

Sphingolipids

The sphingolipids are a group of several lipids which have important functions, although they are found in smaller quantities than are the other lipids. Their structure has similarities with the fatty acids in that they have a long hydrocarbon tail. However, they differ in that instead of a carboxyl group, as in fatty acids, sphingolipids have amino ($-NH_2$) and hydroxyl ($-OH$) groups. Conjugation of the amino group with glucose yields cerebrosides. Sphingolipids are important components of the myelin in Schwann cells in the peripheral nervous system.

Carbohydrates

The carbohydrates found in cells are all based on simple sugars—hydroxyaldehydes or hydroxyketones (*Figure 2.7*). These sugars are reducing agents. This property is used in detection procedures, notably Fehling's test.

Glucose (*Figure 2.7*) is the most important naturally occurring carbohydrate, as cellular metabolism is centred on this sugar. Other sugars (fructose, mannose and galactose) occur extensively but none is metabolized as readily as is glucose. The six

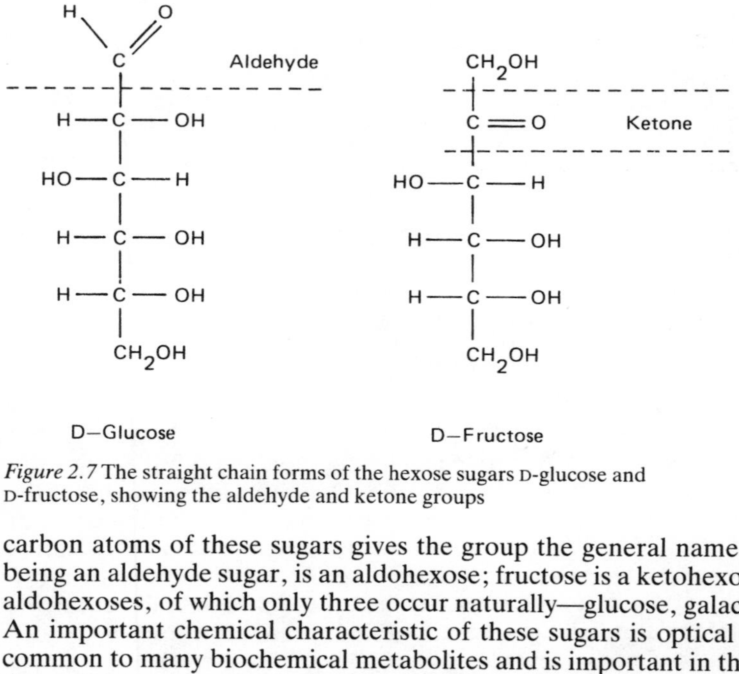

Figure 2.7 The straight chain forms of the hexose sugars D-glucose and D-fructose, showing the aldehyde and ketone groups

carbon atoms of these sugars gives the group the general name hexoses. Glucose, being an aldehyde sugar, is an aldohexose; fructose is a ketohexose. There are eight aldohexoses, of which only three occur naturally—glucose, galactose and mannose. An important chemical characteristic of these sugars is optical isomerism. This is common to many biochemical metabolites and is important in the understanding of the actions of small molecules in biology. Optical isomerism occurs when a molecule has a non-superimposable mirror image, and is of most importance in biochemistry when a carbon chain is attached to four different chemical groups. Under these conditions, a carbon atom is described as asymmetric. In *Figure 2.8* the chemical groups attached to the central carbon atom are represented by W, X, Y and Z. 8(1) is the mirror image of 8(2) and they cannot be superimposed on each other. If group X were the same as group Y, 8(1) and 8(2) would remain mirror images but the two molecules would be identical.

The chemical reactions of the two optical isomers are in most cases identical, and chemical synthesis usually results in an equal mixture of both. This is known as a racemic mixture. Separation of the two forms yields compounds having 'optical activity' associated with this type of isomerism. A solution of an optically active solute is able to rotate the plane of polarized light which passes through the solution. One isomer will rotate the light a few degrees to the left and the other an equal amount to the right. Hence the descriptions laevorotatory and dextrorotatory. Dextrose is the glucose isomer which rotates the polarized light to the right. A conventional shorthand to denote which molecule is being described is either (+) or (*d*) for dextrorotation or (–) or (*l*) for laevorotation. Dextrose is therefore either (+)-glucose or (*d*)-glucose.

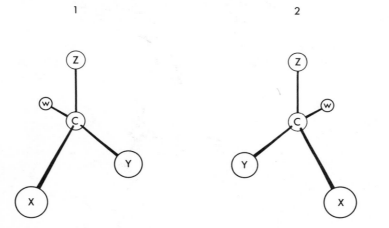

Figure 2.8 Optical isomerism. The central carbon atom (C) is attached to four different atoms W, X, Y and Z. Two different arrangements of these are possible because of the tetrahedral orientation of the carbon valencies. Arrangement 1 is the mirror image of 2. If 2 is rotated anticlockwise about the Z–C axis so that the position of W of 1 matches that of 2, the positions of X and Y on 1 are reversed on 2

Some confusion can arise from an independent notation of optical isomerism. This refers not to the light-rotating properties but to the spatial arrangement of the chemical groups attached to the asymmetric carbon atoms. The notation used for the two forms is L and D. The chemical reasons for the assignment of this notation are beyond the scope of this chapter. It should, however, be noted that this notation has nothing to do with the direction of light rotation. Naturally occurring glucose is dextrorotatory and belongs to the D-series, yet natural fructose, which also belongs to the D-series, is laevorotatory. Cellular chemistry has a distinct preference for particular optical isomers. In mammalian tissues the carbohydrates belong to the D-series and amino acids which have an asymmetric carbon atom belong to the L-series—e.g. L-Dopa.

Many large carbohydrates are found both in the cell membrane and within the cell itself. These large molecules (polymers) consist of chains of much smaller molecules. Starch and glycogen are polysaccharide chains of repeating glucose units. Both starch in plants and glycogen in muscle and liver are relatively insoluble and are storage forms of glucose. The insolubility of starch allows the cell to store large amounts of glucose without affecting the concentration of cell contents. Short-chain soluble saccharides also occur in nature—e.g. sucrose and lactose. Both of these are pairs of hexose molecules, sucrose being glucose and fructose and lactose being glucose and galactose.

Amino acids

Amino acids are molecules which possess amino ($-NH_2$) and carboxylic acid ($-COOH$) groups. Although several types of these compounds are found in living tissues, the name is usually used to refer to the 20 naturally occurring alpha amino acids. These can be isolated from all tissues or from the hydrolysis of proteins. The Greek letter α refers to the position of the amino group relative to the acid group (*Figure 2.9*). This notation is used to name the carbon atoms of the main carbon chain, starting with the α-carbon adjacent to the carboxyl group. The α-carbon atom of alpha alanine (*Figure 2.9*) has four different groups attached to it and therefore the amino acid occurs as two optical isomers, L and D. However, in most life forms, with the exception of a few bacteria, the alpha amino acids all belong to the L-series. Of the 20 alpha-amino acids occurring naturally, only glycine is not optically active.

The alpha amino acids are metabolized in a variety of ways. Some are oxidized and contribute to the energy production of the cell. Also, some are incorporated into small molecules—e.g. nucleotides and neurotransmitters. However, in most tissues the metabolism of alpha amino acids is closely linked with protein metabolism. Proteins are unbranched chains of amino acids. These polymers are formed by way of peptide bonds between the alpha amino and alpha carboxylic groups of adjacent amino acids (*Figure 2.10*). The formation of the bond eliminates water. Thus, hydrolysis of the peptide bonds of protein yields a mixture of the component amino acids.

Although the peptide link always produces unbranched chains of amino acids, two chains may be joined by a cystine 'bridge'. This is formed between two molecules of the amino acid cysteine, one in each peptide chain. Cysteine is a sulphydryl ($-SH$) amino acid which may be oxidized with a second cysteine molecule to form cystine (*Figure 2.11*). The two peptide chains of insulin are held together in this way.

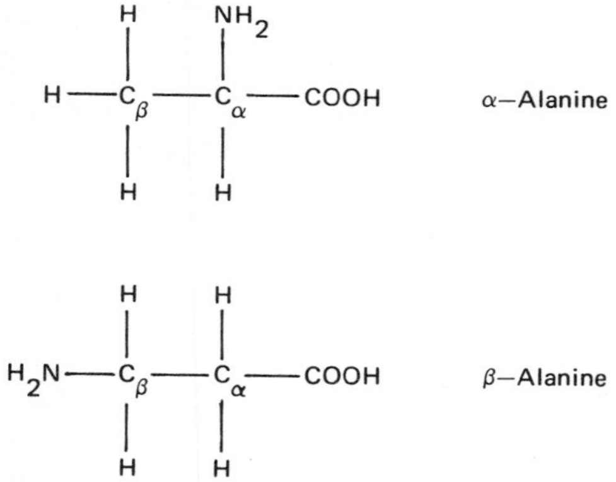

Figure 2.9 α-Alanine and β-alanine

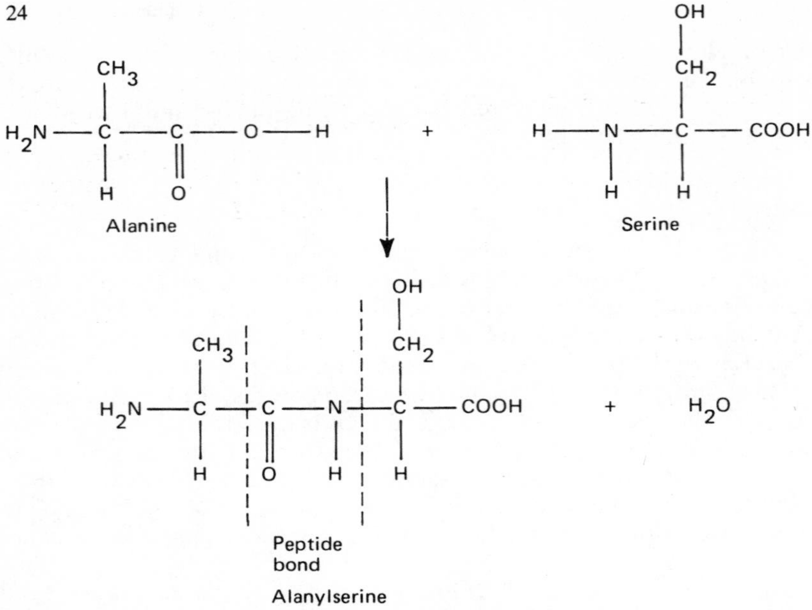

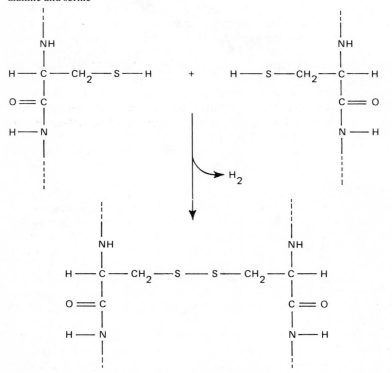

Figure 2.10 Formation of a peptide bond by the condensation of two alpha amino acids, alanine and serine

Figure 2.11 Formation of a cystine 'bridge' between two cysteine molecules within peptide chains

Other amino acids

Several other amino acids not normally found in proteins are found in animal cells. Orthinine and citrulline are alpha amino acids which are not found in proteins but which are important components in the metabolism of nitrogen compounds via the urea cycle. Other important alpha amino acids include the thyroid hormones, tri-iodothyronine (T_3) and thyroxine (T_4), which are derived from tyrosine. When

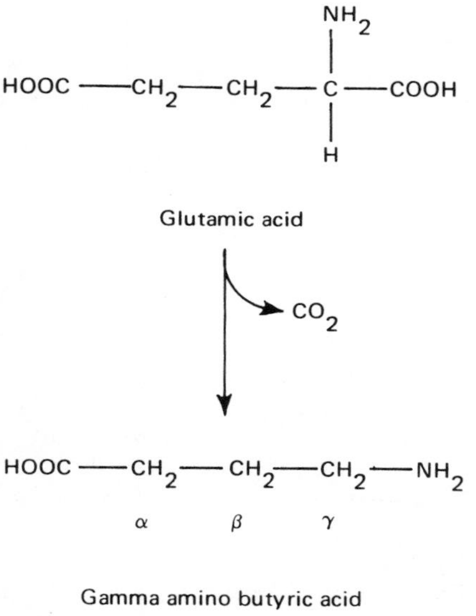

$$HOOC-CH_2-CH_2-\underset{\underset{H}{|}}{\overset{\overset{NH_2}{|}}{C}}-COOH$$

Glutamic acid

$\longrightarrow CO_2$

$$HOOC-\underset{\alpha}{CH_2}-\underset{\beta}{CH_2}-\underset{\gamma}{CH_2}-NH_2$$

Gamma amino butyric acid

Figure 2.12 Biosynthesis of gamma aminobutyric acid (GABA)

glutamic acid is decarboxylated, an amino acid is produced which has an important function as a neurotransmitter. This is gamma aminobutyric acid (GABA) (*Figure 2.12*).

Coenzymes

The three principal classes of metabolites—lipids, carbohydrates and amino acids—provide the fuel for cells, together with the components necessary for building their physical structure. These interconversions are carried out by the cell's enzyme machinery with the aid of a number of essential cofactors. These are known as coenzymes and their presence is required to convert some enzymes into the active form.

Some vitamins are incorporated into the structure of coenzymes, providing a link between nutritional status and biochemical activity. However, it must be remembered that coenzymes are found in all tissues and are not confined to those in which a particular deficiency is first observed.

The specialist function of most coenzymes is to transfer atoms or groups of atoms from one molecule to another. Although the donor and the recipient molecules may vary widely, in most cases each coenzyme only transfers one atom or group of atoms. Of the dozen or so major coenzymes which have been identified, those playing the central role in the cell are the *adenine nucleotides*.

Adenosine phosphates

Adenosine monophosphate (AMP) is a phosphate ester of adenosine (*Figure 2.13*). When the phosphate group is attached to another phosphoric acid molecule by an acid anhydride linkage, adenosine diphosphate (ADP) is produced. Similar addition of a further phosphoric acid molecule yields adenosine triphosphate (ATP). There is an important chemical difference, which has functional consequences, between the phosphate ester linkage in AMP and the phosphate

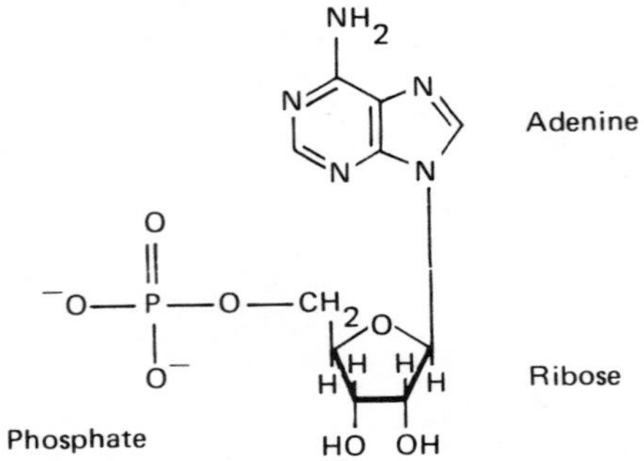

Figure 2.13 Adenosine monophosphate (AMP)

anhydrides of ADP and ATP, despite the fact that all are formed by the removal of a molecule of water. The chemical energy required to form the ester bond is relatively small. However, acid anhydride formation requires a considerable input of energy, with release of energy on hydrolysis of the anhydride. In ATP the energy requirements for the making and breaking of the phosphate anhydride provide a mechanism for the transfer of energy between biochemical reactions.

The general method of energy transfer in biochemical reactions is:

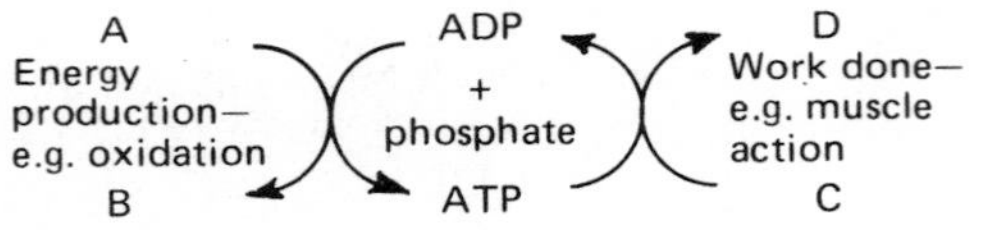

Metabolite A is oxidized to B, which leads to release of energy. The reaction mechanism allows a portion of the energy to be used to synthesize ATP from ADP and phosphoric acid. The ATP from this reaction can be used to provide the chemical energy to drive another metabolic step elsewhere in the cell. This energy transfer, using ADP, is analogous to the hydrogen transfer, using NAD, described previously (*see* page 17).

The utilization by the cell of a single energy transfer molecule for most of its metabolic conversions has many advantages, chief of which is that all metabolic fuels are converted to a single product, which allows energy-requiring processes to draw on a single pool. This allows a diverse variety of molecules to provide the energy for an equally diverse variety of functions. Another slightly more subtle advantage is in terms of the control of the metabolism. As the total amount of adenosine phosphates is reasonably constant, it follows that if the proportion of ATP increases, oxidation reactions linked closely with ADP availability are curtailed. This provides a coarse control of metabolism.

A fourth adenine nucleotide has recently been identified. This is adenosine 3',5'-monophosphate, usually known as cyclic AMP because of the ring formed

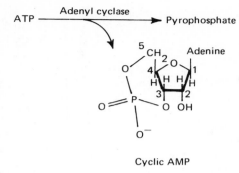

Figure 2.14 3′,5′-cyclic adenosine monophosphate (cyclic AMP) and its synthesis from ATP, with the enzyme adenyl cyclase. The numbers on the ribose ring structure indicate the numbers used in the nomenclature of cyclic AMP

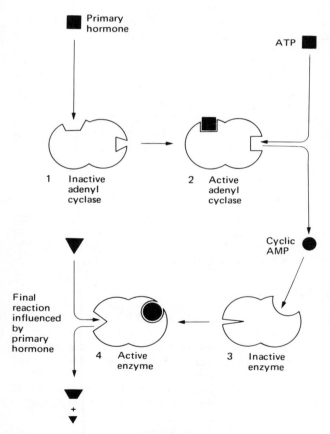

Figure 2.15 Cyclic AMP as a metabolic relay. (1) The primary hormone binds to an inactive form of the enzyme adenyl cyclase and converts it to an active form; (2) the active enzyme converts ATP to cyclic AMP; (3) cyclic AMP activates an enzyme, which; (4) catalyses a metabolic reaction

between the sugar and the phosphate molecules (*Figure 2.14*). Unlike other coenzymes, cyclic AMP does not appear to take part in transfer reactions but operates by activating certain enzymes. In the absence of cyclic AMP, these enzymes would either be unreactive or have very low activity. A consistent pattern of cyclic AMP involvement in many cellular reactions has emerged. The coenzyme appears to act as an 'intermediate hormone' or 'second messenger' (*Figure 2.15*). When a primary hormone reaches its target cell, a reaction occurs with a hormone receptor. This reaction activates the enzyme adenyl cyclase and increases the amount of cyclic AMP in the cell, which proceeds to activate further enzymes of this reaction sequence. Neurochemical transmission is believed to operate in this way. The neurotransmitter is the primary hormone and the cyclic AMP is intermediate in the process of depolarization of the postsynaptic membrane.

Nicotinamide adenine dinucleotide (NAD)

This coenzyme was known previously as diphosphopyridine nucleotide (DPN) and coenzyme 1. Its structure includes one molecule of AMP and also the vitamin niacin (nicotinamide). A deficiency of nicotinamide results in pellagra. However, a dietary deficiency of nicotinamide alone is unlikely to cause this condition, as nicotinamide is a product of the metabolism of the amino acid tryptophan.

NAD is a hydrogen transfer molecule which participates in oxidation reactions (*see* page 17). $NADH_2$, which is the reduced form, can be reoxidized by transferring the H_2 to other metabolic intermediates. However, a larger proportion of the reoxidation occurs in mitochondria. Mitochondrial oxidations are reactions in which a series of hydrogen transfer molecules, including the cytochromes, are successively reduced. Their reoxidation is associated with the conversion of ADP to ATP. Ultimately the H_2 which started on the $NADH_2$ molecule reacts with molecular oxygen to produce water. The overall scheme is

$$NADH_2 + \tfrac{1}{2}O_2 + 3ADP + 3phosphate \longrightarrow NAD + H_2O + 3ATP$$

This mitochondrial reaction is the link between the redox reactions and the energy-requiring processes of living tissues, many of which are not themselves redox reactions. In this way, oxidation of food sources such as glucose initially produces $NADH_2$, which leads to the conversion of ADP to ATP.

Nicotinamide adenine dinucleotide phosphate (NADP)

This coenzyme is a phosphorylated derivative of NAD and is also a hydrogen transfer molecule. Whereas NAD is involved in catabolism and mitochondrial oxidation, yielding ATP, NADP is mostly concerned with providing a reducing power for many synthetic reactions (anabolism). A notable example is in the synthesis of fatty acids. A few catabolic oxidations produce $NADPH_2$ in order to supply synthetic processes. The glucose oxidation reactions of the pentose phosphate pathways use NADP as a hydrogen transfer cofactor, and this pathway is active in adipose tissue.

Enzymes

It has already been described how many organic chemical reactions are reversible and how, when the reaction is completed, an equilibrium mixture of both reactants and products is obtained. Often associated with this is a slow rate of reaction, which can mean that equilibrium may still not be achieved after hours or even days. However, a slow reaction may be accelerated by addition of a suitable catalyst. To return to the example of ester formation from acetic acid and ethanol, this slow reaction can be speeded up by the addition of a relatively small amount of sulphuric acid to the mixture. The acid performs as a catalyst by activating the acetic acid, which then more readily reacts with the alcohol. At equilibrium the sulphuric acid can be recovered unchanged and the equilibrium mixture of ethyl acetate, water, acetic acid and ethanol will yield the same value for the equilibrium constant (K) (*see* page 16) as would have been observed in the absence of the sulphuric acid. To summarize, the main characteristics of a catalyst are that they activate one or several of the reactants, that they are present in smaller quantities than the main reactants, that they can be recovered unchanged from the equilibrium mixture and that they do not affect the composition of the final equilibrium mixture.

Enzymes are biological catalysts, and the reactants controlled by the enzymes are known as the enzyme *substrates.*

In addition to their catalytic activity, enzymes have a second important function. This is the ability to select the substrates from the cell contents and direct the formation of particular products. In the example cited above, ethyl acetate and water are the only products that might be expected. However, there are many reactions in which a number of different products may be formed from the same reactants. The contents of a cell might undergo a variety of wasteful reactions were it not for the directing influence of the enzymes.

Enzymes normally catalyse only one type of reaction—oxidation, decarboxylation, etc. The substrate selected by the enzyme may vary, so that a group of similar molecules may be handled by the same enzyme. For example, a single enzyme may catalyse the transamination of a number of amino acids, although the rates of reaction may be different for each amino acid.

NOMENCLATURE OF ENZYMES

As increasing numbers of enzymes are isolated and characterized, it has become necessary to provide them with a descriptive name. The enzyme catalogue (EC) system currently in use indicates the principal reactants, the enzyme reaction type and the catalogue number—e.g. alcohol: NAD oxidoreductase EC 1.1.1.1. The first three numbers of this catalogue number indicate the type of reaction and the fourth is the number of the enzyme in the catalogue. In addition, trivial names are used for many enzymes, as in the above example, which is commonly known as alcohol dehydrogenase. Trivial names are normally constructed by the addition of the suffix -ase to the reaction type, which is preceded by the principal substrate.

ENZYME STRUCTURE

Enzymes are proteins which either are soluble in the cytoplasm or form insoluble complex protein conglomerates. They may also be associated with or even embedded in the cell membranes. Protein molecules are chains of amino acids, and their overall shape is in dynamic equilibrium with the cell environment. For enzymes this has great significance. The mechanical flexibility of the enzyme protein allows it to wrap itself around a substrate, which makes possible the creation of an independent chemical environment in which the reaction may take place. Changes in the cell environment may prevent this 'envelope' effect of the enzyme and affect its catalytic activity. For example, small molecules not directly involved in the enzyme-controlled reaction may indirectly affect the reaction rate by changing the shape of the protein. In addition to the general effectors such as pH, many metabolites have potent specific effects on certain enzymes and perform a delicate control function of enzyme activity.

A peptide chain of the enzyme molecule is made up of amino acids. The chemical side-chains provided by these amino acids equip the protein with a number of chemical functions. Some side-chains have a tendency to prefer a non-aqueous environment. Collectively, within a protein a number of such side-chains can create a water-repelling or hydrophobic region. In contrast, several side-chains, particularly those which are ionized, prefer an aqueous environment and are therefore hydrophilic. These forces contribute to the internal structure and overall shape of the protein molecule, and, in addition, are important to the catalytic activity of the enzyme.

Enzyme catalysis occurs at a specific point in the protein molecule. The reaction may take place at or near the surface or within the protein. The location is known as the active site of the enzyme. This region is most sensitive to chemical damage, whereas only a minor disruption of enzyme activity may occur if sections of the non-catalytic region are removed.

ENZYME ACTION

The main processes of enzyme catalysis are: (1) diffusion of substrates to the enzyme surface; (2) reversible location of substrates on the active site; (3) reaction of substrates within the enzyme to form products; (4) reversible disengagement of products from the active site; (5) diffusion of products from the enzyme surface. Both (1) and (5) are independent of the enzyme, depending on the diffusion rate of the substrate and products within the reaction medium. This process is usually more rapid than enzyme catalysis. Steps (2)–(4) are the processes involved in enzyme action. The overall rate of reaction through these will be limited by the slowest component in the sequence and is the rate-limiting (or rate-determining) step.

The main factors determining the location of a substrate on the active site of an enzyme are: (1) the molecular shape and chemical function of groups of the substrate, and (2) the shape and the chemical function of the active site. Successful attachment of substrate to the enzyme requires that these two factors complement each other. The simple analogy of a lock, representing the enzyme, and a key, representing the substrate, is useful in illustrating this. Some keys will not fit a lock at all; some may enter the lock but not turn; others may turn with difficulty; and the correct key will turn with ease. Similarly, some molecules are not substrates for an enzyme, and others merely enter an active site and occlude it. The remaining analogies represent substrates of the enzyme with varying degrees of activity. After the precise orientation of the correct substrate in the active site, reaction can take place—i.e. the key can turn. This happens because the reactive parts of the enzyme and substrates are located in exactly the right places.

A variety of forces may locate the substrate and preserve the enzyme–substrate complex. Often a collection of individually weak forces combine to be effective. Both covalent and ionic bonds may be formed, perhaps strengthened by a change in the active site microenvironment induced by formation of the complex.

The forces involved in locating the substrate in the correct position on the enzyme may also be involved in the catalytic activity. The chemical forces between the enzyme and the substrate may weaken hitherto stable bonds in the substrate and cause them to break. Further direction of a reaction pathway by chemical groups on the enzyme and/or proximity of a similarly activated coreactant leads to completion of the reaction. The specificity of the enzyme reaction is controlled by the enzyme only allowing certain substrates to enter the active site and by having the reactant located specifically. In this way, only one chemical route is allowed.

To summarize, the main points of enzyme action are: (1) specific location of substrates, leading to (2) weakening of chemical bonds, facilitating reaction; (3) close proximity of interacting groups, allowing (4) specific reaction to occur, with (5) an overall increase in reaction velocity.

ENZYME INHIBITORS

The rate of a biochemical reaction depends on the amount of active enzyme present. Consequently, variation of the concentration of active enzyme by the cell can modify the rate of a particular reaction. The phrase 'active enzyme' is used because the total amount of enzyme available to the cell may be constant. The important change is the proportion of enzyme molecules which are in an active catalytic state. Metabolites which resemble the usual substrate or product, or perhaps the product itself, may occupy or otherwise occlude the active site of the enzyme. Some of the enzyme molecules will be inhibited and the rate of reaction will be reduced. It is possible that some of the enzyme molecules are normally inhibited, so that changes in the level of inhibitor can either reduce or increase the normal reaction rate.

This type of enzyme inhibition is characterized by the inhibitor directly affecting the access of the substrate to the active site. However, another type of inhibition has been recognized where the inhibitor is attached to the enzyme at a specific site, which is not directly connected with the active catalytic site. Because the inhibitor is located at another place on the molecule, this type of inhibition is described as allosteric. When the allosteric inhibitor is located in its specific receptor site on the enzyme, the protein shape is changed and the highly organized structure of the active site is affected. The consequent reduction in the affinity of the enzyme for the substrate reduces the catalytic rate. Similarly, an allosteric activator can change the structure of the active site, to enhance the affinity of the enzyme for the substrate.

METABOLIC CONTROL OF ENZYME ACTIVITY

The purpose of enzyme inhibition and activation mechanisms is to provide the cell with a metabolic control system. In this, activities of key enzymes in metabolic pathways are affected according to the needs of the cell, providing a sensitive mechanism for the control of metabolism.

The metabolic signal for initiating the control mechanism is usually the concentration of one of the metabolites of a reaction sequence. Feedback inhibition is typical (*Figure 2.16*). This allows a reasonably constant concentration of the final product to be maintained and prevents the wasteful production of the first metabolite in the series, which might otherwise be used by other pathways. This principle is independent of the length of the pathway, which may consist of only

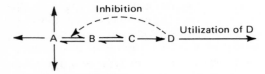

Figure 2.16 Feedback inhibition. A represents a
metabolite at the junction of three pathways. Feedback
inhibition by D of the first enzyme of the pathway to its
synthesis controls the steady state concentration of the
product. This prevents the unnecessary consumption of
A, which has to supply three pathways. Also, an
uncontrolled increase in D may allow it to reach a toxic
level in the cell, perhaps by overactivity of subsequent
reactions\

one step. In this case the product feedback inhibits the enzyme responsible for its
own formation.

When the demands on a particular pathway exceed the ability of these control
mechanisms, the cell may be encouraged to synthesize more enzyme (induction) or
reduce synthesis (repression). This is generally in response to relatively large
changes in substrate availability.

ENZYME INHIBITION AND DRUG ACTION

The usual biochemical effect of a therapeutic drug is to inhibit an enzyme. This may
result in cell death (antibiotics and cancer chemotherapy) or the attenuation of an
overactive process (beta-adrenergic blockers). Whereas direct stimulation of an
underactive enzyme by a drug is rare, the correct strategy can lead to the
potentiation of a biochemical effect.

A simple strategy is to encourage the activity of a pathway by preventing the
removal of an essential intermediate by a competing pathway. In depressive illness
a dominant hypothesis has been one which suggested that the neurotransmitter
amines are deficient in some neurons. The relevant amines are synthesized from
amino acids and excess amine is removed by the enzyme monoamine oxidase
(MAO):

$$\text{Amino acid} \longrightarrow \text{Amine transmitter} \xrightarrow{\text{MAO}} \text{Oxidized amine}$$
$$\downarrow$$
$$\text{Neurotransmission}$$

A series of monoamine oxidase inhibitors (MAOIs) are now available as antidepressants. By reducing the oxidation of the amines, the MAOIs lead to
accumulation of the amine transmitter in the terminals of neurons, this increasing
the release of the neurotransmitters.

A similar manoeuvre is employed with the tricyclic antidepressants, where, of
two competing actions, one is inhibited in order to increase the activity of the other.
When an amine is released into the synaptic cleft, the time allowed for it to attach
itself to a postsynaptic receptor is limited by re-uptake of the amine across the
presynaptic membrane. Tricyclic antidepressants inhibit this presynaptic re-uptake,
allowing the amine to remain in the synaptic cleft and thus prolong postsynaptic
stimulation.

Energy production by the cell

All animals require food, and failure to eat leads to both behavioural and physical changes, even in the short term. Utilization of food for energy is obvious during muscle activity, but other less obvious cellular processes throughout the body and in the brain are consuming energy for metabolic work. Much activity in cells is devoted to the oxidation of food to provide the energy necessary for these important functions.

The first step is digestion, in which a variety of large molecules are broken down into smaller units. The smaller units of carbohydrates, lipids and amino acids are processed by the liver. A number of the amino acids together with carbohydrates, are converted to the polymer of glucose, glycogen. The glycogen store can be released in a controlled way, in accordance with blood glucose level. Some of the amino acids are used to synthesize body proteins. The lipid is stored in fat cells throughout the body and used as required both for membrane synthesis and as a metabolic fuel. This organization results in the cellular fuel being stored as two main components. Glycogen is hydrolysed to glucose and the hydrolysis of fats yields the fatty acids.

Glycogen or glucose metabolism produces a readily available supply of ATP, whereas lipids are generally mobilized during fasting. Muscles, having a requirement for bursts of energy, draw on their glycogen stores, and the brain has an almost exclusive requirement for glucose.

A summary of the catabolism of glucose and fatty acids is shown in *Figure 2.17*. Oxidation of these leads ultimately to the synthesis of ATP from ADP. The

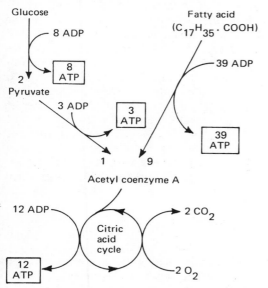

Figure 2.17 A summary of the major pathways of ATP production in the cell. The mols of ATP assume complete oxidation of NADH, etc. The numbers by the arrowheads indicate the amount of product from one substrate molecule, e.g. complete oxidation of stearic acid yields $39 + (9 \times 12) = 147$ ATP

chemical energy of ATP is then used to 'drive' the cellular activities. In muscle ATP enables protein fibres to contract, and in neurons the ion differential across the membrane is maintained by ATP.

An important feature of both glucose and fatty acid catabolism is that both require energy in the form of ATP for initiation of the catabolic process. Glucose is phosphorylated to glucose-6-phosphate, and the fatty acids, after a multistep process involving ATP, are attached to coenzyme A to produce fatty acyl coenzyme A. Both steps provide a metabolic 'gate' which enables the cell to control the amount of catabolism according to its needs.

The first phase of glucose catabolism is glycolysis, the final product being lactic acid. This pathway has a small yield of ATP, but it has the advantage of being anaerobic. In muscle this is important for providing ATP at a rate faster than oxygen can be supplied for aerobic respiration. At rest, when an energy supply from other sources is available, lactate may be converted back to glucose by a process which is largely a reverse of glycolysis with a few additional reactions. This process is gluconeogenesis. The alternative fate of lactic acid is conversion first to pyruvic acid, which after a multistep oxidation is converted to acetyl coenzyme A. Acetyl coenzyme A is also the product of the oxidative breakdown of the fatty acids. The long chains of even numbers of carbon atoms are broken down by a stepwise transfer of molecular units containing two carbon atoms from the fatty acid to coenzyme A.

Acetyl coenzyme A is the fuel for the citric acid cycle of oxidation, which takes place inside the mitochondria. The initial step is the reaction of oxaloacetic acid with acetyl coenzyme A to produce citric acid. This is followed by a series of oxidative steps yielding $NADH_2$. The two carbon atoms of the acetate which entered the cycle are evolved as carbon dioxide. Subsequent conversions of the rest of the molecule derived from citric acid lead to oxaloacetic acid becoming available for further condensation with acetyl coenzyme A. The primary energy carrier derived from the citric acid cycle oxidations is $NADH_2$. In the mitochondria $NADH_2$ is oxidized by a stepwise process to regenerate NAD and ultimately to produce water by combination of the hydrogen with molecular oxygen. The electrons associated with the hydrogen of $NADH_2$ are transported along a series of respiratory pigments which include a flavin enzyme, quinone and a number of cytochromes. These are sensitive to respiratory poisons, the reaction of cytochromes with cyanide being the best-known. As the electrons are passed between the respiratory pigments, some chemical energy is made available. At three points in this chain the energy is used to phosphorylate ADP to produce ATP, which has led to the description of this process as oxidative phosphorylation.

Biopolymers

A polymer is a large molecule consisting of chains of smaller molecular units joined together. The simplest biopolymers are the starches, in which the molecular unit is glucose. Glycogen, abundant in liver and muscle, has a molecular weight of between 300 000 and 100 000 000. This represents between 2000 and 600 000 glucose molecules per glycogen molecule. Unlike glucose, the large glycogen polymers are insoluble in the cell contents. This means that large amounts of glucose may be stored in the form of glycogen without affecting the concentration and osmotic pressure of the cytoplasm.

Other polysaccharides have been found in various tissues in which monosaccharide units other than glucose are found. These are present particularly in cell membranes and mucopolysaccharides.

Although the polysaccharides have extremely important functions in the body, the two groups of biopolymer on which the cell depends most are the nucleic acids and the proteins. The nucleic acids provide the genetic information necessary for cells to reproduce themselves, and proteins are the physical expression of that information.

Nucleic acids

The nucleic acids are polymers of nucleotides. The general structure is a 'backbone' of alternating sugar and phosphate, with each sugar having an organic base as a side-chain. Two nucleic acids are found in most cells—deoxyribonucleic acid (DNA) and ribonucleic acid (RNA).

DEOXYRIBONUCLEIC ACID (DNA)

DNA is found in the cell nucleus and is the genetic material of the cell. Within it is the chemical information necessary to direct all the protein synthesis taking place inside the cell.

The nucleotides found in DNA have the general structure

organic base————deoxyribose————phosphate

Four organic bases—adenine, guanine, cytosine and thymine (*Figure 2.18*)—

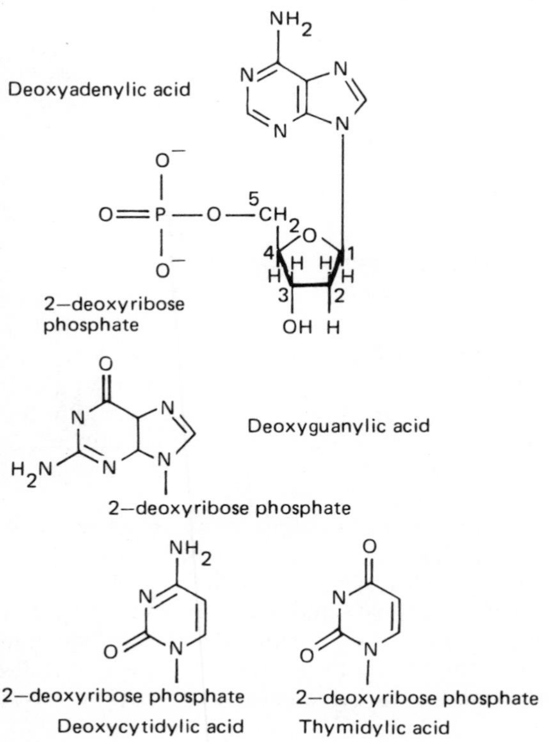

Deoxyadenylic acid

2—deoxyribose phosphate

Deoxyguanylic acid

2—deoxyribose phosphate

2—deoxyribose phosphate
Deoxycytidylic acid

2—deoxyribose phosphate
Thymidylic acid

Figure 2.18 Deoxyribonucleotides compare with the ribonucleotide adenylic acid in *Figure 2.13*

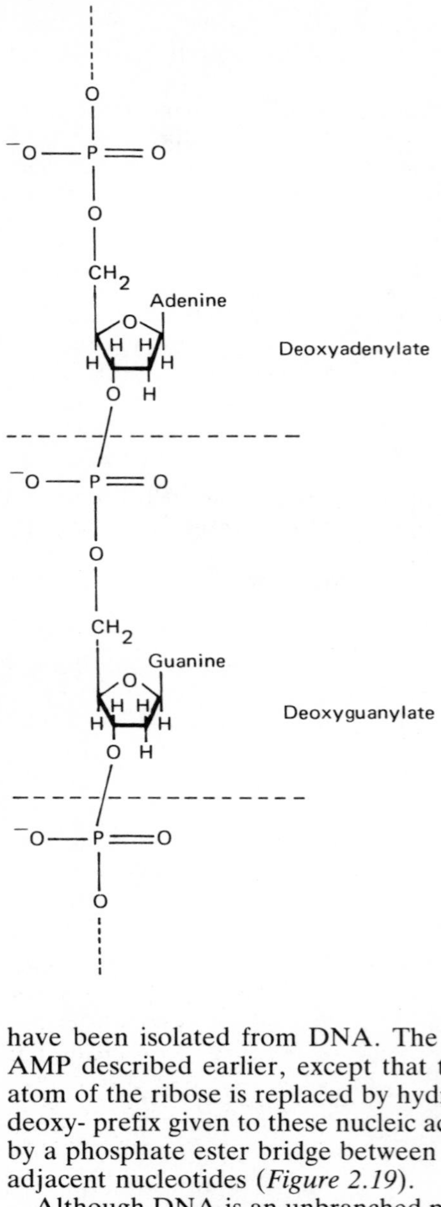

Figure 2.19 Repeating nucleotide monomers of the DNA polymer

have been isolated from DNA. The deoxyadenylic acid is identical with that of AMP described earlier, except that the hydroxyl group on the number 2 carbon atom of the ribose is replaced by hydrogen. This loss of oxygen is described in the deoxy- prefix given to these nucleic acids. Formation of the nucleic acid polymer is by a phosphate ester bridge between the 3- and 5-hydroxyls of the ribose sugar of adjacent nucleotides (*Figure 2.19*).

Although DNA is an unbranched polymer, in mammalian cells it exists as a pair of complementary strands wound around each other in the form of a right-handed double helix. The association of the two strands is achieved by the organic bases of one strand forming a weak and reversible chemical bond with a base on the other strand. Each base has an obligatory partner—adenine with thymine and guanine with cytosine (*Figure 2.20*). The genetic information is carried in these molecules by means of a code using the order of the four organic bases in one of the DNA strands.

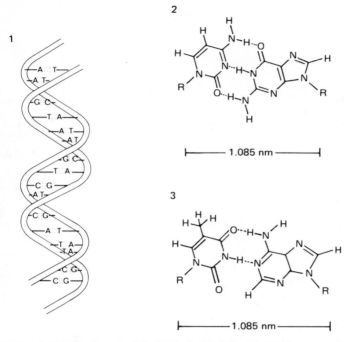

Figure 2.20 (1) A diagram of the DNA double helix. The two interwound ribbons represent repeating sugar-phosphate 'backbones', which are cross-linked by the paired bases. (2) The bases cytosine and guanine arranged to show the hydrogen bonding (indicated by dotted lines) found in DNA. The letter R is where the base joins the nucleic acid backbone. The association of these two bases gives an inter-chain distance of 1.085 nm which is also found in (3) the hydrogen-bonded bases thymine and adenine

DNA replication

On cell division the genetic material of the cell must be replicated so that each daughter cell contains a copy of the chromosomes. The chemistry of DNA provides the mechanism necessary for gene replication. The critical feature is the obligatory base pairing of alanine with thymine and of guanine with cytosine. This means that when two complementary strands of DNA are separated and two double helices re-created by use of the free nucleotides in the cell, the products must be identical with the original DNA double helix. The replication process is shown schematically in *Figure 2.21*.

RIBONUCLEIC ACID (RNA)

The major chemical differences between RNA and DNA are that in RNA the sugar is ribose not deoxyribose, the thymine base is replaced by uracil (*Figure 2.22*) and RNA molecules are single strands. The base-pairing characteristics are similar, except that adenine pairs with uracil.

The function of RNA is to decode the genetic information of DNA in order that

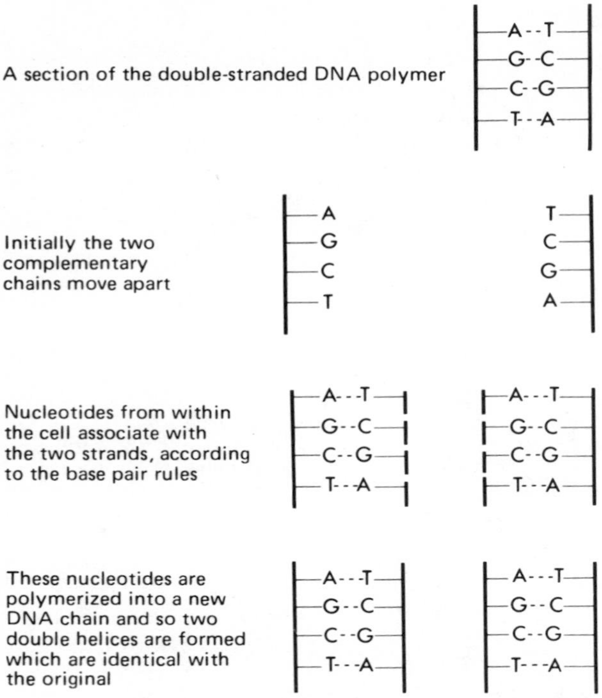

A section of the double-stranded DNA polymer

```
—A--T—
—G--C—
—C--G—
—T--A—
```

Initially the two
complementary
chains move apart

```
—A        T—
—G        C—
—C        G—
—T        A—
```

Nucleotides from within
the cell associate with
the two strands, according
to the base pair rules

```
—A--T—      —A---T—
—G--C—      —G--C—
—C--G—      —C--G—
—T--A—      —T--A—
```

These nucleotides are
polymerized into a new
DNA chain and so two
double helices are formed
which are identical with
the original

```
—A--T—      —A---T—
—G--C—      —G--C—
—C--G—      —C--G—
—T--A—      —T---A—
```

Figure 2.21 Replication of DNA using the base pair rules: A = adenine with T = thymine; G = guanine with C = cytosine

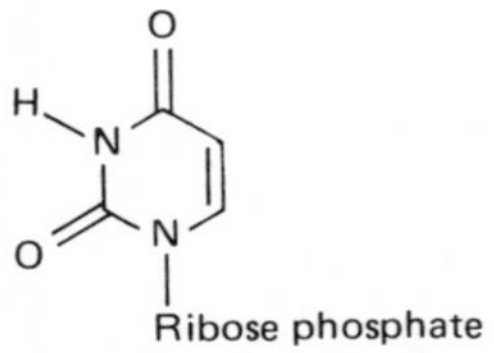

Ribose phosphate   *Figure 2.22* Uridylic acid: compare with AMP (*Figure 2.13*)

proteins may be correctly synthesized. Two different forms of RNA molecule are used in this process—messenger RNA and transfer RNA.

Messenger RNA (mRNA) is a single strand of RNA which is an RNA copy of a section of one strand of a DNA molecule. The information within this section will be sufficient to synthesize a protein molecule. In the cytoplasm of the cell there are particulate enzyme structures known as ribosomes, which carry out the chemical tasks of translation of the nucleic acid code into protein molecules. The ribosomes recognize the starting point of the mRNA code and work their way along, decoding and assembling the protein molecules.

A second type of RNA molecule essential to this process is transfer RNA (tRNA), which also is a single-stranded molecule but is folded upon itself with the aid of internal base pairing. The function of tRNA is to collect free amino acids from the cytoplasm and locate them on the mRNA template in order that ribosomes may link the amino acids to the protein chain.

The triplet code and protein synthesis

Each amino acid has at least one tRNA molecule to which it is specifically attached for the transfer process. On these RNA molecules there is a group of three adjacent unpaired bases. These bases locate themselves by pairing with the complementary bases on the mRNA. In this way each group of three bases in the mRNA represents the coding for one amino acid. The triplet of bases on the mRNA is called the codon and the triplet on tRNA is called the anticodon. The translation process is shown schematically in *Figure 2.23*.

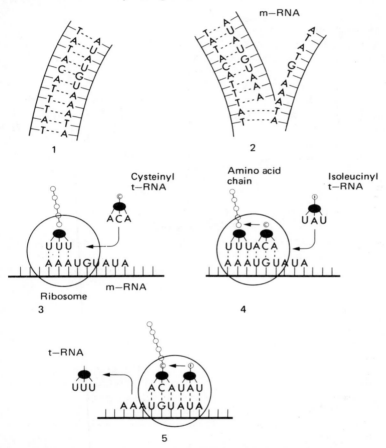

Figure 2.23 DNA-directed synthesis of proteins. (1) A short section of the DNA double helix containing the bases adenine (A), thymine (T), guanine (G) and cytosine (C). (2) Separation of the two DNA chains to allow transcription of the genetic code into messenger RNA (mRNA). In mRNA the thymine is replaced by uracil (U). (3) mRNA becomes attached to a complex protein ribosome in the cytoplasm. This combination translates the genetic code into a protein 'message'. (4) A transfer TNA (tRNA) molecule, carrying a specific amino acid (cysteine in this example), pairs three of its bases with three on the mRNA. This locates the cysteine molecule adjacent to the growing protein chain. (5) The protein chain is coupled to the cysteine molecule and the tRNA (UUU) is released to collect another amino acid. Meanwhile the next tRNA molecule, this time carrying isoleucine, enters the ribosome

Since each of the three positions in the codon can be filled by one of four bases, there are $4 \times 4 \times 4 = 64$ possible triplets.

As only 20 amino acids are used in protein synthesis, this means that even with chain-initiating and chain-terminating codons, there are codons to spare. It is found that several amino acids are coded by more than one codon. For example, leucine, arginine and serine are each coded by six codons.

Mistranslation of the code at any stage would lead to the wrong protein being synthesized unless the fault happens to provide one of the alternative codons for the correct amino acid. In *Figure 2.23*, if the first base of the illustrated mRNA is changed from U to C, the amino acid coded would be arginine, not cysteine. Another possible form of mistranslation would be if the first base in the sequence were ignored. In *Figure 2.23*, if the sequence was read beginning GUA instead of UGU, the coded amino acid would be valine, and all subsequent amino acids would be similarly miscoded. This would produce a 'nonsense' protein.

Genetic diseases are caused by changes, often single changes, in the DNA base sequence. As described above, a single change in the base sequence would be sufficient to produce an abnormal protein, with one amino acid substituted for another. Although proteins are large molecules, the effect of changing one amino acid can have great significance. Sickle-cell anaemia has been shown to result from a substitution of valine for glutamic acid in the beta chains of haemoglobin.

Proteins

DNA in the nucleus of a cell has the information necessary to direct the synthesis of all proteins produced by the cell. The proteins have both structural and enzymic roles. Structural proteins contribute to the formation of cell membranes, which not only form the cell boundary, but also form subcellular organelles. Many enzymes are associated with these, as in mitochondria, but others are also freely soluble in the cytoplasm.

PROTEIN STRUCTURE

The synthesis of proteins under the direction of the nucleic acids leads to a linear chain of amino acids. This is known as the *primary structure* of the protein. The amino acid side-chains of the proteins have particular chemical characteristics, and their interactions allow the protein to adopt a particular alignment. This is the *secondary structure* of the protein. Three types of secondary structure appear to dominate the proteins. The chains may coil into an alpha helix or lie alongside each other in the form of a pleated sheet. Alternatively, no order arrangement may be preferred by the protein chain and it may exist as a random coil. A single protein may include all these types of structure at different points along the molecule.

The next stage of structural organization is folding of the coils and sheets into the *tertiary structure*. It is at this level that enzymes acquire their functional capacity. The tertiary structure provides the clefts of the active site of enzymes, the shape of which depends on the folding of the entire molecule.

When a number of separate protein molecules aggregate to form a single functional unit, the construction of this unit is known as the *quaternary structure*.

Although the tertiary structure required for enzyme activity is probably one of many structures that might be taken up by a protein molecule, it seems that the primary structure has a great deal to do with directing the ultimate shape of the protein. Some enzymes have been allowed to redevelop their tertiary structure after the original folding pattern was disrupted. The subsequent identification of significant amounts of enzyme activity in the reconstituted protein showed that the primary structure must have influenced the folding process.

Cell membranes

For many years membrane structure was not of great interest, as it was thought that it was 'once formed' and simply provided a cell enclosure. The advent of radioactive tracer techniques demonstrated that components of the cell membrane were in dynamic chemical equilibrium with the cell contents. The steady turnover of membrane components stimulated further interest. It became clear that many enzymes were bound to membranes and that the fixed location of these enzymes was essential to the functions they carried out. Oxidative phosphorylation, in particular, uses some of the physical characteristics of the mitochondrial membranes to co-ordinate electron transport and ATP synthesis.

In neurons the cell membrane is a major functional structure. Axon filaments provide a means of electrical signalling throughout the body, including complex cerebral activity. In the resting state axon membranes separate different ion concentrations inside and outside the cell. Potassium concentration inside the neuron is around 20 times higher than sodium concentration; outside, the relationship is reversed. This leads to a potential difference across the membrane. Signal conduction initiated by a neuroreceptor occurs when permeability of the membrane is increased. Sodium and potassium ion concentrations equalize and the resting potential is reduced. Diminution of the resting potential, known as depolarization, causes permeability changes in the vicinity of the neuromembrane. Depolarization progresses along the length of the fibre, completing signal transmission. Recovery of the resting potential after transmission is achieved by an ATP-driven ion pump in a membrane which re-creates the ion difference.

Membrane structure

The selective permeability of neuronal membranes is a characteristic of all biomembranes. They consist largely of non-polar lipid, which repels charged particles, so that ions do not pass freely across and usually require specific transport mechanisms to do so. However, the simple lipid envelope is elaborated with an ionic surface to allow it to be compatible with the aqueous cell medium.

Although membranes are complex, they are constructed from simple molecules. Primarily, membranes are an association of lipids and proteins. Proteins are synthesized from amino acids under DNA direction, and the lipids are a collection of relatively small molecules described previously (pages 18–21). Most of these have the schematic structure shown in *Figure 2.24*. The hydrophobic tail may be flexible, as in the triglycerides and phospholipids, or rigid, as in cholesterol. The

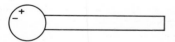

Figure 2.24 The simplified structure of lipids found most abundantly in membranes. It consists of a hydrophilic 'head' which frequently has ionized groups and a hydrophobic hydrocarbon 'tail'. This may be the flexible carbon chain of fatty acids or the rigid ring structure of cholesterol

hydrophilic head can be the strongly ionic amino phosphate of the phospholipid or the weakly polar hydroxyl group of cholesterol.

In an aqueous medium lipid molecules tend to aggregate, so that the hydrophobic tails coalesce, allowing the hydrophilic heads to form a polar coat to the particle. The chemical interactions providing the forces which allow these aggregations are those which are utilized in providing a stable membrane structure.

When membranes are treated with a polar stain, a cross-section appears as a dark–light–dark sandwich when examined with an electron microscope. This is consistent with the currently accepted general view of membranes (*Figure 2.25*), in which the polar regions of the lipid face the aqueous medium and the hydrophobic region forms a barrier.

Some membrane proteins assist in the selective permeability of the membranes. The chemical characteristics of enzyme substrate binding can be applied to transport mechanisms (*Figure 2.26*). For this to take place, proteins must be

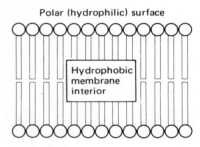

Figure 2.25 Lipid membrane. Cross-section of a hypothetical model of a lipid membrane. In this simple form the membrane would consist of two layers of lipid molecules arranged with their polar 'heads' forming the outer surfaces in contact with the aqueous cell medium

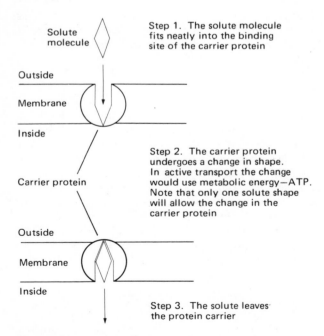

Figure 2.26 A simple model for protein-carrier mediated transport

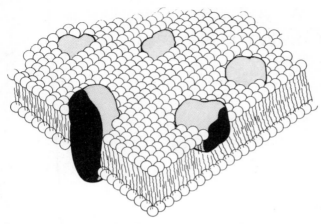

Figure 2.27 The fluid mosaic model of biological membranes proposed by Singer and Nicholson. In this model the matrix of the membrane is composed of lipid molecules orientated so that their polar heads form the membrane surface. Embedded in this lipid are molecules of protein having polarity characteristics similar to those of lipid molecules. Those parts of the protein molecule which are embedded within the membrane would consist of amino acids with neutral non-polar side-chains, whereas in the aqueous phase they would be ionic. From *Science, N.Y.*, **175**, 723 (1972)

embedded in the lipid structure. A membrane model of this type has been suggested which accounts for many of the physical and chemical characteristics of membranes (*Figure 2.27*). This suggests that some proteins are relatively loosely associated with the surface and others embedded in the surface, presumably including the membrane-bound enzymes. These are in addition to the transport proteins which connect both membrane surfaces.

Chapter 3

Cells of the central nervous system

Neuroglia

It is tempting to think only of neurons when discussing cells of the CNS. Certainly at the present level of knowledge neurons are the most interesting and important units in the brain. A change in function within neuroglial cells as the undetected basis of some behavioural disorders, however, cannot be discounted. Neuroglia are non-excitable cells which form a major component of brain and spinal cord. Histologists have recognized several types of glial cell—astrocytes, oligodendrocytes, ependymal cells and the microglia. Astrocytes have very small cell bodies and long, very fine processes which pass between the neurons and into fibre tracts. Oligodendrocytes have fewer cell processes but come into close apposition to neuron cell bodies and axons. Astrocytes and oligodendrocytes are found in both grey and white areas of the brain and the spinal cord. Ependymal cells do not have such a wide distribution, since they line the surface of the cerebral ventricles and the canal of the spinal cord. The lining is formed from a single layer of squamous or columnar cells. The microglial cells are small, with very short processes, and contain many lysosomes. It is thought that they may function as tissue macrophages and assume the role of scavenger cells when nervous tissue is damaged. They are often referred to as gitter cells.

The functions of glial cells are not fully understood. They probably provide mechanical support and, in the case of the oligodendroglia, act as electrical insulators. When the nervous system is damaged, the glial components can act as phagocytes and can form a type of scar tissue. Ependymal cells are involved in the transport of substances into and out of the cerebrospinal fluid. Possibly of greater importance than is at present believed is the role of glia in regulating the biochemical environment of neurons. This seems to be of particular importance in the brain, where processes of neurons can be great distances from the control of the cell nucleus. It will be shown later that a particularly widespread and important neurotransmitter in the brain is gamma amino butyric acid (GABA). This amino acid causes a strong depression of cell excitability when applied artificially, but this depression lasts only a few seconds. In an experiment to study the activity of glial cells, tiny amounts of radioactively labelled GABA were injected into the brain into the immediate environment of neurons. Thin sections of brain were then cut and coated with photographic emulsion. The radioactivity in the GABA causes silver crystals to form in the photographic emulsion. It was discovered that much of the radioactivity (and therefore much of the GABA) was contained in the glial cells. It thus seems that the glia is responsible, in part at least, for the very short half-life* of this powerful inhibitory substance in the extracellular fluid of the brain. Nothing is known yet about any changes in the function of glial cells in psychiatric illness.

Neurons

Neurons are excitable cells which are specialized for the reception, integration, conduction and transmission of information, which is in all cases coded in units of nerve impulses. There is considerable variation in the shape of neurons but they all present some features in common. Around the nucleus there is a mass of cytoplasm which forms the *soma*. From the soma project processes of variable length. These

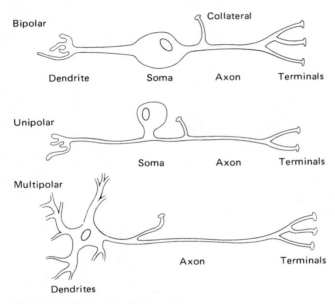

Figure 3.1 Different forms of neuron

may be classified into two groups: *axons* and *dendrites*. Dendrites usually have a wide base and progressively taper and branch away from the soma. Axons, on the other hand, although originating in a small conical expansion of the soma, *the axon hillock*, do not taper progressively and are much less branched than are dendrites. There is only one axon, usually to each neuron, and it may be very long, sometimes as much as one metre. A few side-branches of the axon may occur a short distance from the soma and these are called *axon collaterals*. Axons often end in a large number of very fine branches, each with one or more small swellings called *terminals*.

*Half-life = the period of time in which concentration or activity of a substance diminishes to half of its initial value.

The classic idea of neuronal function is that coded information is collected by the dendrites and channelled to the soma, and the integrated result of this input is conveyed away by the axon towards the terminals. The terminals lie in close apposition to another cell. Outside the CNS the terminals may be applied to glands or muscles, but inside the CNS the terminals lie close to other neurons. The gap, or *synapse*, between the two cells is the site of transmission of impulses from cell to cell. This simple concept of the shape of a neuron is very useful, but it is important to remember that there are many variations. It is common to see neurons classified into three types—unipolar, bipolar and multipolar (*Figure 3.1*). The term simply refers to the number of processes emerging from the soma. *Figure 3.1* reveals a problem with the classification of dendrites and axons, however. The unipolar neuron has, like the other neurons, receptive sites at one end and axon terminals at the other. Is the process to the left an axon or a dendrite? It looks like an axon, and, in cells of this type, functions like an axon. We shall leave these semantic arguments to others and call it an axon, but this is not apparently in accord with the generalization made above that neurons function by collecting coded information at the dendrites and integrating the information at the level of the soma. The unipolar neuron of the dorsal root ganglia thus have axons conducting action potentials from peripheral receptors directly into the CNS. However, nearly all neurons of central and autonomic nervous systems are multipolar.

Subcellular structure of neurons of the CNS

Neurons have a very similar range of organelles and inclusions to other cells in the body. The cytoplasm is surrounded by the *cell membrane*. This appears to consist of two monomolecular layers of phospholipid. These layers are penetrated by large protein molecules which are free to move about within the membrane. It is difficult to explain all the properties of membranes with such a simple structure, and various alternatives have been proposed. It is most likely that membranes change their structure under different physiological conditions or with different methods of fixation before microscopic examination. The factors controlling these changes and the nature of the structural alterations are not known. The membrane can transport small molecules actively into or out of the cell and transports large molecules into the cell by the process of *pinocytosis*, whereby the membrane invaginates and creates a small vacuole containing some extracellular material. The opposite process of *exocytosis* involves the ejection of large organic molecules from the cell. The most obvious characteristic of the membranes of excitable cells is the maintenance of the membrane potential of approximately 70 mV (inside negative). This is discussed in detail later, but involves the pumping of potassium ions into, and sodium ions out of, the cell by an active process utilizing ATP.

Inside the cell membrane, within the cytoplasm, is an extensive system of interconnecting, membrane-lined channels. This is the *endoplasmic reticulum*. The endoplasmic reticulum essentially divides the intracellular space into two compartments—that inside the system of channels and that outside. The products of cell metabolism and synthesis are stored and transported inside the system of channels, and the enzymes, ribosomes and small molecules are located outside the channels. The membranous surface of the endoplasmic reticulum is where many of the cellular enzymes are attached, and therefore they are conveniently located close to their substrates and the storage or transport system of the cell. Two types of endoplasmic reticulum can be seen—smooth and rough. Rough endoplasmic reticulum has many *Nissl bodies* attached to it, imparting the rough appearance. Nissl bodies are accumulations of *ribosomes* which contain protein and RNA acid. Characteristically, neurons have high concentrations of Nissl bodies, as have other cells in the body where intense protein synthesis and secretion (including neuro-transmitter release) occurs. Within the CNS, the most active neurons, such as the anterior horn cells, have the greatest concentration of Nissl granules. Apparently neuronal activity and neurosecretion require high levels of protein synthesis. Protein is needed for the maintenance and repair of all cells, but neurons are very active, with a high metabolic rate; they are large, with many processes; and they require proportionately greater synthesis of protein. Neurons also secrete subst-ances from axon terminals and synthesize enzymes which manufacture these secretory products. Much of the protein is required to maintain these metabolic processes. Smooth endoplasmic reticulum is the site of many other cellular synthetic activities.

Mitochondria are large organelles of up to $4 \mu m^*$ in length. They are composed of a smooth outer membrane and a very folded inner membrane to which many enzymes adhere, particularly those concerned with oxidative metabolism and ATP formation. Within the lumen, ribosomes, RNA and DNA are found. Occasionally mitochondria are attached to, and are continuous with, the endoplasmic reticulum. They accumulate in metabolically active parts of the cell, and therefore are found in the soma and axon terminals but rarely in the axon itself. *Lysosomes* and the *Golgi apparatus* are also formed from the endoplasmic reticulum. Lysosomes are membrane-bound spheres, rich in proteolytic enzymes, and may be formed by budding off from the endoplasmic reticulum. The Golgi apparatus consists of stacks of smooth endoplasmic reticulum and is involved with the production of secretory materials. Lysosomes and the Golgi apparatus are highly metabolically active and contain many enzymes.

Neurons contain a high density of *microtubules* and *microfilaments*. These are small tubes of protein which have a skeletal function, supporting the cell contents and maintaining its shape. They also have an important function in the transport of substances within the cell. This is particularly important in neurons, where the axon is a great distance from the soma and the terminal is a highly active part of the cell. Two types of transport along axons have been observed. A slower transport, at 1–3 mm/24 h, involves the bulk flow of axoplasm. A second, fast transport of about 100 mm/24 h, transports certain proteins and some other materials. It is this fast transport which involves microtubules, because chemical agents which disrupt the protein of the microtubule also disrupt the fast axonal transport.

Many other inclusions may be seen in neurons. Discussion of the synaptic vesicles has been left to page 68. The function of many organelles is unknown but has become the focus of much research. Biochemical investigations of organelle function often involve the disruption of the cell structure and differential centri-fugation of the homogenized tissue. In this technique the cell contents are placed in the top of a tube which contains layers of sucrose solutions of increasing density. As the heaviest solution is at the bottom of the tube, centrifuging does not mix up the solutions. The organelles will pass through the different solutions until they enter a layer with a density similar to their own. As many of the organelles have different densities, this technique separates them into bands. The band containing the

---

$^*\mu m$ = micrometre, one-millionth of a metre or 10^{-6} m.

organelle under study can be selected and its biochemistry studied. It is unsatisfactory that the initial disruption of the organized structure of the cell may alter the functioning of the organelle, but there are problems of this type with every technique.

An alternative method exists for studying cellular function. Some chemical reactions within cells give rise to a coloured or fluorescent end-product. If the reaction takes place in a thin slice of brain tissue, the slice may then be examined under the light microscope and the distribution and concentration of this product examined. This technique avoids disruption of the cell structure, but usually has to be fixed by precipitation of the proteins. This fixing process is probably more disruptive than the homogenizing required for the previously described technique. For years histologists have used this principle to stain tissues, but recently the reactions used have become very specific and have revealed, for example, the precise locations of enzymes within cells. The technique has also played a major part in revealing the presence of highly localized neurotransmitter systems in the brain.

An improvement in the technique of microscopy which has been extremely useful is the development of the electron microscope. The ability of electron radiation to pass through structures of different composition varies in exactly the same way as light varies in its ability to penetrate. The important difference between light and an electron beam is that the latter enables greatly enhanced resolution of the image to be achieved. Detailed structure may be seen which is not visible with the light microscope. This means, however, that the total field of view is very small and the section viewed is very thin. It is necessary, therefore, to correlate the structures studied with the electron microscope with studies using the light microscope so that the relationships between adjacent structures can be understood.

The physiology of neurons

Neurons, like all cells in the body, have a very large number of chemical reactions occurring within them. Most of these processes are not unique to neurons but form the bases of the life process in all cells. In this section only those aspects of neuronal physiology which are of special relevance to an understanding of neuronal function will be described. It is important to remember, however, that dysfunction of nervous tissues frequently occurs as the result of a disturbance of general metabolism and the breakdown of a chain of synthetic reactions which are not unique to neurons.

The plasma membrane of neurons has properties which enable a potential difference of some 70 millivolts (mV; 10^{-3} volt) to be developed across it. This membrane potential is found in many cells of the body and is usually quite stable. In excitable cells, however, it is not stable, and if they are stimulated, the membrane potential will suddenly reverse. This reversal will last for a very brief time only, and is called the action potential. The action potential flows away from the point of stimulation, in all directions, until most of the plasma membrane has been invaded. When the terminals of axons are invaded by an action potential, a chemical is released which can excite (or inhibit) other neurons. The following section examines these special characteristics of excitable cells in some more detail.

THE MEMBRANE POTENTIAL

Although membrane potentials are not unique to excitable cells, it is clear from the summary above that a proper understanding of the forces generating the potential is essential to an understanding of neurophysiology. The plasma membrane, surrounding the neuron, is 'porous'. Molecules and ions can pass into and out of the cell through very small pores in the membrane. Although it is impossible to see these pores, calculations suggest that they have a diameter of 0.4–0.5 nm. Many molecules are larger than this and have difficulty in passing through the membrane. Of course, larger molecules do pass into the cell, but do so more slowly, either by dissolving in the lipid of the membrane itself or because the membrane invaginates and envelops a small volume of extracellular fluid which contains the large molecules. Normally, however, any molecule and ion larger than 0.4–0.5 nm cannot traverse the membrane rapidly. Analysis of extracellular and intracellular fluids of neurons reveals that, apart from water, the most common ions of around this size are sodium $(Na^+)^*$, potassium (K^+) and chloride (Cl^-). It would be expected that these would all pass through the membrane with ease, and experiments can be conducted to determine whether this is so. If radioactively labelled Na^+, K^+ and Cl^- are injected into a neuron and the cell suspended in extracellular fluid for a time, the extracellular fluid can be examined to determine whether the radioactivity has diffused out of the cell. Such experiments have demonstrated the ease with which K^+ and Cl^- pass through the membrane. Na^+ also comes out of the cell, but it does so much more quickly than expected. The experiment can be done the other way around—i.e. the radioactively labelled ions are in the extracellular fluid and their appearance inside the cell is followed. Again K^+ and Cl^- cross the membrane with ease but Na^+, this time, enters the cell slowly. Thus, Na^+ passes out of the cell with great facility but enters it with difficulty. Finally, labelled Na^+ can be added to the inside of the cell together with a metabolic poison such as dinitrophenol which blocks energy-consuming processes. Under these circumstances Na^+ leaves the cell slowly.

The conclusion is that an energy-consuming process pumps Na^+ out of the cell. When this is poisoned, Na^+ pass through the membrane with difficulty. The explanation for the difficulty Na^+ experience in passing across the membrane lies in the size of the ions. They are hydrated ions, always, in aqueous solution, being surrounded by molecules of water tightly attached by electrical forces. This makes the diameter of the Na^+ much larger than that of K^+ and too large to pass freely through the pores in the membrane:

Ion	Diameter (nm; 10^{-9} metres)
Cl^-	0.38
K^+	0.40
Na^+	0.59

If Na^+ is being pumped out of the cell and can only diffuse back with difficulty, it might be expected that the inside of the cell has a low concentration of Na^+.

*The symbol Na^+ is employed throughout this text as a shorthand for 'sodium ions' or 'some ionized sodium'.

Analysis of intracellular and extracellular fluids shows that this is so and that K^+ and Cl^- are distributed unevenly as well (*see Table 3.1*).

TABLE 3.1. Differences in the concentration of principal ions in mammals (all values are in milliequivalents/litre)

Ion	Extracellular	Intracellular
Cl^-	120	4
K^+	4	155
Na^+	140	12

Other experiments with radioactively labelled ions and poisons show that there is a metabolic pump which transfers potassium into the cell. Furthermore, the sodium pump and the potassium pump either are closely linked or are the same pump, because if K^+ are not available for transfer then Na^+ are not extruded from the cell. It should be noted that there is little evidence for a chloride pump in mammalian neurons, although chloride is actively transported across their membranes in other species. However, the results of some experiments in mammals seem to be explicable only if Cl^- also are pumped out of the cell.

To summarize so far, experiments lead to the conclusion that Na^+ are relatively impermeable to passage across the cell membrane and are pumped out of neurons; K^+ are relatively permeable but are continually pumped into the cells. As might be predicted, extracellular Na^+ concentration is high and intracellular K^+ concentration is high. Chloride does not seem to be pumped and yet is unevenly distributed. In *Figure 3.2* the representation of the ion distributions around a nerve cell shows

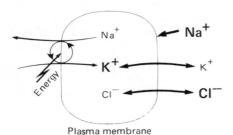

Plasma membrane

Figure 3.2 Electrolyte distribution across the cell membrane. For details, see text

by the size of the lettering that K^+ is highly concentrated inside the cell and Na^+ and Cl^- concentration are high outside the cell. To the right of the diagram the arrows reveal that the permeability of Na^+ through the membrane is poor but that K^+ and Cl^- can pass with relative ease. To the left is shown the energy-consuming metabolic pump transferring Na^+ out of and K^+ into the cell.

How do these ion distributions explain the membrane potential? As these ions are charged particles, an uneven distribution of ions on either side of the membrane may lead to an uneven distribution of charges on either side of the membrane. However, measurements show that the intracellular and the extracellular fluids are electrochemically neutral. In other words, as far as can be practically determined, there are just as many positively charged ions as there are negatively charged ions in either fluid. The intracellular fluid contains many very large negatively charged ions (proteins and phosphate ions) which cannot penetrate the plasma membrane and are not included in *Figure 3.2*. The charges on these ions balance the high concentration of K^+ inside the cell.

To explain the membrane potential, diffusional forces must be considered. For instance, K^+ will tend to diffuse down its concentration gradient, from the high intracellular concentration, and move out of the cell. When it does so, the positive charges must move with the ions. The large-sized negatively charged particles cannot pass through the membrane; therefore, the inside of the cell would have slightly too few positive charges and would become negatively charged. The negative charge inside the cell prevents the escape of more than a small fraction of K^+ and attracts Na^+, but these are unable to pass the membrane freely and cannot enter the cell to neutralize the negative charge. Cl^- can penetrate the membrane easily, but the negative charge on the ions is repelled by the negative charge inside the cell. Any Cl^- that enter would increase the negative charge inside the cell. Thus, it is the ability of K^+ to diffuse through the plasma membrane, and carry charges with them, that causes the inside of cells to be negatively charged. It is wrong to think of the membrane potential as a *direct* result of activity of the energy-consuming Na^+/K^+ pump. If this pump is poisoned, the charge remains across the membrane for some considerable time, although eventually it will wane as the concentration of ions slowly equilibrates.

The membrane potential of neurons is about $-70mV$, the inside of the plasma membrane being negative. The factors controlling the diffusion of ions which give this particular value have to include the electrical forces of repulsion between similarly charged particles and of attraction between unlike charges. When the inside of the cell possesses a certain charge, no more K^+ will diffuse out, because the attraction between the positively charged ions and the negatively charged solution will be too great. It can be thought of as two forces: A, the force of diffusion, pushing K^+ out of the cell; and B, an electrical force, holding potassium back inside the cell. When these two forces are equal (and they are, of course, opposite), a state of equilibrium will result and the net flow of ions will be zero (*Figure 3.3*).

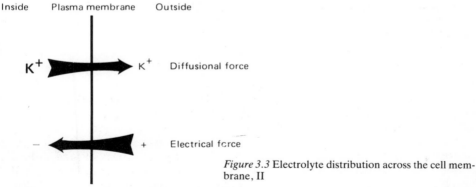

Inside   Plasma membrane   Outside

K^+ ⟶ K^+ Diffusional force

− ⟵ +   Electrical force

Figure 3.3 Electrolyte distribution across the cell membrane, II

When these forces are precisely balanced for all the diffusible ions around the plasma membrane, the membrane potential will be quite stable.

These processes are described precisely by the Nernst and Goldman equations. The Nernst equation enables the calculations of the membrane potential expected if only one ion is involved:

$$E = K \log \frac{\text{ionic concentration on one side}}{\text{ionic concentration on the other side}}$$

where E is the equilibrium potential difference across the membrane and K is a constant depending upon temperature, valency of ions, etc. (at 37°C, $K = 60$). By use of this equation and the known concentration of ions inside cells and in extracellular fluid, the potentials at which the diffusional and electrical forces would be in equilibrium can be calculated:

Na^+ +60 mV
Cl^- −70 mV
K^+ −90 mV approximately

(The negative signs indicate that the inside of the cell is negative.) The experimentally measured membrane potential is about −70 mV. Only chloride is at equilibrium, across the cell membrane at the membrane potential. It has been suggested up to now that Na^+ ions are impermeable and do not influence the polarization of the membrane. This is qualitatively true, but measurements reveal that although Na^+ are 50 times less able to penetrate the membrane than K^+, they can still do so slightly. Therefore, Na^+ will have an effect on the polarization of the membrane in proportion to its permeability. Thus, Na^+ movement will tend to make the inside of the cell positive and K^+ movement to make the inside more negative. The actual membrane potential will be somewhere in between. Where in between these extremes is revealed by the Goldman equation:

$$E = K \log \frac{\text{permeability} \times \text{concentration of ion A (outside)} + \text{permeability} \times \text{concentration of ion B (outside)} + \ldots}{\text{permeability} \times \text{concentration of ion A (inside)} + \text{permeability} \times \text{concentration of ion B (inside)} + \ldots}$$

where E is the membrane potential and K is a constant depending upon temperature, etc. Obviously, the net influence of any ion upon the membrane potential is very dependent not only upon the difference in concentration of the ion across the membrane, but also upon the permeability of the ion through the membrane. If the basis of the membrane potential is grasped, then much of the remaining electrophysiology of neurons becomes easily understood.

THE ACTION POTENTIAL

It has already been stated that a membrane potential is a characteristic of many cells of the body. Neurons (and muscle cells) are unusual in that they are excitable cells. The membrane potential of excitable cells is not stable and can show sudden brief reversals of the membrane potential, known as action potentials.

Figure 3.4 provides a graph of the action potential as a change in voltage across the plasma membrane plotted against time. This is the usual way of presenting the action potential, because the cathode ray oscilloscope automatically creates this graph when it is used to study action potentials. *Figure 3.4* shows that an action potential from a neuron or nerve fibre of mammals lasts for a little less than a millisecond, is roughly triangular in shape and involves a reversal of the membrane potential. These elements imply that the action potential is not very variable in form, and this is essentially true. It is commonly called an 'all or none' event, which indicates that an action potential is unlikely to occur in a partial or graded form but will always, within a few per cent, have the characteristics illustrated. In some muscles, and in invertebrate species, a considerable range of action potential shapes and sizes are encountered, yet in human neurons this is not so.

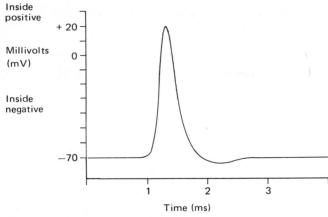

Figure 3.4 The action potential

Ionic basis of the action potential

A number of factors cause the membrane potential of excitable cells to be unstable. A revealing experiment involves the addition of radioactively labelled Na$^+$ to a dish of artificial extracellular fluid and suspending a large nerve in the dish. After some time the nerve is removed and washed, and the radioactivity in the nerve is determined. As may be expected from the relative impermeability of the nerve cell membranes to Na$^+$, rather little radioactivity is found inside the nerve. If the same process is repeated, but this time the nerve is regularly stimulated so that action potentials pass along it, then it is found to have a larger amount of radioactivity inside. Analysis of the total amount of sodium inside the axon would show little change in the internal concentration of sodium, but some of the sodium is now radioactive. It may be concluded that the passage of action potentials involves the entry of Na$^+$ into the cell. Other experiments reveal that the permeability of the plasma membrane to sodium alters during the action potential. Some of the most elegant experiments ever done have demonstrated this fact and left little doubt that the following account is true.

The Goldman equation shows that the equilibrium potential for Na$^+$ is +60 mV (inside positive). The recorded membrane potential is –70 mV, however, because the permeability of the membrane to K$^+$ is high and the permeability to Na$^+$ is low. Na$^+$, therefore, have little effect on the resting membrane potential. The forces acting on Na$^+$ (*see Figure 3.2*) are an *inward* diffusional force and an *inward* electrical force. At the onset of the action potential, the membrane suddenly becomes permeable to Na$^+$ and a vigorous inrush of Na$^+$ results. The charges carried with the sodium cause the inside of the membrane to become positively charged. The permeability change to Na$^+$ is best thought of as an opening of Na$^+$ channels through the membrane to above 0.6 nm (*see* table on page 49). It is further suggested that the opening of the channels is itself sensitive to the potential gradient across the membrane, and a fall in potential beyond a critical value causes the opening of the channels.

The permeability of the membrane to sodium is very short-lived (*Figure 3.5*). The forces acting on K$^+$ at the peak of the action potential are additive: the electrical forces repel positively charged ions from the inner surface of the

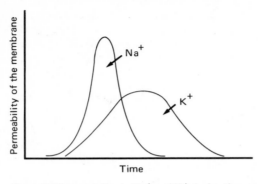

Figure 3.5 Permeability to Na$^+$ and K$^+$ during the action potential

membrane and the diffusional force for K$^+$ is an outward force. K$^+$, therefore, rapidly leave the cell. The transfer of positive charge out of the cell causes the inside to become negative again, and the membrane potential is recovered. The process of K$^+$ flux is assisted by an increase in the permeability of the membrane to K$^+$.

The increased permeability of the membrane to K$^+$ outlasts the action potential by a millisecond and causes a small overshoot of the membrane potential immediately after the action potential (*Figure 3.4*).

Conduction of the action potential
Action potentials pass along axons, which have a superficial resemblance to insulated wires. Conduction of the action potential is fundamentally different from

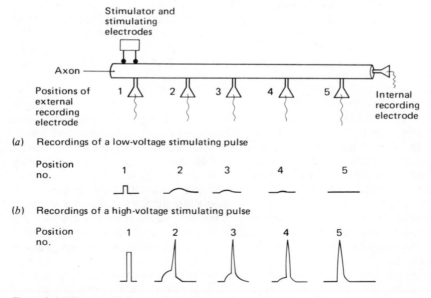

Figure 3.6 'All or none' characteristics of the action potential

conduction in a wire, however, and some useful contrasts can be drawn between the two. An electrical impulse passed along an insulated wire progressively loses voltage (as happens in any wire telephone or telegraph system), whereas an action potential has an amplitude at the end of an axon equal to its amplitude at the beginning. Electrical impulses pass through wire at close to the speed of light, but action potentials are conducted comparatively slowly along axons.

An experiment can be done with a single axon laid over two wires (*Figure 3.6*). Records of the transmembrane voltage are made at various distances from the wires. If a brief low-voltage pulse is applied to the wires, no action potential is initiated and nothing may be recorded some distance from the stimulating wires. Close to them, however, a small, short, depolarization of the membrane is recorded.

If the voltage applied to the stimulating wires is increased, the small local depolarization increases in amplitude until, suddenly, the full action potential appears superimposed upon it. When the action potential is recorded close to the stimulating wires, the process continues along the whole length of the axon. It seems that a small depolarization of the membrane is insufficient to generate the action potential but, above a critical value, a larger depolarization triggers the opening of the sodium channels and elicits the 'all or none' action potential. This is the basis of the generation and propagation of the action potential in non-experimental conditions.

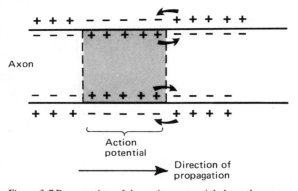

Figure 3.7 Propagation of the action potential along the axon

Figure 3.7 shows an action potential moving along an axon, the small arrows representing the currents that must flow inside and outside the plasma membrane. These currents will reduce the membrane potential ahead of the action potential, until the critical level is reached and the Na^+ pores open. It is this which results in the continual movement of the action potential along the axon.

The action potential does not change direction and pass back along the axon, because the membrane is in a stable condition for a short period after recovery of the membrane potential. The Na^+ pores are resistant to reopening shortly after closing for a time known as the refractory period, lasting approximately 0.5 ms.

The opening and closing of Na^+ channels and other processes underlying the action potential take a measurable time to occur, and the action potentials progress slowly along the axons. The rate of conduction can be measured by placing stimulating wires at one end of an axon and recording from several points at increasing distance from the end (*Figure 3.8*).

When the stimulus is applied to the left-hand end of the axon, an action potential is generated and a small artefact is conducted along the nerve at approximately the speed of light. This artefact can be detected by all the recording stations along the length of the nerve, and precisely locates the moment when the action potential was initiated. By measuring how long one has to wait for the action potential to arrive, the conduction velocity can be calculated. In the example, the conduction velocity is 50 metres per second (m/s).

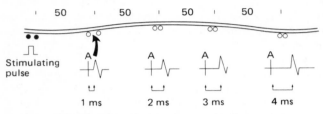

Figure 3.8 Rate of conduction of the action potential. Distances in mm; A = stimulus artefact

The biphasic (upward, then downward) nature of the recorded action potential is due to the potential arriving first at one recording wire and then at the second wire of the recording electrodes. Owing to the normal arrangement of the recording circuit, this leads to a biphasic signal.

Action potentials are conducted over a wide range of velocities in different axons in both peripheral and central nervous systems. Velocities as low as 0.5 m/s and as high as 110 m/s occur in man and other mammals. The size of axons varies a good deal, as does the complexity of the surrounding tissues.

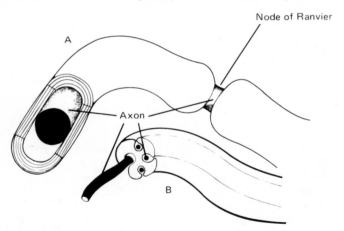

Figure 3.9 This diagram shows a myelinated axon (A) and a group of unmyelinated axons (B). Both are surrounded by protective sheaths. The illustrated nerves are peripheral and the sheaths are formed by Schwann cells. In the central nervous system a similar protective function is carried out by oligodendrocytes. Note that axons vary in diameter, thickness of the protective sheath, structure of the protective sheath and the closeness with which the sheath is applied to the axon. The nodes of Ranvier only occur in those fibres which have thick closely applied sheaths

The range of types of fibre is considerable, varying from large-diameter axons, with closely applied thick layers of protective sheath, to small poorly protected axons. *Figure 3.9* shows a myelinated axon (A) and a group of unmyelinated axons (B). Both are surrounded by protective sheaths. The illustrated nerves are peripheral and the sheaths are formed by Schwann cells. In the CNS a similar protective function is carried out by oligodendrocytes. Axons vary in diameter, in the thickness of the protective sheath, in the structure of the protective sheath and in the closeness with which the sheath is applied to the axon. The nodes of Ranvier only occur in those fibres which have thick closely applied sheaths. Large-diameter axons conduct action potentials more quickly than do small axons. Those axons covered with thick layers of Schwann cells, interrupted occasionally by nodes of Ranvier, conduct more quickly than would be expected from their axon diameter alone. Cells with no protective Schwann cell sheath conduct slowly. These two factors, diameter and sheath, explain the range of conduction velocities encountered.

The protective sheaths around axons contain myelin, which is a good electrical insulator. The external currents in *Figure 3.10* cannot flow easily in myelinated

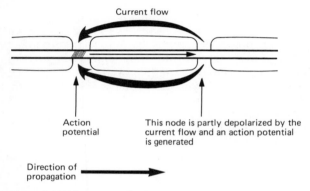

Current flow

Action potential

This node is partly depolarized by the current flow and an action potential is generated

Direction of propagation

Figure 3.10 Saltatory conduction

axons and action potentials are not propagated along them in the same way as previously described for unmyelinated axons. Action potentials can only develop at the nodes of Ranvier, and the extra-axonal currents flow outside the myelin sheath. This current flow is sufficient to depolarize the next node along the fibre to its critical value, so that it then develops an action potential.

Because the action potential 'jumps' from node to node, this form of propagation is known as *saltatory conduction* (from the Latin *saltare*, to leap). It is faster than in unmyelinated axons by up to 50-fold, because between nodes of Ranvier the currents travel at approximately the speed of light. It is also more efficient in metabolic terms, since only small bits of the axon are depolarized and correspondingly small amounts of Na^+ and K^+ move across the membrane.

It is because of saltatory conduction that many neuronal processes in the human CNS can operate so rapidly.

Chapter 4

Transmission between neurons

Introduction

In Chapter 3 the typical neuron of the central nervous system (CNS) was shown to have an axon which divides into several terminal branches. At the end of each branch a terminal swelling was closely applied to another neuron. There are many variations on this basic theme. Sometimes an axon will be repeatedly applied to several cells. Each time the axon approaches another cell, it swells into a terminal but then continues on to form several more synaptic contacts. Terminals are applied to many different regions of cells. They are found on dendrites, on the cell body and also on the area where the axon forms from the cell body. The terminal may be applied to a flat portion of a cell membrane or may lie on a projection from the surface known as a spine. There are also axo-axonic contacts where one terminal makes contact with another (*Figure 4.1*). Considerable variation can be

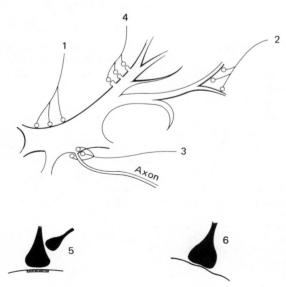

Figure 4.1 These schematic diagrams illustrate the considerable variation found in synapses within the central nervous system. Terminals may be: 1, axonal somatic synapses; 2, axonal-dendritic synapses; 3, axon-hillock synapses; 4, dendritic spine synapses; 5, axo-axonal synapses; tight, or electrical, synapse (note the narrow gap between presynaptic and postsynaptic neurons)

58

detected in the fine structure of the terminal regions, the most striking being the so-called tight junctions where particularly close contact between two cells occurs and the terminal is lacking some of the special features usually associated with them. This confusing variation is such an essential feature of neurotransmission in the CNS that it is necessary to bear in mind that the account which follows is typical but cannot be applied in a simple way to all neurotransmitter systems.

Excitatory transmission

In the mammal neurotransmission has been studied most extensively on the motoneuron (anterior horn cell). These cells are large—approximately 70 μm in diameter—and are innervated by different axons which enter the spinal cord through the dorsal roots. The motoneuron axons leave the CNS through the ventral roots. Several techniques are used to study them. Most information has come from

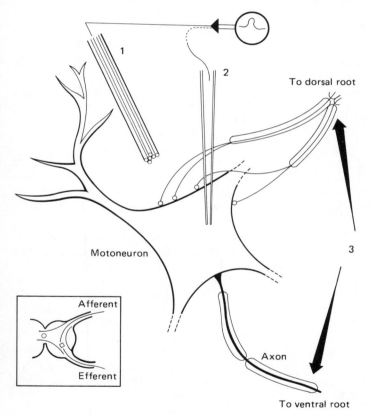

Figure 4.2 The diagram indicates three major techniques for studying the physiology of neurotransmission in the motoneuron. (1) Shows the tip of a five-barrelled glass micropipette lying in the extracellular space close to a motoneuron. One barrel of the pipette is filled with an electrolyte solution and action potentials generated by the motoneuron can be detected by the pipette, amplified and displayed, as shown, on an oscilloscope. (2) Shows another micropipette actually within the motoneuron, and (3) indicates points where the incoming or outgoing axons may be electrically stimulated

those where the cell is penetrated with the tip of a very fine micropipette made from a glass tube. The tip of the pipette is too small to damage the cell extensively, and the cell membrane apparently 'seals' around the pipette wall, so that the integrity of the cell is maintained. Thereafter, with some good fortune, it continues to function normally. The pipette is filled with an electrolyte solution which enables the electrical potential inside the cell to be recorded. The experimental layout is as in *Figure 4.2*.

Before the pipette has penetrated the cell membrane, the amplifier records the difference in voltage between the fluid in the pipette and the contact with the extracellular fluids of the animal. When the tip of the pipette lies in extracellular fluid, no voltage difference is observed on the oscilloscope screen, but as the pipette penetrates a motoneuron, a voltage of −70 mV is suddenly obtained. This is the potential across the cell membrane of the motoneuron. As described in Chapter 3, the inside of the cell is always negatively charged. It is now possible to stimulate the dorsal roots, thus creating action potentials in the afferent axons, and to record the effects of these on the membrane potential of the motoneuron (*Figure 4.3*).

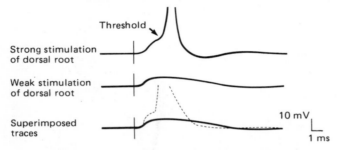

Figure 4.3 The effects of strong and weak stimulation of dorsal roots on the membrane potential of a motoneuron. In the lower part of the figure the two traces are superimposed

Weak stimulation of the dorsal roots causes a small depolarization of the cell membrane which lasts for 5 ms or so. Even weaker stimulation produces a smaller depolarization, and stronger stimulation produces a larger depolarization. If the depolarization reaches a critical value (threshold), an action potential is triggered. These graded depolarizations of the membrane are called excitatory postsynaptic potentials (e.p.s.p.s). It can be shown that weak stimulation of the dorsal root evokes an action potential in only a few of the many axons with terminals applied to the motoneuron, and activity in only a few terminals is insufficient to cause an e.p.s.p. large enough to trigger an action potential. Stronger stimulation evokes action potentials in many different fibres and an e.p.s.p. results which reaches threshold and an action potential is generated. As stated above, action potentials, unlike e.p.s.p.s, are not graded. They obey the 'all or none' law.

Inhibitory transmission

The experiment described in *Figure 4.2* does not always reveal e.p.s.p.s. During the excitation of motoneurons of an antagonist muscle, a quite different type of postsynaptic potential will be seen. Instead of a depolarization of the membrane, a hyperpolarization occurs—i.e. the potential across the membrane is increased

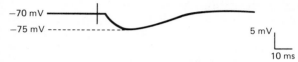

-70 mV

-75 mV

5 mV

10 ms

Figure 4.4 The inhibitory postsynaptic potential (i.p.s.p.)

(interior becoming more negative) above its usual level. The membrane potential thus moves further away from the threshold at which an action potential can be initiated. More e.p.s.p.s are now required to bring the potential down to threshold and evoke action potentials. Thus, action potentials are less likely to occur during inhibitory postsynaptic potentials (i.p.s.p.s). I.p.s.p.s have a longer duration than e.p.s.p.s, lasting for 10–20 ms (*Figure 4.4*).

Ionic bases of synaptic potentials

It is possible with some nerve cells from invertebrate species to bathe the outside of the cell body membrane with fluids lacking some of the ions normally present in extracellular fluid. Micropipettes can be used to inject ions into mammalian cells and thus alter the relative concentrations of ion across the membrane. The effects that these treatments have on the synaptic potentials leads to the conclusion that postsynaptic potentials, like the action potential, are the result of changes in the permeability of the cell membrane to ions.

The e.p.s.p. is a depolarization of the membrane. Either Cl^- leave the inside of the membrane or Na^+ enter. Altering Cl^- concentration on either side of the membrane has little effect, and it has been concluded that the e.p.s.p. results from an increase in permeability of the membrane to Na^+ which flow into the cell, reducing the inner negativity. Altering K^+ concentration also alters the e.p.s.p. however, so the permeability of the membrane to K^+ must change also. If K^+ did not flow out of the cell as Na^+ entered, the e.p.s.p. would be much larger than it is (*Figure 4.5*).

The i.p.s.p. is relatively unaffected by changes in Na^+ concentrations on either side of the membrane, and it is concluded that this ion does not participate. Alteration of K^+ and Cl^- concentrations has a marked effect, however. Increase of the membrane permeability to K^+ (opening of K^+ channels) allows the efflux of positive charge, which results in the hyperpolarization of the membrane. The ability of Cl^- to flow through the same, or adjacent, channels in the membrane reduces the size of the i.p.s.p. (*Figure 4.5*). The effect of these ion fluxes can be understood in greater detail by reference to the Goldman equation (*see* page 52).

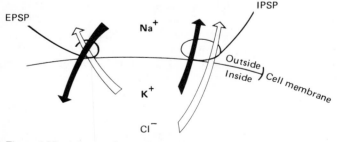

Figure 4.5 Ionic bases of synaptic potentials

The integration of excitation and inhibition by neurons

Some invertebrate species have very large neurons, so that micropipettes can be placed into different parts of the cell. This technique has been used to find out that synaptic potentials are largest immediately beneath the synaptic terminals and that, as the pipette is moved away from the synaptic region, they become smaller. This suggests that the potentials are not propagated like action potentials but give rise to currents which flow through the fluids of the cell, just as current flows through a piece of wire. The cell membrane in the region of the axon hillock is much more sensitive to the flow of these currents than is any other part of the cell, and it is at the axon hillock that the action potential is generated (*Figure 4.6*).

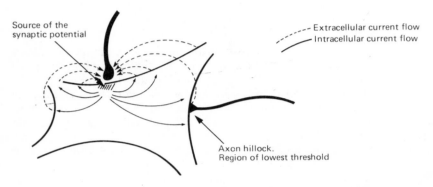

Figure 4.6 Current flow resulting from partial depolarization of a small part of a cell membrane beneath a synaptic terminal

The effect of current flow in reducing the membrane potential to a critical level for generation of the action potential was described in the section on propagation of the action potential along axons (page 55). It may be helpful to refer back to this section. As in the case of the action potential being propagated along a nerve fibre, at the axon hillock the Na$^+$ channels of the membrane are opened by the small drop in membrane potential caused by the e.p.s.p. developing elsewhere in the neuron.

The role of the axon hillock as the site of action potential initiation has an interesting implication for the integrative functions of nerve cells. The axon hillock is bombarded by a wide range of influences from thousands of terminals all over the soma and dendrites of the neuron. It is the additive resultant of all these influences which determines whether an action potential is produced. A relevant experiment is illustrated in *Figure 4.7*.

Stimulation of excitatory axon A evokes a very small e.p.s.p. because the terminals are applied to the cell wall out on a dendrite. The e.p.s.p. is generated at some distance from the soma and the axon hillock, and has a much smaller effect on them than on the excitatory terminals of axons B or C. These both have terminals on the cell soma and generate very large e.p.s.p.s when they are stimulated. However, neither is large enough to reach the threshold for initiation of action potentials. D and E axons are both inhibitory and their stimulation causes an i.p.s.p. As both have terminals located close to the soma, the i.p.s.p.s are of similar size.

The interaction between the synapses is particularly interesting. Simultaneous stimulation of axons A and B evokes e.p.s.p.s which are additive. The large e.p.s.p. from B adds with the small e.p.s.p. from A to give a total which exceeds the threshold depolarization at the axon hillock, and an action potential is initiated. Stimulation of axons B and D evokes an e.p.s.p. and an i.p.s.p. These add to give a small complex wave on the membrane potential which does not come near to initiating an action potential. The depolarization is much smaller than when B was stimulated alone.

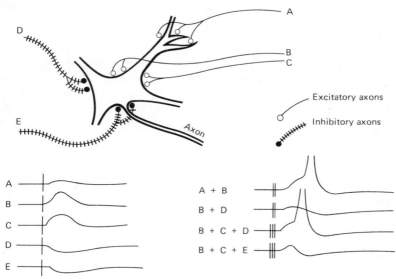

Figure 4.7 Some experiments on the interaction of synapses

Stimulation of B, C and D evokes an action potential, because B and C both give rise to large e.p.s.p.s and the i.p.s.p. from D is insufficient to lower its amplitude to below threshold. However, axon E produces a considerable suppression of the large e.p.s.p.s to well below threshold. This may seem surprising in view of the similarity of the i.p.s.p. amplitudes evoked from D and E. The explanation lies in the location of the terminals of E. They are placed very close to the axon hillock, which is maximally influenced by their activity. Terminals in this location often seem to be inhibitory and have such a potent effect that they may be thought of as 'turning the cell off', effectively overriding other influences upon it. The complex nature of interactions between afferent inputs to cells can be understood partially by this experiment, but it must be realized that even this is a simplification.

The example of *Figure 4.7* does not include an excitatory input which, by itself, is sufficient to evoke an action potential. Although there are synaptic contacts between cells capable of simply relaying action potentials from one cell to another, much activity in afferent pathways evokes e.p.s.p.s which are subthreshold. Although they do not evoke action potentials, they increase the excitability of the cell, and make it more likely that a subsequent e.p.s.p. will do so. It is particularly important that transmission in the CNS be *not* thought of as a process of one action potential leading to another on a different cell. It is much more accurate to think of a cell receiving many excitatory inputs and action potentials occurring when several inputs are active simultaneously. This concept stresses the process of integration which occurs at cells and helps to develop an understanding of the brain as a decision-making organ.

Presynaptic inhibition

There is a form of inhibition in the CNS of mammals which is very different from the postsynaptic inhibition which has just been described. This is known as presynaptic inhibition, and its presence is demonstrated by the following experiment (*Figures 4.8, 4.9*).

Stimulation of input A evokes an e.p.s.p. but stimulation of B has no apparent effect on the postsynaptic cell. Nevertheless, when B is stimulated some time before A, the e.p.s.p. produced by A is very much reduced in size. There are several possible explanations for this result, but in some tissues from invertebrates it has been possible to demonstrate that stimulation of B evokes the depolarization

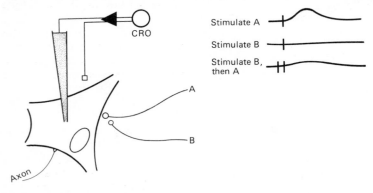

Figure 4.8 Presynaptic inhibition, I

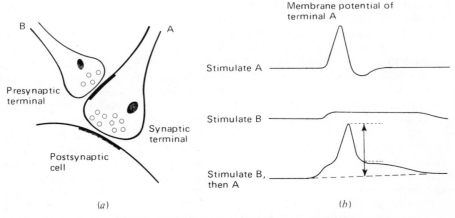

Figure 4.9 Presynaptic inhibition, II. The arrow in the lower part of (b) indicates the normal height of the action potential on terminal A. Depolarization of terminal A by activity in terminal B reduces the amplitude of this action potential

of terminal A. Many experiments have led to the following conclusion. Histologists have reported the existence of axo-axonic synapses where one axon seems to terminate on another axon, close to its terminal. An action potential in the first terminal evokes an e.p.s.p.-like depolarization of the second terminal such that when an action potential arrives at the second terminal, it is reduced in size.

It seems that the amplitude of the excitatory postsynaptic potential is somehow related to the amplitude of the action potential arriving at the synaptic terminal. This can be explained briefly by stating that the release of the chemical transmitter from the synaptic terminal is proportional to the voltage change induced by the action potential (i.e. the 'height' of the action potential). Normally the membrane potential is $-70\,mV$ and the action potential peak has a value of $+40\,mV$—i.e. a total change of $110\,mv$. Partial depolarization of the synaptic terminal to, for example, $-50\,mV$ will cause an action potential to have an amplitude of only $90\,mV$. This is because the ion fluxes which determine the peak of the action potential cause the peak amplitude to be $+40\,mV$ whatever the starting point. It can be demonstrated experimentally that release of neurochemical transmitter substances is significantly less with this reduction in the amplitude of the action potential.

Presynaptic inhibition of this nature is probably a widespread phenomenon in the mammalian CNS. It provides the opportunity of reducing the effectiveness of one excitatory input to a cell without altering the excitability of the cell to other synaptic drives. There is a particularly interesting role for presynaptic inhibition in the control of pain (see below).

The chemical nature of neurotransmission

The best-known synapse in the body is the neuromuscular junction between the axons of motoneurons and the voluntary muscle fibres. The chemical nature of neurotransmission was discovered during experiments with this tissue, and many of the principles discovered apply equally to the neuromuscular junction and to synapses between neurons in the CNS. However, there are differences which must not be overlooked. The neuromuscular junction is never inhibitory in mammals; there is little opportunity for the integration of different afferent inputs; and the high safety factor ensures that one action potential in nerve gives rise to one action potential in muscle. The neuromuscular junction is a rather simple synapse.

If a muscle and the nerve innervating it are removed and placed into an oxygenated fluid of the body, several experiments can be performed which come close to proving the chemical nature of the neurotransmission process. Addition of acetylcholine to the fluid will cause a powerful contraction of the muscle. Electrical measurements will show that these contractions are due to repeated invasion of the muscle, but not the nerve, by action potentials. This effect of acetylcholine can be prevented by addition of D-tubocurarine to the bath. This substance, the active constituent of curare, blocks the action of acetylcholine without preventing action potentials travelling along the nerve or along the muscle. Administration of curare to the intact animal causes paralysis. It was concluded from these observations that the nerve secretes acteylcholine and that the muscle responds to the chemical. This has been confirmed by many different experiments. It has been shown that very small amounts of acetylcholine forced out of very fine glass pipettes will evoke action potentials on muscle, but only if the tip of the pipette is close to the point where the nerve lies against the muscle. The muscle is sensitive to acetylcholine only in the junctional region. Elsewhere acetylcholine is without effect. When the nerve is stimulated repeatedly for long periods, the concentration of acetylcholine in the bath fluid increases in proportion to the number of action potentials which arrive at the junction. Microchemical techniques also have revealed the presence of acetylcholine in the junctional region and that, during periods of intense activity of the nerve, the amount of acetylcholine can be reduced. These experiments were all difficult to perform for the first time. The technique took a long time to develop all the facets needed in a successful experiment. For example, acetylcholine is destroyed by the neuromuscular junction almost as quickly as the nerve can secrete it. The demonstration of the release of acetylcholine is convincing only when the degrading enzyme, cholinesterase, is destroyed. The experiments were difficult with the neuromuscular junction; those with synapses within the CNS are considerably more so.

One of the most intriguing techniques for the study of chemical transmission in the brain is micro-iontophoresis. A bundle of glass tubes is heated in the middle and pulled rapidly outwards to form a multibarrelled pipette (*Figure 4.10*). The fine end of the pipette does not seal off but the hole through each tube remains patent. The tip is very small, being 4–6 μm across, compared with the diameter of many cortical neurons of 20–40 μm. The tubes are filled with ionized solutions. One or more contain salt. These barrels are connected to amplifiers and an oscilloscope, and record the action potentials from active neurons which lie close to the tip of the pipette. These are extracellular records, and the potentials will be small, between 200 and 1000 μV. Ionized drug solutions are placed into the other barrels. A positive charge placed on top of the drug solution will cause the ejection of positively charged ions from the tip of the pipette and the attraction, away from the tip, of negatively charged ions. If acetylcholine (+), chloride (−) is in the pipette barrel, then acetylcholine (+) ions will move out of the electrode into the extracellular environment of the neurons lying close to the tip of the pipette. *Figure 4.11* shows how such a pipette can be used to study transmission of impulses in anterior horn cells (motoneurons) in the spinal cord.

This technique has also established that neocortical neurons are extremely sensitive to minute quantities of acetylcholine. The acetylcholine antagonist dihydro-β-erythroidine, applied before a pulse of acetylcholine, is able to block the effects of iontophoretically applied acetylcholine. The antagonist also prevents the cell responding to electrical stimulation of the midline thalamic nuclei. This suggests that stimulation of these nuclei causes the release of acetylcholine from afferent fibres onto postsynaptic receptors for acetylcholine. It is suggested that the transmission between the presynaptic fibres and the neocortical neuron is *cholinergic*. The cell is excited by electrical stimulation of many different pathways, however, and transmission at many of them is not affected by application of dihydro-β-erythroidine, which suggests that the cell has many different transmitters released onto it from different afferent fibres.

Further proof of the cholinergic nature of this transmission is required. Does activity in the afferent pathway cause the release of acetylcholine? A cortical cup is used. This is a small ring of Perspex sealed onto the surface of the exposed cortex with grease and filled with artificial cerebrospinal fluid. Every five minutes the fluid is removed and assayed for acetylcholine. If the enzyme cholinesterase is added to the fluid and the midline thalamic nuclei stimulated, acetylcholine appears in the cortical cup.

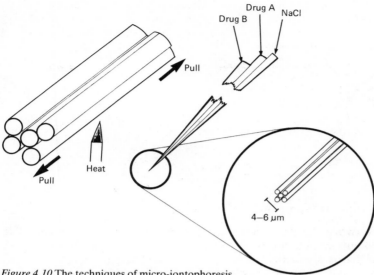

Figure 4.10 The techniques of micro-iontophoresis

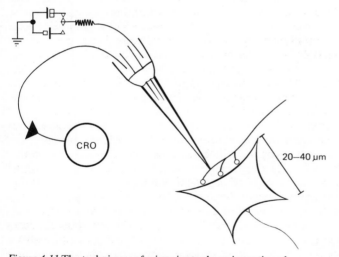

Figure 4.11 The techniques of micro-iontophoresis continued

These experiments, and many others giving quantitative measures of transmitter release and activity, are quite convincing. Acetylcholine is believed to be one of the transmitters between the thalamus and the neocortex. The experiments are difficult to conduct, however, and need to be repeated for each of the many pathways converging onto cortical cells, for all the cellular areas of the brain and for each of the chemicals that have been suggested as possible transmitters in the brain. This is a daunting prospect indeed, and explains why, at so many synapses, the neurotransmitters are still unidentified.

Figure 4.12 is a diagram of the synaptic terminal under the electron microscope, which shows that terminals do not make contact with cells. There is a gap or

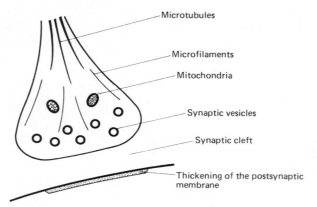

Figure 4.12 The synaptic terminal (diagrammatic)

synapse of 20 nm between the presynaptic and the postsynaptic membranes. The terminals contain many mitochondria which synthesize ATP among other things and it is concluded that many of the processes in axon terminals consume energy. Terminals usually contain synaptic vesicles, which are small round or oval sacs which cluster near to the synapse. Two experiments identify their function. Sucrose gradient ultracentrifugation was described on page 47. If homogenized brain is centrifuged in this way, a layer can be found which contains *synaptosomes*. These are the axon terminals and a small piece of the postsynaptic membrane. If these are subjected to osmotic shocks (i.e. are placed in a solution of low osmotic pressure), the synaptosomes rupture, spilling their contents. Centrifugation of this material provides a layer containing relatively pure synaptic vesicles which contain a particularly high concentration of neurotransmitter. It is likely, therefore, that the synaptic vesicles act as stores for transmitters.

Confirmation of this is provided by studies using the venom of the black widow spider. If the neuromuscular junction is studied with the isolated preparation described earlier, addition of the venom will cause vigorous contraction of the muscle. This is accompanied by the appearance of acetylcholine in the bathing fluid. The venom has caused the release of acetylcholine from the nerve ending. After a few minutes the contractions cease. Then the terminal region of the nerve is devoid of synaptic vesicles. It may be inferred from this experiment that the release of acetylcholine from the terminal involves the disruption of the synaptic vesicles. Precise quantitative studies using microelectrodes inside the postsynaptic cell to record depolarizations have provided good evidence that depolarizations are quantal in nature. That is to say that the smallest depolarization recorded with the minimum transmitter release is a unit, or quantum. All bigger depolarizations are $2 \times$, $3 \times$ ... $10000 \times$ this unit of depolarization. It is suggested that the unit of depolarization is the result of one quantum of transmitter. It is very tempting to believe that one quantum of transmitter is contained in one synaptic vesicle.

Although the process of transmitter release is not well understood, three facts support an interesting hypothesis. Calcium ions (Ca^{2+}) are required for the release of transmitter; Ca^{2+} enter axon terminals when these are invaded by action potentials, and the terminals contain two proteins called neurin and stenin. These proteins resemble the proteins, actin and myosin, found in muscle cells, proteins which require calcium ions to display their unusual interaction. It is proposed that the synaptic vesicles are coated with stenin and the microfilaments with neurin. In the presence of calcium, neurin and stenin interact in a ratchet-like way to roll the vesicle down the microfilament into contact with the presynaptic membrane. This is also coated with neurin and the synaptic vesicle ruptures into the synaptic cleft. This process is activated by the ingress of calcium, which occurs principally during the action potential. If Ca^{2+} leaks slowly into an axon terminal in the absence of an action potential, this would account for the spontaneous release of small amounts of transmitter sometimes seen. The whole process of interaction of Ca^{2+} with neurin and stenin is extremely reminiscent of that between calcium and the ratchet between actin and myosin which forms the basis of the contraction of muscle.

Transmitter is replenished in two ways. The basic method seems to be the synthesis of transmitter in the cell body and its migration in vesicles down the axon to the terminal. This can be seen in studies where nerve fibre tracts are cut in the CNS or where peripheral nerve trunks are tightly ligatured. Histochemical staining and microscopic examination a few days later shows that transmitter is concentrated close to the ligature on the same side as the cell body. It is believed that the granules are transported down the microtubules.

The second and probably dominant method of renewing transmitter occurs in the terminal itself. This usually contains all the enzymes required for synthesis of the transmitter from its substrate. This enters the terminals from the extracellular fluid. In other cases the neurotransmitter released by a previous action potential is rapidly taken back into the terminal and stored for future release.

Synaptic vesicles are lost when transmitter is ejected into the synaptic cleft. It seems possible that the membrane surrounding the vesicle fuses with, and becomes a part of, the terminal membrane. Evidence for this comes from the observation that intense activity of nerve terminals leads to swelling. Re-formation of the synaptic vesicles could occur by a mechanism revealed by experiments with horseradish peroxidase. This substance is easily stained and will not penetrate membranes. If it enters a cell, it must do so by a process of pinocytosis (the invagination of the cell membrane and the capture of some of the extracellular fluid). During intense nervous activity horseradish peroxidase placed into the extracellular fluid enters terminals. It is seen at first in coated vesicles (CV) which move to the centre of the terminal to coalesce into terminal cisternae (CIS). The cisternae then bud off simple vesicles (V) which contain both horseradish peroxidase and transmitter. This mechanism explains both the origin of vesicles and why, if vesicles fuse with the terminal membrane, this does not become hugely swollen (*Figure 4.13*).

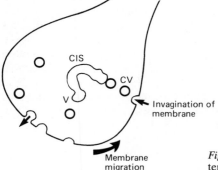

Figure 4.13 Synaptic vesicles and the re-use of terminal membrane

The e.p.s.p. resulting from the arrival of a single action potential at excitatory terminals lasts for 5–10 ms (*Figure 4.3*). This very brief effect of the transmitter implies that its life in the synaptic cleft is very brief. In the neuromuscular junction acetylcholine is inactivated by cholinesterase, an enzyme which splits the transmitter into acetate and choline. Neither of these substances will occupy the acetylcholine receptor, so this process terminates the postsynaptic activity. Choline re-enters the presynaptic terminal and is utilized in the synthesis of new transmitter.

There are degrading enzymes for all the transmitters but they are not all as active as is cholinesterase, and an alternative method of inactivation exists. This is the re-uptake of modified transmitter into the presynaptic terminals. The uptake process is extremely effective in limiting the time spent by the transmitter in the synaptic cleft. It also reduces the energy utilized in the transmitter synthesis, as the transmitter taken up is restored for future use.

The postsynaptic actions of transmitters are governed by the law of mass action. The postsynaptic effects are proportional to the concentration of transmitter, and factors such as temperature have the expected effect. Receptors for the transmitter lie on the postsynaptic membrane, presumably occupying the area which shows a postsynaptic thickening (*Figure 4.14*). The transmitter molecules and the receptor

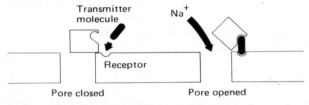

Figure 4.14 A gross oversimplification of the action of transmitters on the postsynaptic membrane

molecules show an affinity for each other which is probably based upon mutually 'satisfying' shapes, sizes and electrostatic charges. It is convenient to explain the interaction between transmitter and receptor in terms of similarity of shape, but this is clearly a diagrammatic oversimplification.

The diagram is useful because it helps to bring together the relationship between receptor occupation and alteration of Na^+ and K^+ conductance in the postsynaptic membrane.

There is some evidence that many transmitters (e.g. noradrenaline) do not act directly upon the ion channels but act via cyclic nucleotide systems (*Figure 4.15*). The enzyme adenyl cyclase is associated with the postsynaptic receptor for the neurotransmitter. When the receptor is occupied, the enzyme is activated. This causes the conversion of ATP molecules (adenosine triphosphate) to cyclic AMP (cyclic adenosine monophosphate). Cyclic AMP is a cofactor for protein kinase enzymes which phosphorylate proteins in the cell membrane. Perhaps the phosphorylation alters the configuration of the proteins which traverse the lipid membrane. This may create a pore through which sodium or potassium ions may flow. It should be noted that this is but one of many possible roles of cyclic AMP (or of cyclic guanosine monophosphate (GMP), which may be similarly produced). Protein kinase enzymes and phosphoprotein phosphatase enzymes within the cell's cytoplasm play important roles in activating further enzyme systems, perhaps affecting many aspects of the cell's metabolic activity over a considerable time

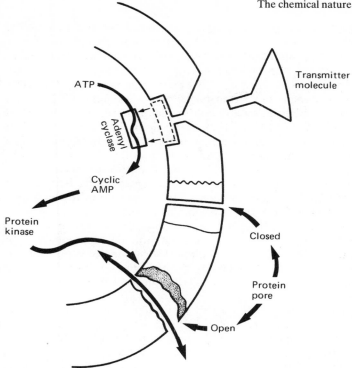

Figure 4.15 Although still a simplification of a proposed postsynaptic action of neurotransmitters, this scheme illustrates the level of complexity more realistically

period. It is highly speculative, but action of a transmitter substance which starts nucleotide cyclase activity and produces cyclic AMP or GMP may possibly be the basis of a chemical or metabolic change in the neuron which is concerned in the 'storage of memory traces' and thus of learned behaviour.

Quite apart from such speculation, and from this mechanism being one aspect of the postsynaptic response to a transmitter released from presynaptic terminals when action potentials reach them, nucleotide cyclases may be activated by other factors. The most important of these are the many peptide hormones known to affect behaviour as well as various physiological functions. It is generally accepted now that these hormones affect their target cells throughout the body in this way. Peptide hormones affecting mental behaviour will be described in more detail in Chapter 8. It is enough here to state that such effects are probably mediated through the nucleotide cyclase mechanism. The cyclic nucleotides in these reactions function as second messengers.

A wide range of chemical reactions may occur at the receptor on the postsynaptic membrane. Antagonists of neurotransmitter action may occupy the receptor without opening the ionic channel. The presence of the antagonist effectively holds the channel closed by denying the transmitter access to the receptor. Some antagonists are called competitive antagonists, because their effectiveness is proportional to their concentration and the transmitter and antagonist compete for occupation of the receptor. Other antagonists form an irreversible combination with the receptor, which means that they have very powerful and long-lasting effects even when administered in low concentrations. Many antagonists of neurotransmitters have shape and charge distributions on the molecule which resemble those of the transmitter (*see* below). They always differ from the transmitter, however, in a way which presumably prevents the opening of the ionic pores. It is a characteristic of many neurotransmitter receptors that close matching of shape or charge characteristics is necessary before occupancy of the receptor site occurs. Slight modification of the molecular shape profoundly reduces the effectiveness of the chemical. This means that the postsynaptic receptors of one synapse are unlikely to be affected by neurotransmitter from an adjacent synapse or by compounds circulating in the extracellular fluid. Such receptors are referred to as having a high degree of specificity. An example of this type of specificity is well known. As will be shown later, some nerve terminals release noradrenaline onto postsynaptic receptors. Adrenaline circulating in the blood has relatively weak effects on some of these postsynaptic receptors but strong actions on others. This is due to slight differences in the structure of the postsynaptic receptors which alters their affinity for adrenaline. Therefore, the circulating hormone can act powerfully at only some synaptic sites, mimicking the transmitter. Pharmacologists distinguish two main types of noradrenaline receptors, called alpha and beta receptors. A discussion of these occurs later.

This principle of specificity, which applies to most neurochemical transmitter systems, means that it is theoretically possible to influence transmission with drugs at one set of synapses without altering transmission at other synapses. In practice, this proves to be difficult, as the antagonists always have 'side-effects'. Many of these unwanted side-effects are not true side-effects, however, but a direct result of antagonizing the neurotransmitter. For example, administration of a vasodilator which blocks alpha-adrenergic receptors leads to failure of ejaculation, an unwanted side-effect. Both vasodilation and the failure of ejaculation are direct results of the antagonism of noradrenaline at postsynaptic receptors. Obviously, ejaculation failure is a side-effect because it is an unwanted effect, but pharmacologically it is not due to lack of specificity of the drug.

Autoreceptors and autoregulation (*Figure 4.16*)

At some synapses in the CNS, notably those employing noradrenaline, dopamine and 5-hydroxytryptamine as transmitters, autoreceptors have been described. These are on the presynaptic membrane—i.e. the axon terminal that liberates the transmitter substance. Some of the transmitter binds to these presynaptic terminals. This binding then reduces the subsequent liberation of the transmitter when further action potentials reach the terminal and reduces the formation of further transmitter. This process has been termed 'autoregulation', since release of transmitter regulates its own further release, in a negative direction. This effect of the autoreceptors is believed to be mediated by reducing the calcium ion available for transmitter release. Specific blocking of autoreceptors can be achieved, and this enhances the turnover of the transmitter substance and the firing rate of the postsynaptic cell.

One of the consequences of autoreceptor action being the reduction of transmitter release is that the density of the postsynaptic receptors may increase. This tends to restore the sensitivity of the postsynaptic neuron, so that it responds normally to the reduced quality of transmitter released when the presynaptic terminal receives impulses. It is now being suggested that an enhancement of autoreceptor activity has thus the effect of raising the sensitivity of the postsynaptic neuron to the transmitter.

It is reasonable to hope that when sufficient is understood about the complexities of the many transmitter systems in the brain, highly specific antagonists or potentiating agents will be found which have very discrete actions upon particular

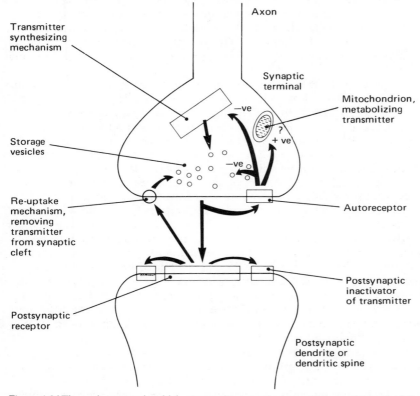

Figure 4.16 The various ways in which a transmitter may be removed from a synaptic cleft, and may interfere with its own production through presynaptic autoreceptors

aspects of brain function. It is certain that only a small proportion of these systems can at present be affected by drugs, and yet sufficient examples are available to illustrate how future progress can be achieved.

The central nervous system neurotransmitters

Before describing the neurotransmitters individually, we may pause and consider the survival value of the evolutionary development of different types of chemical with similar functions. It is difficult simply to list the facts, because so many of the actions of the transmitters are unknown. However, we can speculate with a fair degree of conviction. The first advantage of a range of chemical transmitters has been referred to already. The secretion of hormones such as adrenaline into the blood stream results in the activation of some of the postsynaptic receptors in the body. If these synapses are part of a functional system, then a generalized tonic action upon these synapses will alter the behavioural state of the animal. The 'flight or fright' reaction (following excitation of the alerting reaction centres due to activation of parts of the sympathetic outflow by adrenaline release) is a good example of such an action of a circulating hormone having obvious survival value. Actions of this type are only possible in organisms which have evolved different transmitter systems subserving different functions. Similar reasoning makes it easy to imagine the evolutionary development of two different neurotransmitter chemicals mediating excitation and inhibition. The primitive animal may have easily modified and maintained its levels of excitability by altering the levels of circulating hormone.

There is some evidence that the time course of the effects of the various transmitters is very different. For example, glutamate (an amino acid, but also a transmitter) is extremely fast-acting when applied to postsynaptic receptors, and substance P (a polypeptide transmitter) has a rather slow action on its receptors. The optimal functioning of some systems in the brain is best achieved by transmitters which have a slow but very prolonged action. Other systems use transmitters with fast but very brief actions on receptors. It is likely that the 'slow' transmitters are operating through the cyclic nucleotide system, perhaps as much on general neuronal metabolism as on membrane ionic permeability.

The time course of the postsynaptic effect of transmitters is influenced by several factors, the kinetics of the transmitter–receptor interaction being only one. Others include the activity of enzymes which inactivate the transmitter and the time course of the chemical reactions inside the postsynaptic cell which were triggered by the transmitter. Refer to *Figure 4.14*, which shows a postulated link between receptor occupation and opening of ionic pores in the membrane. If these chemical reactions are rapid and brief, then the apparent action of the transmitter will be brief. It is suspected that some transmitters trigger changes in the chemistry of the postsynaptic cell which are very prolonged—so prolonged that these chemical changes may form the basis of learning and memory.

It is almost hopeless to try to understand how the brain works before a complete list of transmitters is known. Regrettably, most neuroscientists suspect that many more transmitter substances remain to be identified, and there is an intense search for new chemical transmitters taking place at present. A set of criteria have come to be accepted as the guide to the degree of confidence one may have in any proposal that a new chemical joins the list of established transmitters. These criteria are:

(1) LOCATION *The substance must exist in the CNS.* Clearly, if the chemical does not exist in the brain in its natural state, it would be unlikely to be a transmitter. It is possible, however, that a problem lies with the chemical techniques for extracting and identifying the chemical, which may only be present in minute quantities.

    The substance must exist in the terminals of nerve, protected from enzymic degradation, possibly in synaptic vesicles. This criterion is often very difficult to satisfy. Complex microtechniques are required which do not completely disrupt the structure of the brain. Histochemical microfluorescence (page 78) has been very successful for some transmitters and immunofluorescence for others. This latter technique involves preparing a protein (a ligand) which binds in a highly specific manner to the proposed transmitter. The protein can then be made to fluoresce under the microscope.

Considerable doubt is currently being expressed over the need for transmitters to be stored in synaptic vesicles. Very many are, but do they all need to be? This is an unanswerable question, and perhaps the presence of transmitters in synaptic vesicles should not be considered essential.

Location of associated enzymes. Enzymes for the synthesis of the transmitter should also be located in the cell body and terminals. Transmitters are very potent substances and are usually synthesized very close to their site of action. Similarly, enzymes for the breakdown of the transmitter into inactive metabolites should be identified close to the synaptic terminals. Absence of any of these enzymes places doubt on the proposed neurotransmission role for any chemical. It must be remembered that many hundreds of chemical substances can be found in nerve terminals. They are not all neurotransmitters.

(2) RELEASE To be effective, neurotransmitters must be released into the extracellular fluid. Electrical stimulation of the afferent pathway should cause detectable quantities of the substance to appear in fluids bathing the cell. There are many ways of trying to demonstrate this. The cortical cup technique has been described previously. Such very small amounts of transmitter are released and the activity of enzymes inactivating the transmitter are so great that this is very difficult to do. Sometimes it may be considered sufficient to show that if transmitter synthesis is inhibited, electrical stimulation of the afferent pathway causes depletion of stores of transmitter in the nerve terminals. This is not so convincing, however, as there are many jobs done by chemicals in the terminal which are used up during intense nervous activity. Even if release is demonstrated, it must be remembered that many products of metabolism diffuse from cells into the extracellular fluid and then into the blood stream. Increased activity of cells leads to the increased production of waste products.

(3) IDENTITY OF ACTION *Is the proposed transmitter active on the postsynaptic membrane?* The substance must affect receptors on the postsynaptic membrane in such a way as to change the excitability of the cell. Furthermore, the concentration of substance required to have these effects must be similar to the concentration which can be achieved by neuronal release. Of course, many substances which are not transmitters are known to affect nervous activity even when applied in small concentrations. These substances are not found in nerve cells nor are they released by nerve stimulation.

Does the postsynaptic activity of the proposed transmitter resemble the effects of nerve stimulation? The final proof that the proposed substance is actually a neurotransmitter comes from experiments which show that the quantitative aspects of the postsynaptic effects of nerve stimulation closely resemble the effects of applying the substance artificially. It is best if the substance being applied is very pure and preferably synthesized in the laboratory.

The technique of micro-iontophoresis has been described previously. It enables the physiologist to determine whether the amplitudes of postsynaptic potentials are the same for the endogenous transmitter (synthesized by the animal) and for the exogenous transmitter (synthesized in the laboratory). The effects of the two substances on the opening of ionic channels may be compared. Lastly, the pharmacology of the two substances may be compared. If an antagonist is known which blocks the effects of the synthesized chemical, it must block the effects of nerve stimulation.

The next sections deal with the best-known of the neurotransmitters in the CNS in more detail. The outlines presented for each transmitter must be supplemented by reference to other chapters in this book.

Acetylcholine

Acetylcholine is probably the best-known of the neurotransmitters. This is because it is found in the peripheral system, where it may be easily studied. It is the transmitter at the neuromuscular junction, being released by the end plate termination of axons from the anterior horn cell on to striated muscle. Acetylcholine is also a transmitter in the parasympathetic part of the autonomic nervous system and the preganglionic nerves of the sympathetic nervous system (*see* Chapter 7).

In the CNS many sites of acetylcholine action have been described, but it is likely that many more remain to be discovered. It must be remembered that the study of transmission in the CNS presents severe technical problems which slow the rate at which information may be gathered.

SYNTHESIS AND DEACTIVATION

The enzyme choline acetylase catalyses the transfer of activated acetate from the carrier coenzyme A (CoA), to the precursor of the transmitter, choline:

$$\text{Acetyl CoA + choline} \xrightarrow{\text{Choline acetylase}} \text{Acetylcholine + CoA}$$

Choline is present in foods and can be synthesized in the body. It enters the cell from the circulation. The availability of choline is the factor that limits the rate of acetylcholine formation. When acetylcholine is released into the synaptic cleft, it is split into choline and acetate ion by the enzyme acetylcholinesterase, which is contained by the postsynaptic membrane. The choline so formed is reabsorbed into the presynaptic terminal, when its presence accelerates the formation of more acetylcholine.

Acetylcholinesterase is also found in the presynaptic terminal. It has the function of destroying the acetylcholine which is produced in excess of the storage ability of the synaptic vesicles. Once acetylcholine enters the vesicles, however, it is protected from enzymic degradation.

Acetylcholine is not all stored in the nerve terminal in the same way. Some is available for release immediately upon arrival of the nerve impulse and some appears to be in a depot from which the available store may be replenished. This is suggested by careful analysis of experiments in which it is observed that rapid trains of action potentials release more acetylcholine per action potential at the beginning of the train than is released by the later action potentials. The total amount of acetylcholine in the terminal does not change, however, which shows that the stores may be replenished by synthesis at a rate equal to the release of acetylcholine.

It is likely that the morphological counterparts of the available and the depot stores for acetylcholine are not identifiable with confidence, but it is possible that they consist of those vesicles close to the synaptic membrane being the available store and those further from the store being the depot. This is supported indirectly by experiments which show that radioactively labelled choline enters terminals and then enters vesicles which lie close to the synaptic membrane. Nerve stimulation releases a high proportion of the radioactively labelled acetylcholine.

There is evidence that acetylcholine in the frog neuromuscular junction is bound to proteins and packed into the vesicles with ATP, and some acetylcholine is bound to proteins in the cytoplasm. It is not clear whether this is an artefact of the disrupting effects of the experiments themselves or whether the extravesicular acetylcholine has a physiological function. It is interesting to note, although pointless to debate the accuracy of the observation here, that it is estimated that between 12000 and 21000 molecules of acetylcholine may be contained in each vesicle.

CHOLINERGIC RECEPTORS AND THEIR PHARMACOLOGY

Receptors stimulated by acetylcholine usually lead to the excitatory depolarization of the postsynaptic cell. There are a few reports of cells in the brain being depressed by application of acetylcholine; so if there are inhibitory receptors, there are not many of them.

There are two types of receptor (both excitatory)—*nicotinic* and *muscarinic*. Nicotine is a highly potent mimic of acetylcholine on the nicotinic receptor and muscarine acts similarly on the muscarinic receptor. Antagonists have different potencies on the two receptor sites. Atropine is an effective blocker of the muscarinic receptor but much less active on nicotinic receptors. D-tubocurarine is an antagonist of peripheral nicotinic receptors but does not penetrate the blood –brain barrier and has no effect in the CNS (*see* below, however, for micro-iontophoretic experiments with this drug).

The distribution and action of the two types of receptor can be studied by using the antagonists as experimental tools. D-tubocurarine causes paralysis, which leads to the correct assumption that acetylcholine receptors on striated muscle are nicotinic. Atropine does not cause paralysis but alters transmission at cholinergic synapses in the intestine, which suggests that muscarinic receptors are found in the autonomic nervous system (ANS). The action of atropine in dilating the pupil supports this fact. Atropine also causes changes in the electroencephalogram wave form recorded from the cortex. Low-voltage desynchronized activity becomes a high-voltage, slower, more synchronized wave form, which indicates the relative inactivation of cells in the neocortex (i.e. blocking of the excitatory effects of acetylcholine). This suggests that muscarinic cholinergic receptors may be found in the brain. However, micro-iontophoresis experiments, where micropipettes record from single brain cells while small quantities of drug are ejected into their environment, suggest that most acetylcholine receptors in brain and spinal cord are nicotinic. It is a very thought-provoking fact that the different physiological roles of these nicotinic and muscarinic receptors remain obscure. The pharmacology of cholinergic synapses in relation to brain–behaviour functions will be referred to in the chapter on psychoactive drugs.

Noradrenaline

Noadrenaline is the transmitter at postganglionic sympathetic nerve terminals. These terminals are readily accessible for experimental investigation, and there can be no doubt that in these peripheral structures noradrenaline is the neurotransmitter. It is very likely to be the transmitter at many synapses in the CNS also, but much less is known about its actions there.

LOCATION

The location of noradrenaline in nerve cells may be studied with the technique of histochemical fluorescence microscopy. Tissues cut into thin sections and fixed with dry formaldehyde vapour fluoresce when irradiated with light in the ultra-violet wavelengths. Tissues containing adrenaline, dopamine and 5-hydroxytryptamine also fluoresce when treated in this way. The catecholamines produce a green fluorescence and the indoleamines a yellow colour. It is difficult to discriminate between the catecholamines, but this may be achieved by selectively interfering with the synthesis of one or other transmitter by pharmacological means. Noradrenaline has been shown to occur very largely in nerve terminals where the concentration may reach very high levels between 1000 and 3000 µg/g. The amine is largely bound within granules in the synaptic terminals. The granule is a dense-cored synaptic vesicle, and there is evidence that stimulation of axons causes depletion of granules, which suggests that they may be extruded into the synaptic cleft on arrival of the nerve impulse. These granules also contain ATP, protein and the enzyme dopamine β-hydroxylase. As stated earlier, ATP and protein are assumed to be molecules to which the transmitter binds. The presence of dopamine β-hydroxylase probably indicates that dopamine is converted to noradrenaline within the granule. The granule stores and protects noradrenaline from destruction by the enzyme monoamine oxidase (MAO), which is present in mitochondria in the terminal.

THE SYNTHESIS AND DEGRADATION OF NORADRENALINE

The enzyme catechol-O-methyl transferase is located in the membrane of the presynaptic terminal and is able to destroy noradrenaline released into the synaptic cleft. It is not primarily responsible for terminating the postsynaptic actions of noradrenaline, however. A very powerful uptake pump exists on the membrane of the presynaptic terminal. This is capable of pumping noradrenaline from a very low extracellular concentration into the much higher intraneuronal concentration. The noradrenaline re-enters the cytoplasm of the terminal and may be destroyed by mitochondrial MAO but may re-enter the storage granules for subsequent release. This is an efficient system which avoids an energy-wasting process of degradation and subsequent resynthesis of transmitter.

Phenylalanine and tyrosine (p-hydroxyphenylalanine) are the precursor amino acids for both noradrenaline and dopamine, the former being converted to tyrosine in the liver. When tyrosine enters nerve terminals, a second hydroxyl group is added to the benzene ring component of the molecule by the enzyme tyrosine hydroxylase. The resultant material is dihydroxyphenylalanine, or DOPA. This is decarboxylated to produce dopamine, to which a further hydroxyl group is added at the β-position on the side-chain to give noradrenaline. The enzyme mediating this reaction is known as dopamine β-hydroxylase.

THE CELL SYSTEMS WHICH CONTAIN NORADRENALINE

Under normal circumstances fluorescence microscopy reveals only the noradrenaline contained in axon terminals. Elsewhere in the neuron the concentration of noradrenaline is too low. Any newly synthesized noradrenaline which cannot immediately enter the storage granules is liable to be degraded by MAO. This can be prevented, however, by drugs which inhibit this enzyme, thus enabling cytoplasmic levels of noradrenaline to rise, and cell bodies and axons then fluoresce. In this way, the cell systems within the brain which contain noradrenaline have been mapped (*Figures 4.17, 4.18*).

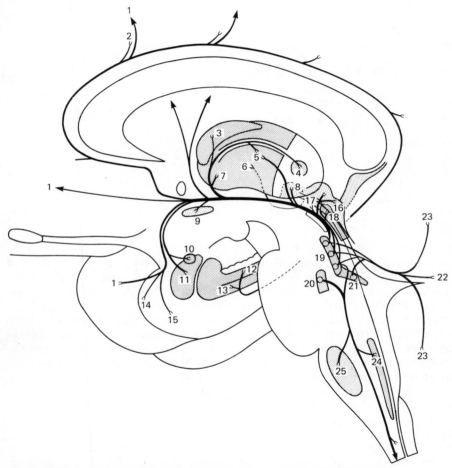

Figure 4.17 The noradrenergic system: 1, neocortex; 2, cingulate cortex; 3–8, Thalamus; 9, substantia innominata; 10, 11, 12, 13, hippocampus; 14, 15, olfactory cortex; 16, 17, midbrain; 18, dorsal raphé nucleus; 19–21, locus coeruleus; 22, 23, cerebellum; 24, V nerve nucleus; 25, olive. The noradrenergic system also connects cell bodies in the midbrain and hindbrain to the reticular system of the midbrain, the hypothalamus, the limbic system and the olfactory bulb

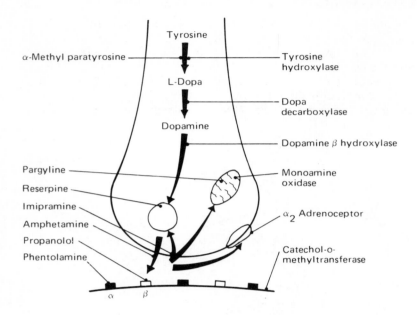

Figure 4.18 Schematic diagram of a few of the basic principles of noradrenaline synthesis and drugs which affect it

The cell bodies containing noradrenaline are found in the pons and the medulla of the brain. Axons from these cells ascend via the median forebrain bundle and make monosynaptic contact with the neocortex, the cerebellar cortex, the limbic system and the hypothalamus. There are also axons which descend to the spinal cord. One of the major nuclei with noradrenaline-containing cell bodies is the locus coeruleus. Possibly all the densely packed cells in this nucleus contain noradrenaline, and a very large number of axons ascend to terminate in several regions of the forebrain. A single cell may give rise to as many as 500 000 terminals. Obviously, the noradrenergic system of cells has a very widespread influence on the activity of cells in the forebrain.

NORADRENERGIC RECEPTORS

In the peripheral nervous system noradrenaline is released by the sympathetic system onto two types of noradrenergic receptor. Alpha noradrenergic receptors mediate the excitation of smooth muscle cells around blood vessels, where beta receptors do the same in heart muscle. Beta receptors are also found on smooth muscle cells of the bronchi and intestines when noradrenaline causes relaxation. There is, therefore, no clear relationship in the sympathetic nervous system between excitation and inhibition and alpha and beta types. In the CNS the postsynaptic actions of noradrenaline are very controversial. Some laboratories report that the iontophoretic application of noradrenaline into the extracellular environment of many different types of neuron only causes inhibition; other laboratories report mixed excitatory and inhibitory responses of cells. One laboratory reports that excitation by noradrenaline in neocortical neurons is due to activation of alpha receptors and that inhibition is due to beta receptor activity. It is hoped that this controversy will be resolved in future years. It is puzzling, however, that so much is known about the presynaptic synthesis, storage, uptake and breakdown of noradrenaline and so little agreement can be reached about its postsynaptic effects. This is generally true for the other catecholamine transmitter, dopamine, and a possible explanation for this confusion is presented below in the section on dopamine.

THE PHARMACOLOGY OF NORADRENERGIC NEUROTRANSMISSION

Alpha and beta receptors in the peripheral nervous system may be distinguished by their different affinities for drugs. Alpha receptors are blocked by the alpha adrenoreceptor antagonist phentolamine, and beta receptors are blocked by propranolol. It must be stressed that these drugs have a greater potency on one of the receptors but at high concentrations can block, or at least partially antagonize, both receptor types. Not all pharmacological experiments are conducted with sufficient care, and the scientific literature is full of misleading statements which result from failing to realize that a drug has a selective action only when it is applied within a narrow range of concentrations. The technique of micro-iontophoretic application of drugs from microelectrodes is the most powerful method for investigating drug action in neurons in the CNS but suffers from the major drawback of being very difficult to quantify. The concentration of drug achieved at receptor sites following the application of a particular iontophoretic current is largely unknown with this technique.

Profound effects on transmission at noradrenaline synapses result from the application of drugs which interfere with the synthesis, storage, release or inactivation of noradrenaline. α-Methyl-p-tyrosine blocks the synthesis of noradrenaline by inhibiting the enzyme tyrosine hydroxylase. The synthesis of dopamine is also prevented by this drug.

Reserpine is a drug of great historical interest to students of psychological illness. It was first administered as a hypotensive agent. A brief rise in blood pressure rapidly followed its administration but this was followed by a prolonged hypotension. Experiments revealed that reserpine interfered with the storage of noradrenaline in synaptic vesicles. Shortly after its administration noradrenaline left the storage granules and entered the cytoplasm. Much of the noradrenaline was metabolized by the mitochondrial MAO, but some entered the synaptic cleft and activated postsynaptic receptors, contracting the smooth muscle of arterioles and causing the brief hypertension. Subsequently, however, newly synthesized noradrenaline was not efficiently stored and protected from MAO, and the noradrenaline content of the presynaptic terminal was very much reduced. Action potentials released much less noradrenaline than formerly and the sympathetic tone of the arterioles was reduced. It was noticed that patients undergoing this treatment showed a marked tendency towards depressive illness, and the catecholamine theory of affective disorder was proposed. This will be discussed fully in a later chapter, but briefly it is suggested that depression resulted from reduced transmission at noradrenaline synapses in the brain. Unfortunately, reserpine was also found to affect dopamine and 5-hydroxytryptamine transmission, so the picture became confused. In any case, the mood change seen in patients taking reserpine acutely is not the same as that of typical affective disorder. Illness occurs after prolonged administration at high dosage and perhaps in vulnerable individuals.

Inhibition of the enzyme monoamine oxidase (by drugs such as pargyline) causes a potentiation of transmission at noradrenaline synapses. The noradrenaline content of the presynaptic terminal rises with this drug, but much of the noradrenaline is unbound and free in the cytoplasm. There are two theories. The first is that the potentiation of transmission results from the 'overspill' of cytoplasmic noradrenaline on to postsynaptic receptors. An action potential will release bound noradrenaline on to receptors already 'primed' and a large post-synaptic response will occur. The second theory is that the high concentration of cytoplasmic noradrenaline causes an increase in the concentration of noradrenaline in the vesicular stores and an increase in the amount of noradrenaline released by the action potential. There is a third theory (speculation perhaps!) which flies in the face of conventional beliefs. This is that noradrenaline is released from the cytoplasm by the action potential and that the synaptic vesicle does not contain the quantum of transmitter. The evidence for this theory is still very poor.

The catecholamine theory of affective disorder has been further supported by the finding that inhibitors of MAO do prove to be therapeutic. However, their therapeutic action is not necessarily linked to their pharmacological action. No evidence has yet been produced to prove this final step in a logical chain of evidence for this theory of affective disorders, and indeed the use of MAO inhibitors in classical affective illness is controversial.

Transmission at noradrenergic synapses may also be potentiated by blocking the pump which removes noradrenaline from the cleft and concentrates it back into the terminal. This process of re-uptake is blocked by the tricyclic antidepressant drugs, which, as their name implies, are useful in the treatment of depression. Imipramine is an early example of these drugs. It can be shown to reduce the rate of accumulation of noradrenaline by the brain and to do so by blocking the uptake receptor on the presynaptic terminal. It was stated earlier that the specificity of drugs is very dependent upon their concentration. Imipramine will block the presynaptic re-uptake receptor but will also block the postsynaptic noradrenaline receptor at slightly higher concentrations. The dose required to potentiate transmission is only slightly lower than the dose which blocks transmission. There is considerable uncertainty associated with the classic interpretation of tricyclic drug action outlined above. It is quite possible that the major effects of the drug on transmission are associated with their postsynaptic actions rather than with their presynaptic actions. This doubt stems from the observation that increased reactiveness of cells to noradrenaline is caused by the presence of imipramine even when all presynaptic terminals have been destroyed. Furthermore, some modern tricyclics and new types of antidepressant have been marketed which do not block uptake or MAO and yet potentiate transmission and give therapeutic benefit. A speculative theory suggests that tricyclics may block the postsynaptic actions of inhibitory and excitatory receptors, both of which may exist on the same postsynaptic membrane. One of these receptors is more sensitive to the drug, however, and in the case where this is the inhibitory receptor, excitatory transmission is potentiated. This example of modern controversy is presented in an attempt to discourage the student from blindly accepting even the most confidently expressed theories in psychopharmacology.

The monoamine oxidase inhibitors (MAOIs) and the other antidepressants do not have effects restricted to noradrenergic systems. The MAOIs block the degradation of dopamine and 5-hydroxytryptamine synthesis and the tricyclics have effects on the uptake of 5-hydroxytryptamine. Acetylcholine is not inactivated by uptake (but by the postsynaptic esterase), yet the tricyclics have blocking actions on the postsynaptic receptors for acetylcholine. Therefore, these drugs have effects which cannot be interpreted purely in terms of changes in noradrenaline neurotransmission.

An invaluable research tool was discovered some years ago when it was found that 6-hydroxydopamine was selectively taken up by terminals of catecholamine neurons. The neurons are then killed by the compound and this enables observations to be made of the behavioural and other effects of degeneration of noradrenaline systems. 6-Hydroxydopamine has to be administered into the brain by local injection, as it fails to enter the brain from the blood supply. Analysis of the catecholaminergic systems (dopamine systems are also affected by the drug) with this agent is far from complete but some valuable insights have been gained already. For example, amphetamine is a well-known drug which has a powerful stimulatory action on behaviour and also upon some cells. It was shown that the cells stimulated by amphetamine received innervation from terminals which contained noradrenaline. It was assumed that amphetamine acted directly upon the postsynaptic receptors of noradrenaline and it was described as an agonist of noradrenaline receptors. Subsequently, however, it was found that if terminals containing noradrenaline were destroyed (for example, with 6-hydroxydopamine), amphetamine was very much less effective. It was shown that amphetamine had its major action on the presynaptic terminal, evoking the release of noradrenaline on to postsynaptic receptors. The synthetic pathway for noradrenaline, the schematic storage site, the process of release, re-uptake and degradation of noradrenaline and sites of action of some drugs are shown in *Figures 15.1* and *15.2*. The diagrams show only the dominant theories and should not be accepted in an uncritical way.

Dopamine

Dopamine is the immediate precursor of noradrenaline. It can be found in all noradrenergic nerve terminals, and interference with the synthesis of dopamine always has effects on the synthesis of noradrenaline. Neurotransmission at dopamine synapses is not found in the peripheral nervous system and its function can only be studied in the relatively inaccessible CNS. It is not surprising, therefore, that for years dopamine neurotransmission was not suspected and dopamine was assumed to act simply as the precursor of noradrenaline.

LOCATION

The histochemical fluorescence technique played a major part in demonstrating that dopamine was selectively stored by a discrete system of neurons, quite separate from the neuron storing noradrenaline. Like noradrenaline, dopamine fluoresces a green colour which is much more intense in nerve terminals, revealing

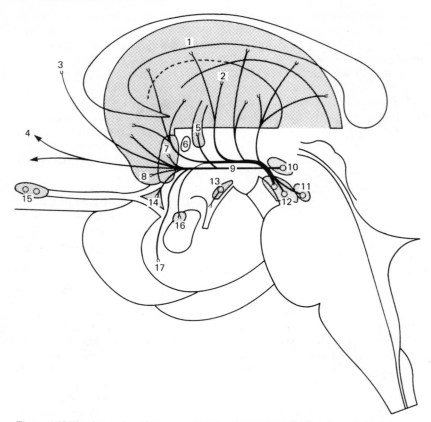

Figure 4.19 The dopaminergic system: 1, 2, corpus striatum; 3, cingulate gyrus; 4, frontal cortex; 5, 16, 17, limbic system; 6, anterior commissure; 7, septal nucleus; 8, nucleus accumbens; 9, mesolimbic tract; 10, nucleus A10; 11, midbrain reticular formation; 12, substantia nigra; 13, infundibular nucleus of hypothalamus (prolactin release inhibiting); 14, 15, olfactory system

that dopamine achieves much higher concentrations in the terminals than in the cell bodies. Inhibition of MAO increases the concentration of dopamine in the cytoplasm of the whole cell, which can then be visualized. *Figure 4.19* shows the distribution of the axons of cells containing dopamine.

It can be seen that dopamine systems are not spread so widely through the CNS as are noradrenaline systems. Basically, they can be subdivided into three principal subgroups. The zona compacta of the substantia nigra contains the cell bodies of axons projecting to the caudate nucleus. A group of cells just dorsal to the interpeduncular nucleus projects to the nucleus accumbens and olfactory tubercle. Finally, a small group of cells in the arcuate nucleus of the hypothalamus send short axons to the median eminence. These latter cells are different in many respects from those of the first two systems and are believed to be involved in neurosecretory control of the pituitary. They may evoke the release of luteinizing hormone. The functions of the nigrostriatal system and the system innervating the limbic lobe structures (nucleus accumbens and olfactory tubercle) are unclear. Certainly, the nigrostriatal pathway is involved in the control of extrapyramidal motor outflow, but it may have other functions. The projection to areas of the limbic system may well have a role in the control of mood. This is implied by the experiments and observations described below, which has made the process of neurotransmission in dopamine cells of fundamental interest to students of behavioural illness.

SYNTHESIS AND DEGRADATION OF DOPAMINE

The synthesis of dopamine follows the same path from the amino acid tyrosine as does that of noradrenaline. In the dopaminergic neurons, however, the last step, the addition of the OH group at the β-position on the molecule, is not performed, so the synthesis stops at dopamine.

Drugs which affect the synthesis of dopamine or its metabolism are those which affect the production of noradrenaline. These have been described in the previous section and will not be repeated in detail here. α-Methyl *p*-tyrosine inhibits the synthesis, reserpine prevents the storage, amphetamine evokes the release and MAOIs slow down the degradation of dopamine.

The tricyclic antidepressant drugs are much less potent in blocking the uptake of dopamine than of noradrenaline. However, benztropine and amphetamine are effective uptake blockers.

DOPAMINE RECEPTORS

Much less is known about receptors for dopamine, owing to the relative inaccessibility of the CNS. Micro-iontophoretic application of the amine into the environment of cells of the caudate nucleus results in mixed excitatory and inhibitory responses, although some laboratories report only inhibitory effects. Stimulation of the substantia nigra evokes responses from caudate neurons which are believed to be monosynaptic. Both inhibitory and excitatory responses may be seen.

One of the problems of studying the pharmacology of postsynaptic receptors is the fact that cells of the substantia nigra are sensitive to the local application of dopamine. These cells do not seem to receive any innervation from axons releasing dopamine. These are likely to be the cells of the substantia nigra which send axons to the caudate nucleus and themselves release dopamine from their axons.

A question mark hangs over the function of these receptors, which do not seem to lie beneath axon terminals and yet will be affected by dopamine and its agonists. A partial answer has come from electron microscope studies, which show that the dendrites of cells in the substantia nigra seem to come into close opposition to other cells and that these dendrites display synaptic vesicles, postsynaptic thickenings and concentrations of mitochondria, all implying a normal neurochemical synapse. Normal, that is, except that the synapse is dendrodendrite in nature. It is possible that these synapses are somehow involved in the regulation of transmitter synthesis or perhaps in the co-ordination of the activity of cells in the substantia nigra. Certainly, the complexity of the systems being revealed is shaking many of the foundations of the long-accepted principles and preventing such simplistic statements as 'the neurotransmitter is inhibitory'.

The receptors which are not immediately subsynaptic are called autoreceptors. Autoreceptors are found on the synaptic terminal, where they 'sense' the extracellular concentration of the neurotransmitter released by the terminal and regulate the synthesis of transmitter taking place in the terminal. It is likely that these receptors act via cyclic AMP and protein kinase, which influences the protein of the enzymes which synthesize the neurotransmitter.

Postsynaptic receptors of dopamine (and autoreceptors) are affected by apomorphine, which is a dopamine agonist. Haloperidol and the newer, more specific, flupenthixol, are antagonists of dopamine. These compounds have relatively specific actions on dopamine receptors and are much less potent upon noradrenaline receptors. Noradrenaline and dopamine molecules bear a close resemblance to each other, and it is no surprise to find that many noradrenaline antagonists are also dopamine antagonists. This has been proved to be a very misleading factor in our understanding of the pharmacology of the antipsychotic drugs. These drugs are good postsynaptic antagonists of noradrenaline and dopamine. However, if a table is constructed in which a range of these drugs is rank-ordered for their potency on noradrenaline receptors and their potency on dopamine receptors, the order is quite different. Add to the table a column rank-ordering the potency of these drugs as tranquillizers and a good correlation is detected between antipsychotic activity and antidopamine activity. The correlation with antinoradrenaline activity is poor. There are other reasons for believing that dopamine transmission is highly relevant in the study of psychosis, but these will be discussed later. However, small doses of antagonists may produce a hypersensitivity of the receptors to dopamine (*see* chapter on psychopharmacology). More recently, detailed studies of these and other drugs have suggested the existence of perhaps four different types of dopamine receptors analogous to the alpha and beta catecholamine receptors.

The role of dopamine neurotransmission in the extrapyramidal motor system was implied above. Parkinson's disease results from a malfunction of nigrostriatal dopamine transmission. The antipsychotics—haloperidol, chlorpromazine, etc.— all tend to worsen the disease and will evoke extrapyramidal symptoms in patients not suffering from motor dysfunction. Post-mortem lesions of the substantia nigra can be detected in Parkinsonian patients, and administration of L-dopa has proved an effective treatment. It is presumed that cell death or some other disruption of nigrostriatal dopamine transmission is the cause of the illness and administration of L-dopa accelerates the synthesis of dopamine in the remaining neurons, enabling sufficient increase in the release of dopamine on to cells in the caudate nucleus for the symptoms to decline.

5-Hydroxytryptamine (also known as serotonin)

5-Hydroxytryptamine (5-HT) is a monoamine like dopamine and noradrenaline. It is not a catechol but an indoleamine. There are marked differences between the synthesis and postsynaptic receptors for 5-HT and the catecholamines which enable 5-HT systems to be selectively disrupted. It is necessary to be very careful in interpreting the effects of these experiments, because many drugs and enzymes affect catechol and indoleamines alike.

No peripheral nerves release 5-HT. However, there seem to be quite specific 5-HT receptors in gut and other peripheral organs. The detailed study of these receptors led to a good understanding of the basic pharmacology of 5-HT before the location of 5-HT neurotransmission systems in the brain.

LOCATION

Differential centrifugation of brain homogenetes located 5-HT concentrated in synaptic vesicles in nerve terminals of the brain. Microfluorescence studies showed that the yellow fluorescent products of 5-HT were found in terminals from many

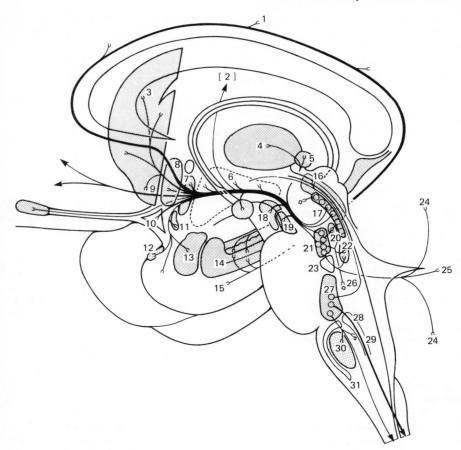

Figure 4.20 The serotoninergic system: 1, cingulate gyrus; 2, neocortex; 3, corpus
striatum; 4, 5, thalamus; 6, 7, hypothalamus; 8, 9, 11–15, limbic system; 10, olfactory
tubercle; 16, periaqueductal grey matter; 17, 21, 23, 27, 28, raphé nuclei; 18, substantia
nigra; 19, interpeduncular nucleus; 20, dorsal tegmental nucleus; 22, nucleus coeruleus;
24, 25, cerebellum; 26, 29, hindbrain reticular formation; 30, inferior olive

regions of the brain. As with noradrenaline and dopamine, cell bodies could be
made to fluoresce by inhibition of MAO and these cell bodies were found in
midline nuclei of the medulla, the pons and the midbrain. These are the various
raphé nuclei. The distribution of systems containing 5-HT is shown in *Figure 4.20*.
A simplified version of the main monoamine neuron systems is given in *Figure 4.21*.

Figure 4.21 includes the distribution of noradrenaline and dopamine to allow
comparison of these systems. The widespread distribution of 5-HT to the neocortex, the limbic forebrain, the basal nuclei, the thalamus, the hypothalamus and the
spinal cord is reminiscent of the distribution of the noradrenaline system. It is
notable that the axons of noradrenaline and of 5-HT run in the medial forebrain
bundle with some of the axons of the dopamine system. This makes possible an
interesting experimental approach. Lesions may be placed by stereotactically

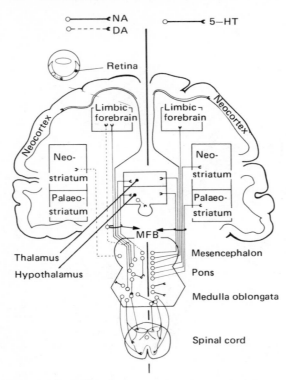

Figure 4.21 Simplified diagram of the main monoamine
neuron systems in the central nervous system

locating an electrode into the medial forebrain bundle and then passing a current of
a few milliamps for several seconds. This burns away the tissue and cuts the
ascending axons. If this is done on one side of the brain only, then comparisons may
be made between the functioning of one side of the brain and the other. The
difficulty with this, as with many other techniques, is that it fails to differentiate
between the various monoamine systems.

5-HT cannot cross the blood–brain barrier, so it is formed *in situ* by neurons
from the precursor amino acid tryptophan, an essential component of dietary
protein. Tryptophan hydroxylase converts the parent amino acid into its 5-hydroxy
derivative (5-HTP). This step in 5-HT synthesis can be blocked by *p*-
chlorophenylalanine, which binds irreversibly with the enzyme. Synthesis of fresh
enzyme by the neuron will then occur, and full recovery of 5-HT levels may take
10–14 days. Normally the concentration of tryptophan available is insufficient to
'saturate' the enzyme. Tryptophan entry into neurons is increased by lithium.
There follows an increased rate of formation of 5-HT. This is short-lived, for less
hydroxylase is then formed and so, despite the increased availability of substrate,
the amount of 5-HTP formed returns to the previous level. Despite this, there is
little evidence that 5-HT itself controls the rate of enzyme production. The final
stage in forming 5-HT, decarboxylation, occurs immediately. A specific 5-HT
decarboxylase exists in serotoninergic neurons, with a higher level of activity than
that of tryptophan hydroxylase, which thus is the rate-limiting enzyme.

5-HT is inactivated by deamination by monoamine oxidase, and the product oxidized to 5-hydroxyindoleacetic acid (5-HIAA), which is transported out of the brain into the blood.

5-HYDROXYTRYPTAMINE RECEPTORS

Like noradrenaline and dopamine, 5-HT receptors in the CNS defy any clear description. In the gut 5-HT causes the contraction of muscle cells; in autonomic ganglia clear depolarizations occur when 5-HT is applied or released within the ganglion; in invertebrates excitatory and inhibitory receptors of 5-HT have been clearly defined. The accessibility and relative simplicity of these structures account for the confidence with which these statements may be made. In the mammalian CNS controversial exchanges occur between laboratories over the nature of the receptor. Micro-iontophoretic application of 5-HT results in the excitation of some cells and the inhibition of others in one laboratory, but in another laboratory only inhibition of cells is seen. No explanation of these differences seems to suffice, and once again a puzzling impasse has to be tolerated until someone discovers what aspect of the difference in technique accounts for the confusion. The various reasons for difficulty of this sort have been discussed in the sections on noradrenaline and dopamine and need not be repeated here.

The actions of 5-HT on postsynaptic receptors may be mimicked by a range of compounds with structures that resemble the structure of 5-HT. These include psilocin (the active compound of psilocybin) and bufotenine (*see* the chapter dealing with schizophrenia). These compounds are hallucinogens. Other compounds are capable of antagonizing the actions of 5-HT. Lysergic acid diethylamide is one of the antagonists of 5-HT in the gut, and, according to several workers, has the same activity in the brain. This compound is also a hallucinogen. Other effective antagonists of 5-HT such as cinanserin are not hallucinogens, however. These data defy summary, except perhaps to deny the strict relationship between an action of 5-HT receptors and hallucinogenic potency. And still, so many substances that are hallucinogenic have actions on 5-HT receptors! It would be nice if 5-HT receptors could be divided into two populations with different susceptibility to different drugs. There are indications that 5-HT may be a neurotransmitter of presynaptic inhibition. The receptors at these sites seem to be resistant to conventional antagonists and to be more susceptible to some adrenoreceptor antagonists. This and other evidence is compatible with the suggestion that a minimum of two and possibly more types of 5-HT receptor exist.

THE PHARMACOLOGY OF 5-HYDROXYTRYPTAMINE TRANSMISSION

The synthesis of 5-HT may be interrupted by administration of *p*-chlorphenylalininine. This compound inhibits tryptophan hydroxylase, preventing the synthesis of 5-HT from tryptophan. Nerve terminals became depleted of 5-HT. Reserpine also depleted nerve terminals of 5-HT. The action of reserpine, as it was with dopamine and noradrenaline, is to prevent the entry of newly synthesized 5-HT into the synaptic vesicles. The resulting depletion of nerve terminals stores depressed transmission at 5-HT synapses. As reserpine affects all monoamines and may cause a depression of mood in man, it was of interest to determine whether the change in mood resulted from an action on 5-HT or catecholamine systems. The depletion of 5-HT with *p*-chlorphenylalanine causes no behavioural depression in rats but reserpine has this effect. Conversely, the inhibitor of noradrenaline synthesis, α-methyl p-tyrosine does depress behaviour in rats. This supports the speculation that reserpine-induced depression is due to depletion of noradrenaline and not of 5-HT. It should again be noted that 'depression' in rats cannot be equated with the syndrome of depressive affective illness, sometimes provoked by long-term administration of reserpine in possibly susceptible individuals.

Synaptically released 5-HT is inactivated primarily by an active presynaptic uptake process. The 5-HT re-enters the synaptic terminal and may be stored for future release or may be degraded by mitochondrial oxidase. This uptake process is blocked by tricyclic antidepressants. Again the question is: Are the effects of the antidepressants due to actions on noradrenaline or on 5-HT synapses? This discussion is presented elsewhere (Chapter 9).

5,6-Dihydrotryptamine is a specific poison when applied locally to neurons containing 5-HT. It seems to work in a manner reminiscent of the action of 6-hydroxydopamine on catecholamine neurons. This drug has made possible the observation of the behavioural effect in animals of specific destruction of 5-HT systems. The question again is whether or not depression of mood or hallucinations in animals are detectable phenomena, comparable with those in man. There are techniques which are indicative, but they do not seem very convincing, one way or the other. There is a stronger case for such things as the role of 5-HT in the control of the temperature and in the regulation of sleep cycles. Body temperature of the rat may be raised by stimulation of the raphe nuclei and the effect may be prevented by prior treatment with p-chlorphenylalanine. Intraventricular injections of microgram amounts of 5-HT will produce a profound elevation of the body temperature of cats and monkeys.

Electroencephalographic (EEG) records give evidence of two major subdivisions of sleep: slow wave sleep, when the subject has hypotonus and a high-voltage low-frequency EEG; and REM sleep, characterized by muscle tone, rapid eye movements (hence REM), dreams and a low-voltage desynchronized EEG. The functions of these sleep periods can only be guessed. It seems that by whatever

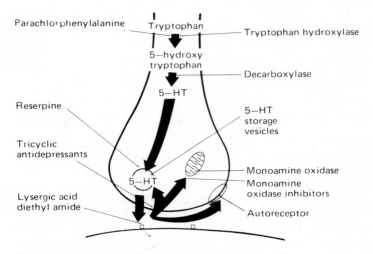

Figure 4.22 A schematic diagram of the basic principles of 5-hydroxytryptamine (5-HT) metabolism and transmission

means 5-HT levels are elevated (intraventricular 5-HT, MAO inhibition or 5-HTP injection) a greater proportion of time is spent in slow wave sleep. Conversely, if p-chlorphenylalanine is given or the raphe nuclei are ablated, a high proportion of time is spent in REM sleep. Catecholamines are also deeply involved in the control of sleep, and it seems likely that the nature of sleep patterns is controlled by the interaction of several neurotransmitter systems.

Gamma aminobutyric acid (GABA)

GABA is an amino acid which was first synthesized in 1883. Its occurrence in the CNS of mammals was not observed until 1950, when it was noted that although very high levels of GABA existed in brain and spinal cord, only very small amounts could be detected elsewhere in the body. GABA's role is that of an inhibitory neurotransmitter acting on the postsynaptic membranes of cells in the brain and it is also a mediator of presynaptic inhibition in the spinal cord.

LOCATION

The concentrations of GABA in the CNS are high, reaching 10 μmol/g, whereas catecholamine and 5-HT concentrations are measured in nmol/g. The highest levels of GABA occur in the substantia nigra, the globus pallidus, the hypothalamus and the spinal grey. Most cellular areas of brain have moderate levels of GABA, but the fibre tracts have the lowest concentrations.

The microdistribution of GABA can be followed from the distribution of the enzyme responsible for its synthesis from glutamate. This enzyme, glutamic acid decarboxylase (GAD), always accompanies GABA and its concentration is related to the concentration of GABA. It has been shown that GAD activity is higher in the grey areas of brain and that synaptosomes have the highest concentration. Synaptosomes, it will be remembered, are 'pinched off' nerve terminals which result from homogenizing brain tissue. Relatively pure, high concentrations of synaptosomes can be prepared by differential centrifugation.

The location of GABA to inhibitory, rather than excitatory, nerve terminals is not so easily achieved. The best evidence that this is the case comes from studies in the cerebellum. The axons of Purkinje cells in the cerebellar cortex make monosynaptic inhibitory connections to several inferior nuclei and the dorsal part of Deiter's nucleus (the vestibular nucleus). The dorsal part of this nucleus synthesizes GABA at 2.5 times the rate of synthesis in the ventral part. When the Purkinje axons are cut, this rate of synthesis is very significantly reduced. Other similar experiments relate GABA synthesis to inhibitory inputs to many nuclei in the brain.

The evidence suggesting that GABA is stored in synaptic vesicles is rather weak and is balanced by evidence that it is stored in the cytoplasm of nerve terminals. The arguments are complex. GABA terminals have postsynaptic effects which are apparently quantal, which suggests release from vesicles. However, preparations of synaptic vesicles by differential centrifugation are reported by some laboratories to contain very little GABA, while the cytoplasm has high concentrations. Other laboratories find the opposite. It may be that GABA is contained in vesicles but that they are easily disrupted by the preparation process and release GABA into the cytoplasm.

Great importance has been attached to the function of GABA in the substantia nigra. Cells containing dopamine in the pars compacta of the substantia nigra project to the striatum via the medial forebrain bundle. These cells may have an important function in the control of extrapyramidal motor function. A GABA pathway with cells in the striatum and the nerve terminals in the substantia nigra is believed to exert a negative feedback control of the dopamine cells. Activity in dopamine cells in the substantia nigra affects cells in the striatum which project back to the substantia nigra and inhibit the dopamine cells. Altered activity of dopamine cells or changed sensitivity of dopamine receptors may be the basis of some motor diseases (Parkinson's disease) and possibly affective disorders. Theoretically, benefit should be derived from any pharmacological intervention which increases the effectiveness of dopamine transmission or which reduces the effectiveness of the GABA-mediated feedback intervention. This latter has proved to be very difficult to demonstrate, possibly because GABA systems elsewhere in the body would also be affected by interference with GABA transmission and the side-effects of the treatment would be too severe. However, the concept of the simple feedback loop has recently been shown to be too simple, because the dopamine cells lie in the pars compacta of the substantia nigra and the GABA feedback terminates in the pars reticulata of the substantia nigra. Much more detail is required of the location of GABA systems in the CNS.

RELEASE AND INACTIVATION

The release of GABA following the depolarization of tissues has been demonstrated clearly. It has usually been necessary to prevent the enzymic destruction of GABA by administration of the GABA-transaminase inhibitor, amino-oxyacetic acid. For example, stimulation of the Purkinje fibre projection of the cerebellum causes a trebling of the amount of GABA collected from perfusates of Deiter's nucleus. Different techniques have been used in various areas of the brain, usually with clear results. What is not so clear is the demonstration that this release is from inhibitory nerve terminals. Again, the arguments are complex and the subject one of controversy. It is likely, however, that although GABA release can be evoked non-specifically from non-neuronal tissue by administration of high potassium or intense electrical stimulation, a proportion of the released GABA comes from nerve terminals. This is revealed by the need for calcium in the extracellular fluids in the tissue and the neural release of GABA is also calcium-dependent, because, at the peak of the action potential, calcium enters the terminal. As discussed before, it is considered that it is calcium which stimulates the extrusion of transmitter.

The enzyme inactivating GABA is intracellular. Synaptically released GABA is removed from the synaptic cleft by a specific GABA uptake mechanism. Demonstration of this uptake is confused by the fact that most tissues are capable of concentrating GABA by an uptake mechanism. At sites where GABA is released, however, the affinity of the uptake receptor for GABA is much greater than that found elsewhere. Nevertheless, a high proportion of radioactively labelled GABA, added to a tissue slice, may subsequently be found in the glial cells surrounding nerve terminals. It is quite likely that the uptake system into glial cells plays some part in the removal of GABA from the synaptic cleft.

SYNTHESIS OF GABA

GABA is formed from glutamic acid, by a specific glutamic acid decarboxylase which removes the carboxyl group adjacent to the α-carbon atom, to which the amine group is attached. The reaction is irreversible and the enzyme requires pyridoxal phosphate as a cofactor. The binding of cofactor to enzyme determines activity of the enzyme. This binding can be blocked or broken by glutamate and adenine nucleotides (?cyclic), so these may affect the rate of GABA formation *in vivo*. It should be noted that 35 per cent only of the enzyme has cofactor bound to it *in vivo*, despite the fact that there is normally sufficient to saturate the enzyme.

GABA is inactivated by a transaminase, which transfers the amine group to α-ketoglutaric acid, forming glutamic acid and succinic semi-aldehyde (SSA), which is rapidly oxidized to succinic acid which enters the Krebs cycle. SSA has not been detected in neural tissues, so avid is its conversion to succinic acid, and so the reverse of the transamination reaction cannot occur.

POSTSYNAPTIC RECEPTORS OF GABA

The iontophoretic application of GABA to cells of the neocortex results in the inhibitory hyperpolarization of the cell body. This hyperpolarization seems to occlude the inhibitory postsynaptic potentials which result from the electrical stimulation of inhibitory pathways, which suggests that the iontophoretically applied GABA occupies the postsynaptic receptors for GABA, leaving none for the synaptically released GABA. Similar experiments have shown that GABA administration mimics the effects of inhibitory pathway stimulation in many cell systems in the brain.

Two substances have powerful antagonistic actions on GABA receptors. These are picrotoxin and bicuculline. Both are powerful convulsants. These facts suggest strongly that GABA is released as an inhibitory transmitter and that its antagonism results in the disinhibition of cell systems, leading to convulsive overactivity in the motor outflow. This conclusion has been seriously questioned by pharmacologists who find that the antagonists are not always specific in their actions on GABA receptors. Obviously, if inhibition is antagonized by these compounds at receptors for transmitters other than GABA, it is not possible to conclude from their actions that GABA is the transmitter. It is likely, however, that the source of the controversy is the dose-dependent specificity of the compounds. High doses will block the effects of GABA, glycine and possibly other inhibitory receptors, but GABA receptors are probably the most sensitive. It is clear that picrotoxin is less specific than bicuculline.

THE PRESYNAPTIC ACTIONS OF GABA

Presynaptic inhibition as a physiological phenomenon has been discussed in Chapter 3. The evidence for GABA being one of the presynaptic inhibitory transmitters in the spinal cord is now quite compelling. The techniques used to study presynaptic inhibition are among the more difficult electrophysiological manipulations and are not presented here.

Iontophoretic application of GABA has been shown to increase the excitability of the central terminals of sensory neurons. This is probably due to depolarization of the primary afferent terminals. This depolarization, by reducing the effective height of the action potential, will reduce the amount of neurotransmitter released by the primary afferent terminal. In this way GABA reduces the excitatory input from peripheral receptors onto cells in the spinal cord.

The primary afferent depolarization produced by GABA and that produced by

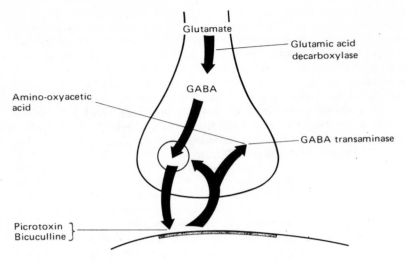

Figure 4.23 The synaptic terminal releasing gamma aminobutyric acid

stimulating the presynaptic inhibitory axons are blocked by administration of picrotoxin or bicuculline (*Figure 4.23*). It can be shown that there is a good relationship between the onset of blockade of presynaptic inhibition and the onset of seizure activity. It is very likely that GABA is a presynaptic inhibitory transmitter in the brain as well as in the spinal cord, but this is difficult to demonstrate.

Further discussion of the actions of GABA will be included in the chapter on psychopharmacology.

Glycine

Glycine is the simplest of the amino acids. It is a powerfully inhibitory neurotransmitter in the spinal cord. It exerts its action on the postsynaptic membranes of cells and has not been shown to have actions on presynaptic membranes.

LOCATION, UPTAKE AND RELEASE

Like GABA, glycine reaches very high levels of concentration in nervous tissue. However, the concentrations in spinal cord are four times those in the brain. Within the cord, concentrations are higher in grey than in white matter and higher in the ventral horn than in the dorsal horn. This latter finding contrasts with that on GABA, which has a higher concentration in the dorsal horn than in the ventral horn and a higher concentration in brain than in spinal cord.

Radioactively labelled glycine is actively taken up by tissue, and autoradiography reveals that the glycine is located largely in synaptic terminals. For years it has been known that synaptic vesicles vary in shape. Some are round and some are flattened. It was suggested that the flattened vesicles were found in synaptic terminals which mediated inhibition, and this seems to be confirmed by the observation that glycine is preferentially taken up into terminals with flattened vesicles. The glycine taken up by these vesicles is available for re-release upon nerve stimulation.

Glycine, like GABA, has both high- and low-affinity uptake systems. It is suspected that the high-affinity system is associated with the complete removal of transmitter from the synaptic cleft and that the low-affinity system is associated with the entry of glycine into all tissues where it is utilized in the general metabolic processes of the cell. In accordance with the preceding statements, it is discovered that only the low-affinity uptake systems can be detected in rostral parts of brain. However, high-affinity uptake can be detected in spinal cord.

The release of glycine has been demonstrated from the spinal cord but not from the brain. Preparations of synaptosomes can be induced to release glycine, and most authors report that the release is calcium-dependent.

It is likely that glycine is not an important inhibitory transmitter in brain but that it has this function in the spinal cord. Strychnine (*see* below) has been used for years as a tool to map the projection of nuclei to different parts of the brain. In strychnine neuronography a small amount of strychnine is placed into a cellular area of the brain. This gives rise to the appearance of 'convulsant' spikes in the EEG of those parts of the brain intimately connected to the primary site. It is shown below that strychnine acts upon glycine receptors. Why, if glycine is not an important transmitter in brain, does the technique work? Either strychnine has a non-specific action on receptors or glycine is an inhibitory transmitter in brain after all. It must be remembered that if a large non-specific low-affinity uptake of glycine in brain is obscuring a small, discrete high-affinity uptake, it could be concluded wrongly that glycine is unimportant in brain.

SYNTHESIS OF GLYCINE

It is unknown whether the dietary glycine is the source of the compound in the nervous system or whether it is synthesized therein. A possible metabolic pathway is from the amino acid serine, requiring tetrahydrofolate in the reaction.

THE GLYCINE RECEPTOR AND ITS PHARMACOLOGY

It has been demonstrated clearly that glycine will hyperpolarize motoneurons. The motoneuron is somewhat more easily studied than many other central neurons, and the data gained by Werman and his colleagues form an excellent example of how the identity of action between synthesized and endogenous transmitter may be compared. For that reason, and because it points out that for many other neurotransmitters such clear information is lacking, the experiment will be described in some detail.

The spinal cord of anaesthetized cats was exposed and a microelectrode was lowered into the ventral horn. The penetration of a motoneuron was indicated by the sudden appearance on the oscilloscope screen (*see* page 60) of the intracellular potential of -70 mV. Stimulation of ventral roots evoked an action potential which conducted antidromically towards the cell body. This was recorded by the intracellular microelectrode and identified the cell as a motoneuron. Side-barrels of the microelectrode contained ionized drug solutions for ejection by micro-iontophoresis. The ends of these drug barrels remained outside the cell as the central recording barrel projected beyond them. Electrical stimulation of some afferent pathways evoked an inhibitory postsynaptic potential (i.p.s.p., hyperpolar-ization). The iontophoretic application of glycine also caused a hyperpolarization. Both the artificially applied putative transmitter and that released at synapses caused a reduction of the resistance of the cell membrane. This means that some ions were able to pass through the membrane more easily in the presence of the transmitter—i.e. ionic channels were opened. To determine which channels were opened, the effective intracellular concentration of chloride ion was elevated by injecting the closely related bromide ion into the cell. (Bromide passes freely through chloride channels, and together they are referred to as halide ions.) Theoretically, if the transmitter had its actions by altering chloride permeability, then halide ions would normally enter the cell, down their diffusion gradient, carrying negative charges into the cell and hyperpolarizing it. If the halide ion concentration inside the cell were raised artificially, however, when the channels opened, ions would diffuse *out* of the cell, carrying negative charges out, and the cell would depolarize. This happened. Both the i.p.s.p. response to nerve stimulation and the response to iontophoretically applied glycine became depolarizing responses when the intracellular halide concentration had thus been raised. Obviously, glycine and the transmitter released by stimulated nerve axon terminals had a very similar action on the postsynaptic cell.

The iontophoretic application of strychnine blocked the effects of both nerve stimulation and iontophoretic glycine. Strychnine was shown to compete with glycine for occupation of the receptor. The elegant clarity of these experiments leaves little doubt that glycine is an inhibitory transmitter of motoneurons.

Elsewhere in the CNS the data are not so convincing. In the brain stem and the hypothalamus glycine has powerful actions on cells and is likely to be a transmitter onto these cells, but in the neocortex few and weak inhibitory actions are found.

Glutamic acid

Glutamate is an amino acid very closely related to GABA structurally and metabolically. It exerts very powerful excitatory actions upon cells in the CNS, and for many years has been considered to be a possible neurotransmitter.

LOCATION, STORAGE AND RELEASE

Glutamate is not localized predominantly in nervous tissue, as is GABA, but is found in most tissues of the body. The concentrations in brain and spinal cord are very high, but only a small proportion is likely to be associated with nerve terminals. The glutamate in nerve terminals is involved in oxidative metabolism and is the precursor of GABA. The problem is whether any is stored as a reasonable pool of neurotransmitter. Several experiments locate glutamate to the cytoplasm of nerve terminals and only a small fraction seems to be present in synaptic vesicles.

Several attempts to demonstrate release of glutamate by nerve stimulation have failed. This failure may be due to the activity of the uptake system or to the assay techniques being insufficiently sensitive to detect the very small amounts released. A convincing demonstration of the release of glutamate from isolated synaptosomes has been published. The release could be evoked by electrical stimulation and by depolarizing the terminals with high-potassium solutions. It is puzzling why such a release proves so difficult to demonstrate *in vivo*.

Nervous tissue is able to concentrate glutamate from the extracellular space. It has been proposed that the uptake of glutamate utilizes the same sodium –potassium ATPase pump as that which pumps the ions across the cell membrane, causing unequal intracellular/extracellular distribution of K^+/Na^+. A conformational change of the carrier in the presence of glutamate is proposed which increases the affinity of the carrier for Na^+. In this way glutamate and Na^+ enter the cell—perhaps enough Na^+ entering to depolarize the membrane and excite the cell. There is no reason why such an uptake mechanism should not be available to a neurotransmitter, but such a system does not specifically argue for a neurotransmitter role for glutamate. The uptake system has a very high affinity for glutamate, however, and this is normally associated with a neurotransmitter role for the substrate.

SYNTHESIS AND DEGRADATION OF GLUTAMATE

Glutamic acid is well known as an amino acid, like glycine. It can be formed by transaminase action on α-ketoglutaric acid, a component of the tricarboxylic acid cycle, and, similarly, it may be deaminated by the same enzyme system. It can also be inactivated by conversion into glutamine, a diamino acid.

THE GLUTAMATE RECEPTOR

In invertebrates special sites on postsynaptic membranes, closely related to synaptic terminals, have been found which are particularly sensitive to local application of glutamate. On these cells, glutamate may also have non-specific actions due to receptors which are diffusely distributed on the cell surface. It is possible that difficulties in demonstrating a synaptic role for glutamate in mammals may be due to the presence of non-specific receptor sites spread over the surface of neurons. These receptors may obscure the effects of specific postsynaptic receptors without in any way denying their presence.

The identification of a specific receptor antagonist of glutamate would help immensely in resolving this difficulty. Three structural analogues have been identified which all seem to have activity in blocking glutamate receptors, but some doubt remains concerning their specificity. There has been one successful attempt to block the action of glutamate with an antagonist which also blocked the effects of synaptic excitation.

There must remain doubt about the role of glutamate as an excitatory transmitter. This doubt is possibly a reflection of the relative paucity of experiments which have investigated its action. Perhaps experimenters are put off by the evident difficulty of working with a substance which has such an important role in the Krebs cycle.

Substance P

This unlikely name was given to a biologically active extract of brain and intestine which was observed in 1934. It was rapidly recognized as a protein-like material, and many experiments were conducted with it. It was not until 1970 that it was isolated and identified as an undecapeptide with a molecular weight of 1420. Since 1974, when the compound became available in purified form, a great deal of accurate information has accumulated, suggesting that substance P is very likely to be an excitatory neurotransmitter in the brain and the spinal cord.

LOCATION, STORAGE AND RELEASE

Substance P has a wide distribution throughout the various organs of the body but is particularly concentrated in the intestinal tract and nervous tissue. Interestingly, the concentration of substance P is greatest in the brains of primitive vertebrates and least in the highly differentiated brains of the advanced vertebrates. This is because the concentration of substance P is highest in the phylogenetically older brain-stems of all species.

The grey matter has much higher concentrations than white matter, and the highest concentrations are achieved in the hypothalamus, the substantia nigra, the globus pallidus, the caudate nucleus, the putamen and various nuclei of the pons and medulla. Moderately high concentrations occur in the spinal cord, particularly in the dorsal roots.

Substance P may be visualized by a fluorescence immunohistochemical technique. This has shown that the fluorescence is associated with nerve terminals. Only one area of the brain—the medial habenula (above the posterior pole of the thalamus)—has been shown to contain nerve cell bodies with substance P. This is reminiscent of the monoamine transmitters, where a small number of discrete nuclei contain the parent cell bodies of most of the terminals in the brain. In the case of substance P, this may be simply because insufficient time has elapsed for the small group of underfinanced research workers to find more. One observation has revealed that the substance P content of the interpeduncular nucleus of the rat declines following ablation of the habenula, which suggests that the axons from the habenula project to the interpeduncular nucleus.

More is known about the distribution of substance P in the spinal cord. Section or ligature of the dorsal root prevents axonal transport, and it has been observed that substance P concentration increases markedly distal to the ligature—i.e. between the ligature and the cell body. This treatment results in a depletion of substance P in the dorsal horn. The fibres in the dorsal root which contain the substance P are the fine unmyelinated C fibres, which conduct slowly. These fibres may be responsible for conducting impulses signalling pain to the CNS.

Little is known about the storage of substance P. If homogenized brain cells are subjected to osmotic shock and centrifuged by a differential gradient technique, the intracellular organelles separate into layers. Substance P seems to be associated with the fraction containing mitochondria—a finding which is difficult to equate with its role as a neurotransmitter.

Substance P is found in several bound forms and a free form in nervous tissue. Reports using different techniques all confirm that electrical and other types of depolarizing stimulation of nerve result in the release of substance P from nervous tissue and that this is calcium-dependent.

SUBSTANCE P RECEPTORS

Very little information is available to date. Substance P may be applied by iontophoresis and has been shown to cause the excitation of cells by depolarizing the membrane. A number of agonists have been found—principally eledoisin and physalaemin, which mimic the central actions of substance P. These agonists are undecapeptides like substance P, and this has led to some attempts to define the structure/activity relationships of the peptides and their receptor. There is as yet no clear conclusion to this work. No generally accepted antagonist of substance P has been found.

Substance P may be present in nerve terminals which signal pain to the spinal cord. Dorsal horn interneurons which respond to noxious stimulation of peripheral receptors are especially sensitive to iontophoretic application of substance P. Indirect evidence of release and quite strong evidence for a transmitter role for substance P comes from the observation that section of dorsal roots leads to denervation supersensitivity of interneurons to peptides. Denervation supersensitivity is a common phenomenon; many receptors to neurotransmitters become much more sensitive following degeneration of afferent fibres.

The above account of substance P suggests that it is a substance of considerable potential interest. It is very likely to be a neurotransmitter, but nothing is known about behavioural changes which might result from the selective blockade of transmission in substance P systems. Only one thing seems quite definite, and that is the basic law, that if a system, process or function can go wrong, it will go wrong, and a human disorder of some kind will manifest itself and be recognized. The possible effects of malfunction of substance P pathways are as yet unknown.

Opioid transmitters

The analgesic and euphoric properties of the opium alkaloids have been known for very many years. The stereospecific nature of the effects and their blocking by selective antagonists, such as naloxone, has suggested that the drugs act at specific receptor sites. Such sites were discovered in the early 1970s with the use of ^{3}H-opiates. Evidence soon followed of endogenous materials normally attached to the receptors, and two pentapeptides, differing only at the C-terminal, were soon found. These are known as methionine and leucine enkephalin. When the amino acid sequence of these was determined met-enkephalin was found to be the same as the N-terminal end of another polypeptide, already isolated and named β-endorphin. This is a 31-peptide fragment of a 91-peptide hormone known as β-lipotrophin and found in the anterior pituitary associated with adrenocorticotrophic hormone.

Although β-endorphin is found in high concentration in the anterior piuitary, it is also, as will be described below, present in many parts of the brain.

SITES OF OPIATE RECEPTORS AND OPIOID TRANSMITTERS

Opiate receptors have been located in the dorsal horn of the spinal cord, in laminae 1 and 2. These receptors appear to be on the terminals of the sensory neurons of spinal nerves. Opiate receptors have also been found in parts of the limbic system, in the globus pallidus, the thalamus and the periaqueductal grey matter. All these are regions where micro-injections of morphine have been found to cause analgesia, and where naloxone, in morphine-dependent animals, causes withdrawal signs (*Figure 4.24*).

The location of enkephalins has been investigated by immunological methods which are unable to distinguish between the methionine and the leucine forms. They are found in the spinal cord dorsal horn, on interneurons synapsing with the sensory neuron terminals bearing the opiate receptors. Their presence in the brain is similarly in small 'interneurons' in the same sites as those already described for opiate receptors. Smaller concentrations do, however, appear elsewhere.

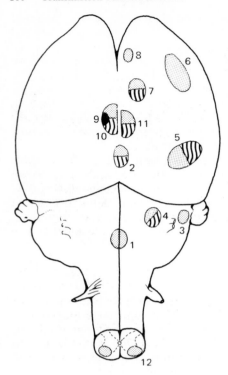

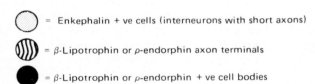

Figure 4.24 Rat brain and spinal cord seen from below. 1 = n raphé magnus; 2 = peri-aqueductal grey; 3 = n parabrachialis; 4 = locus coeruleus; 5 = amygdala; 6 = c striatum; 7 = n accumbens; 8 = lat septum; 9 = arcuate n of hypothalamus; 10 = hypothalamic nuclei; 11 = periventricular n of thalamus; 12 = dorsal horn of spinal cord. This figure was prepared by M.B. Llewelyn, BSc

The distribution of β-endorphin is somewhat different. As well as its high concentration in the anterior pituitary, this compound is also found in the cells of the basomedial and the basolateral hypothalamus, with axons distributed to the anterior hypothalamus, the septum, the periaqueductal grey matter and parts of the pons.

THE ACTIONS OF OPIOID TRANSMITTERS

When they are applied by micro-iontophoresis, the effect of these compounds is usually depressant. One can presume that in the dorsal horn of the spinal cord they act by presynaptic inhibition. In the hippocampus, where opiate receptors have not been detected, application of opioids is said to be excitatory, to the point of inducing hippocampal seizures. The depressant action of the compounds is blocked by pre-treatment with naloxone.

Along with these actions on neuronal activity, all the opioid compounds are described as analgesic, but the degree of activity depends on the mode of administration. Penetration of the blood–brain barrier is uncertain, and the compounds may be inactivated en route to the receptor site. Nevertheless, β-endorphin has been described as having 50–100 times the effect of morphine, on a molar basis, and synthetic derivatives of enkephalin, active when given by mouth, may be up to 30000 times as potent as the naturally occurring enkephalin.

Other behavioural effects seen on animal administration include akinesia, progressing with increased dosage to generalized muscular rigidity, and hypothermia. For this reason the opioids have been described as 'natural neuroleptics', but, in fact, more detailed analysis of the effects show that they are different from those of the synthetic neuroleptic drugs.

OPIATE ANTAGONISTS

Synthetic derivatives of the morphine molecule can be made which antagonize the actions of the parent substance. Naloxone is the best-known and most complete of these antagonists. Other compounds have a mixed effect, blocking some actions of morphine but mimicking others. This implies that there are structural differences between different opiate receptors. Furthermore, the agonistic actions of these compounds may themselves be blocked by small amounts of Na^+. This complicates the search for a morphine derivative which has only analgesic and no euphoric action.

Detailed study of the actions of morphine, of synthetic derivatives of morphine and of other compounds with morphine-like actions, and of their antagonists, is now suggesting that there may be several distinct opiate receptors, each responding normally to only one of the various endogenous opioid polypeptides which have been discovered. This is a field which is being explored currently, and the state of knowledge may be very different in 5–10 years' time. At the time of writing four or five specific receptor types have been proposed, each given letters of the Greek alphabet (kappa, sigma, etc.).

Other peptides that may be neurotransmitters

As well as substance P, endorphin and the enkephalins, various other polypeptides have had neurotransmitter roles ascribed to them. Some have long been recognized as G1 tract hormones and others as having equally specific endocrine roles in other body systems.

This list includes cholecystokinin, vasoactive intestinal polypeptide, thyrotrophin-releasing factor, somatostatin, angiotensin II, neurotensin and bradykinin. All of these compounds have been located in various parts of the CNS, or have been shown to have effects which can be interpreted as the stimulation or inhibition of neurons when artificially administered. Conclusive evidence of their activity as transmitters is still wanting, however. As is the case with peripheral activities of these and other polypeptide hormones, it is likely that these substances act via a cyclic nucleotide system, and so perhaps produce longer-lasting effects on neurons than do the classical neurotransmitters. To speculate, a precise location of these compounds' activities and the physiological events that call them into action might eventually produce the link between the brief events of synaptic transmission and the long-term basis of memory, learning and those patterns of behaviour that we identify as 'disease states'. Some of the compounds on this list are well-known hormones. Their actions will be referred to again in Chapter 8.

Chapter 5

The sensory functions of the brain

Introduction

This chapter and the next two aim to provide a fairly detailed look at the structures associated with the important functions of the brain, so far as they can be determined. Among the subjects covered are sensation and movement, understanding, speech, memory and feeling. Inevitably, and particularly with the last of these subjects, it is necessary to consider how activity usually thought of as 'in the mind' can, through the brain, affect many other systems in the body, both physiologically and even structurally. In this more detailed look at the brain, reference to the gross anatomy of the brain may be helpful. For a psychiatrist, particularly one starting a career now, familiarity with the structure of the brain should become part of everyday knowledge.

It is harder to show the relationship between the intimate details of how nerve impulses are conducted along fibres and, much more important, how they are transmitted between neurons, and the systematic study of the brain's functions. It is comparable to knowing how transistors, conductors, resistors and capacitors work, and yet having no idea of how these components function as parts of the tuner, amplifier, and volume and tone controls of a radio. The sites of the major functional units of the brain are identified (in the same way that one can point to bits of the radio circuitry and say 'this receives radio waves' or 'this amplifies signals'), but, when it comes down to saying how their millions of individual components are linked together and how these linkages result in the unit working in the way it does, then the level of ignorance is extreme. Many years of painstaking work must be done before it will be possible to describe how a particular pattern of impulses arriving at a particular area of the cerebral cortex results in the conscious awareness of having heard the word 'thud' being spoken, and even more years before we will know how that pattern may *not* be generated by sound waves entering the ears, but from some other, abnormally functioning part of the brain. It is an overwhelming task for anybody to attempt to relate structure and function of the brain, and it is vital to remember that only the most superficial study of these topics is possible at present.

103

Specific sensory systems

Various physical and chemical phenomena in the distant or the immediate external environment have the property of stimulating 'receptors' and causing these to emit nerve impulses which travel along nerve fibres and eventually reach the brain. Before describing each system associated with the different types of physical or chemical events, it may help to discuss general aspects, common to them all.

Much has been written about the properties of receptors and the way in which the different physical or chemical modalities to which we are sensitive affect the receptors. In general, receptors act as transducers. In other words, they change one event into another, altering one form of physical or chemical energy into another form. In many cases they also act as amplifiers, the energy content of nerve impulses being greater than that of the signal to which the receptor is sensitive.

Receptors are usually specific to alterations in only one kind of physical or chemical change impinging on them, although this specificity may in some cases not be as complete as the tidy-minded scientist would like. The light receptors in the eyes are not sensitive to sounds, in the ordinary course of events, although a blow on the head—a vibration, if ever there was one—results in 'seeing stars' and steady pressure on the eyeball produces a brilliant and patterned display arising from stimulation of retinal cells. The structure and mode of impulse production in the receptors of the organ of Corti (sensitive to sounds) and those of the semicircular canal (sensitive to head movement) are remarkably similar. It is their location in these different parts of the inner ear and the construction of these parts that gives the receptors their specificity. Also, receptors respond to a far smaller energy input from their 'normal' stimulus than from the abnormal stimuli to which they can be made to respond. Thus, the energy content of light from a real star is far smaller than that of the blow on the head, yet it evokes a comparable response from the light receptors of the eyes.

Another general property of receptors which must be mentioned is the way in which they signal variations in strength of stimulus. This they do by varying the rate of production of impulses. The nerve impulses emerging from a particular receptor and travelling along its associated nerve fibre are always the same size, and they always travel at the same speed. As the strength of the stimulus changes, so does the frequency with which the receptor emits impulses (*Figure 5.1*). It is like a door-bell push button, constructed so that light pressure makes the bell respond with one 'ping' every second and a harder push makes the bell ring ten or twenty times a second. However, each one is still the same ping. There are just more of them in each second when the stimulus is more intense. Receptors 'adapt', at varying rates, to a constantly maintained stimulus. If the door-to-door salesman keeps his finger pressed firmly on the button, the bell's ringing steadily dies down from 50, to 10, to 1 ping each second, and finally it may stop altogether (*Figure 5.2*). With a momentary removal followed by reapplication of the stimulus to the receptor, the response goes back to its original strength. The 'caller' gets a far better response by intermittent pressure on the bell push than if he pressed continuously, without any breaks.

Whatever the stimulus appropriate for a receptor, light waves in the retina, elongation of a muscle or blood vessel's stretch receptor, chemicals of various sorts for other receptors, this stimulus must cause the production of nerve impulses in the emergent nerve fibre. Moreover, as just described, the frequency of generation of these impulses must be related to the strength of the stimulus.

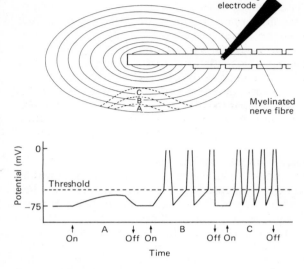

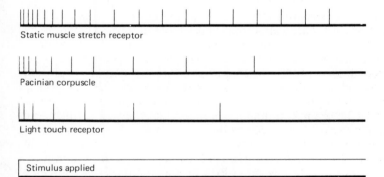

Figure 5.1 The effect of increasing the depth of deformation (A to B to C) of a Pacinian corpuscle (above) on the membrane potential of its nerve fibre, as recorded from the electrode

Figure 5.2 The differing rates of adaptation of three receptors when the appropriate constant stimulus is applied to each

In the example of pressure–deformation-sensitive receptor found beneath the skin, the Pacinian corpuscle, this process is partly understood. This receptor consists of a naked nerve fibre surrounded by many layers of specialized fibroblast-like cells, the whole looking not unlike a microscopic onion (*Figure 5.1*). Pressure upon the corpuscle, changing its shape, results in a reduction in membrane potential of the nerve fibre. The extent of this local depolarization, and perhaps the speed with which it develops, is determined by the amount of deformity, which is, in turn, related to the strength of the impinging stimulus. If the stimulus is strong enough, then the local depolarization is great enough to reach the threshold for impulse generation and an impulse starts and proceeds along the nerve fibre, passing towards the CNS. After generation of an impulse, the fibre returns towards its resting state, but if the stimulus persists, the local depolarization develops again, and causes the generation of a second impulse, and so on, for as long as the stimulus is applied. The more intense the stimulus, the more rapidly the depolarization, called the *generator potential*, reaches threshold, and the higher the frequency of impulse production. Now generator potentials, or their analogues in other receptors, have not been demonstrated in all types of receptor, but the similarity of the above description to that of impulse production in a neuron, stimulated through its excitor synapses, must be such as to lead us to suspect that impulse generation at a receptor proceeds in the same general way as it does in a nerve cell. Adaptation may then be described as a more or less slowly developing loss of production of generator potential.

Finally, the physical or chemical stimulus that evokes the response from the receptor and starts nerve impulses coursing towards the brain must be distinguished from the 'sensation' or the 'perception' which is the conscious experience when these impulses reach certain, not wholly defined areas of the brain, because those two events are quite distinct. Perceptions are usually related to receptor stimulation, but all sorts of changes intervene between them, and there are many opportunities for their modulation and for misinterpretations en route. It is like being a cave-dweller, interpreting events in the outer world by the shadows they cast on the wall.

There is also one general point that should be made about the nerve fibre pathways along which impulses travel from receptors to the cerebral cortex, where they are eventually interpreted. It has been stated that for every sensory modality a path involving three neurons and two intermediate synapses conveys impulses from receptor to brain. In many cases this is now known not to be true, and, in fact, things are more complex and more varied than this simple pattern. The complexities are linked to the ways in which the nervous system 'handles' the incoming formation and allows interaction between the different inputs, so that, perhaps, the important take precedence, although the unimportant are not entirely neglected. Among these complexities is the existence of efferent fibres, conveying impulses away from the brain, either right to the receptors, or to one of the synaptic relays on the pathway towards the brain. It is not known for certain what is the function of these efferent fibre pathways, but it is possible that impulses in them set the sensitivity of the receptors, so that their response to a given strength of stimulus may be varied, and the brain shielded from too great a barrage of information of a trivial nature, but alerted to very low intensities of stimulation from sources of importance to it. It is a common experience that sense of hearing is enhanced in a fog or in the dark.

The mechanics of this handling of incoming sensory impulses by the CNS can be explained by the various types of synaptic activity described in Chapter 3. Thus, an e.p.s.p. that does not cause a cell to 'fire' but makes it more responsive to a weak input from a receptor will raise the sensitivity of the system to that receptor's stimulation. Inhibition, particularly presynaptic inhibition, will, conversely, lower a system's response to stimulation of its receptors.

Cutaneous sensation

It is conventional to regard the skin as the source of four types of sensation—touch (with which pressure and position senses are associated), pain, heat and cold—and to look automatically for distinct receptors associated with each one of these modalities of sensation. There is, however, a continuing conflict of evidence, both scientific and from common sense, that makes nonsense of any dogmatic statements anyone may care to make about this subject. It has, for example, been stated many times that intense heat or cold causes a sensation of pain, because heat and cold damage tissues, as much as does mechanical injury, and some of the chemical products of this damage (perhaps histamine, serotonin or bradykinin) stimulate the specific pain sensory endings. How, then, can the intensely unpleasant itching painful sensation that may result from the lightest touch, particularly on parts of the face, be explained? Tissue damage is far from occurring with this gentlest of mechanical stimulus, but the sensation may be intense and extremely unpleasant. One hypothesis which was designed to get around the confusion is the *pattern theory of sensation*. In this, groups of nerve endings, each associated with its nerve fibre, together form a complex, or *spot*. Any stimulus applied to this spot will evoke its own specific pattern of impulses in some or all of the sensory fibres from the spot, and then these differing patterns are interpreted as the different sensations resulting from the different stimuli.

Be that as it may, cutaneous pain is described as being of two types—the sharp or pricking pain felt rapidly after a stimulus is applied, and a burning sensation which may be detected as much as a second later. Other types of pain are the sustained ache that comes from damaged joints, ligaments, etc., and the cramp or colic-like pains that come from powerfully contracting muscles, among which is the pain of angina pectoris.

From skin, pain afferents are either Aδ or C fibres in type and their endings are thought to be free in the tissues. Heat and cold probably stimulate similar fibres through similar undifferentiated endings. When these fibres enter the spinal cord, via the lateral divisions of the posterior roots of the spinal nerves, they pass into the *dorsolateral fasciculus* (zone of Lissauer), in which branches of these fibres run up or down the cord for one or two segments. These give off many collateral branches which penetrate the substantia gelatinosa and synaptically terminate on its Golgi type II cells. These cells also receive many synapses of axons from adjacent regions of the spinal cord and of fibres that descend from the brain. Their axons eventually enter the chief nucleus of the dorsal horn of the spinal cord, from which arise the classical *second-order* sensory axons (*see Figure 5.4* for some of these local interconnections).

There is thus no simple relaying of impulses from one fibre, conveying them from receptor to spinal cord, to a second fibre which transmits the impulses up the cord to the brain. The interneurons of the substantia gelatinosa receive many other axons from various places in the CNS, not least the sensory cortex of the brain, and then themselves transfer the resultant activity to the cells of the 'second' sensory axons which pass up the spinal cord. The substantia gelatinosa neurons are the supposed sites of the hypothetical *gate* mechanism, whereby some, non-pain, afferent impulses could block the passage of impulses, entering along the pain fibres to the 'second-order' sensory fibres (*Figure 5.3*). The descending fibres from the brain which enter this region, too, may also inhibit these interneurons.

The 'second' sensory axons, activity in which is the resultant of both the impulses entering the spinal cord from the stimulated receptors and the many local and descending influences on these impulses, cross the midline of the spinal cord and enter mainly the lateral spinothalamic tract on the opposite side. Those that enter this ascending tract first, in the sacral part of the cord, are the most lateral

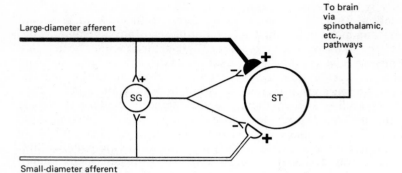

Figure 5.3 Impulses in the large-diameter afferent, from a non-nociceptive receptor, stimulate the S.G. cell. This applies a presynaptic inhibitory brake on all impulses reaching the S.T. cell, so its transmission to the brain is reduced. Impulses in the small-diameter afferent inhibit the S.G. cell and thus remove the presynaptic brake on the S.T. cell. Impulses from the small-diameter fibre, from nociceptive receptors, thus are transmitted by the S.T. cell to the brain

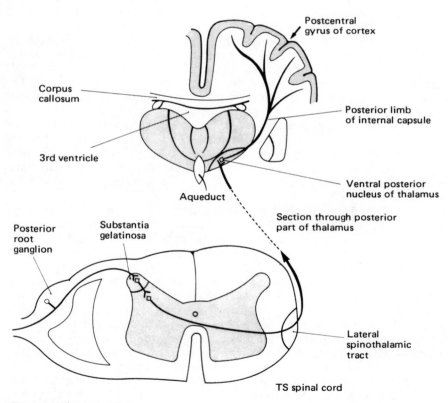

Figure 5.4 The pain pathway

component of the tract, and fibres progressively join its medial aspect as one
ascends through the spinal cord to the cervical region (*see Figure 5.4*). Some
'second' fibres, conveying touch sensation, travel similarly in the anterior spinothalamic tract. In the brain-stem the two spinothalamic tracts on each side merge, and
after passing through the brain-stem as the spinal lemniscus, these axons enter the
ventral posterior nucleus of the thalamus.

A very similar organization is followed by impulses from similar receptors in the
head and the face. The great majority of the afferent sensory neurons are in the
fifth cranial (trigeminal) nerve, but a few are found in the facial, the glossopharyn-
geal and the vagus nerves also. The analogues to the spinal cord posterior horn are
all found in the nucleus of the spinal trigeminal tract (formed from the incoming
sensory axons). The 'second' sensory neurons arising from this nucleus also for the
most part cross the mid-line and ascend through the brain-stem as the trigeminotha-
lamic tract, which ends in the medial part of the ventral posterior thalamic nucleus
(*Figure 5.5*).

Apart from the well-defined somatotopic organization of this region of the
thalamus, it is thought that conscious awareness, with but poor localization, of pain
and temperature sensation arises when impulses reach the region in 'second'

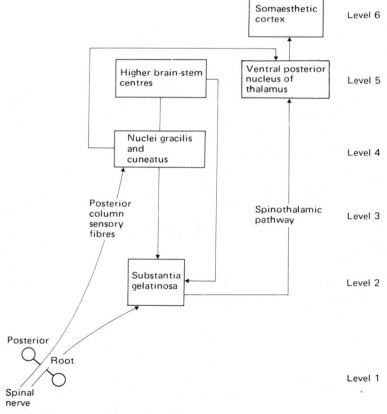

Figure 5.5 Sensory paths and descending paths

sensory neurons. The further description of its projection to the sensory cerebral cortex via the 'third-order' sensory neurons will be described below.

Impulses conveying sensations of touch, pressure and position sense travel from the periphery by a somewhat different route, although in this case, also, the 'second' sensory axons end in the same ventral posterior nucleus of the thalamus. On entering the spinal cord in the medial division of the posterior nerve root, the axons from the mechanoreceptors, mostly Ia and Ib fibres, directly enter the posterior columns of the spinal cord and *ascend on the same side* as their point of entry. The lower fibres, entering the spinal cord first, will be found most medially in the posterior column and the fibres entering further up the cord will join the column from its lateral face. In the medulla these fibres terminate in the nuclei gracilis and cuneatus. In these nuclei there is a similar complex organization to that described in the spinal cord's posterior horn, and from them eventually arise the 'second' axons of this sensory pathway. The nuclei receive, as well as the primary sensory axons, fibres descending from the brain, and from them fibres descend to the posterior horn cells of the spinal cord. Thus, in these nuclei there is a place for the same sort of modulation of the patterns of incoming impulses from the receptors by higher brain centres and interaction between incoming impulses as in the posterior horn cells, with the added complication that activity in these nuclei may itself affect the posterior horn neurons and their output into the spinothalamic path.

The 'second' axons which arise from the nuclei gracilis and cuneatus immediately cross the mid-line and ascend through the brain-stem as the medial lemniscus, to enter the ventral posterior nucleus of the thalamus on the *opposite side of the body* from the point of origin of the sensory impulses.

From the ventral posterior nucleus of the thalamus the 'third' sensory axons project to the somataesthetic area of the cerebral cortex, usually located in the post-central gyrus of the parietal lobe. All sensory modalities from one part of the body—touch, pressure, and perhaps pain and temperature—are referred to the same region of the cerebral cortex, and there is an orderly representation of the body in the gyrus, starting with the foot at the upper medial end and ending with the facial region at its lower and lateral end. The representation on the cortex is related to the density of peripheral receptors, with the hand and facial areas being, of course, far larger than areas for the trunk and limbs generally (*Figure 5.6*). From this cortical 'reception' area in the postcentral gyrus, it is assumed that impulses pass into the adjacent association area in the parietal cortex and that activity passing in this direction is associated with 'understanding' or 'interpreting' the meaning of the incoming information from the receptors. Thus, a person with damage to the post-central gyrus is no longer aware of an object placed, say, in his hand, but damage in the association area results in the recognition that the object is round, flat, cold, hard and heavy, but it is not recognized as a coin of the realm.

As well as these two routes for conveying sensory impulses from specific cutaneous regions to related areas of the cerebral cortex, a third, non-specific, afferent pathway is also now recognized. Partly through the substantia gelatinosa cells and partly directly the smaller spinal nerve root sensory fibres make synaptic connections with cells deeper in the posterior horn of grey matter. Eventually cells at the root of the posterior horn are affected from which *spinoreticular* axons arise. These ascend in the spinal cord in no recognized tract. At all levels in the brain-stem, and in the spinal cord, too, these fibres make synaptic connections with further neurons, until their rostral projections end in the intralaminar nuclei of the thalamus. In the brain-stem the non-specific pathway receives further contributions from both the visual and the auditory systems. At each stage up the CNS, convergence and divergence occur, any cell receiving many afferents and its axon branching to supply many neurons at the next stage. There is no specific laterality in this system. Neurons on one side of the spinal cord project to cells on both sides of the medullary reticular formation, and any one cell of this may project to both thalami. The intralaminar nuclei of the thalamus project diffusely to the sensory cortex and also in a point-to-point way to the corpus striatum. So far as conscious

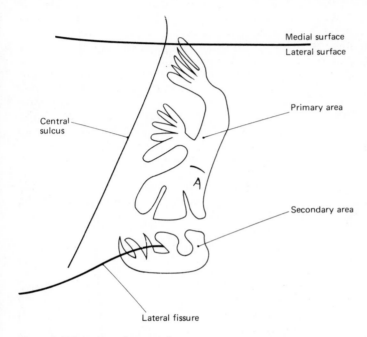

Figure 5.6 The sensory homunculus

awareness is concerned, the pathway mediates what were once called protopathic sensations, poorly localized and poorly defined, but running from itch to agonizing pain. It is also clearly concerned in the arousal mechanism. Thus, damage to the reticular core of the midbrain does not stop evoked potentials arising in the appropriate cortical region but a lesioned animal makes no response to, say, a loud noise. If lemniscal paths are damaged and the central core left intact, however, a noise will provoke a vigorous response, while the cortical area remains unstimulated. It is further suggested that the intralaminar nuclei of the thalamus and the associated reticular formation are involved in the production of the 8–12 c/s and the 18–32 c/s rhythms of quiescent human EEG, and for their replacement with asynchronous, fast low-voltage activity when the subject starts to perform mental arithmetic or attend to some aspect of his environment. It should be noted that opiate receptors, and opioid transmitter-containing axons, are found within parts of this system, both in the spinal cord and in the midbrain. Through the intralaminar nuclei of the thalamus this sensory system is linked to the limbic system of the forebrain, of which these nuclei form a part.

Vision

It seems an impertinence to include a brief summary of our knowledge of all stages of the visual process from the formation of an accurately focused image of the visual field on the retinal receptors, to how these receptors are stimulated to produce impulses, the organization of the impulses which occurs within the retina itself, the transmission of impulses in optic nerves, chiasma and tracts, through the lateral geniculate body to the occipital cortex, and to how, finally, the incoming information is processed there so that what we consciously perceive is a faithful replica (or so we believe) of the 'real' world that originally produced the light rays that penetrate the eye's pupil. Many great textbooks have been written and much research done on each stage in the whole process. Work is still continuing, and statements written here may well be out of date before this book is published. We shall therefore briefly summarize the various processes that occur between light rays impinging on the eyes and the conscious perception of the visual field.

The first is the formation of an accurately focused image of the visual field upon the retinal receptors. This is achieved largely by the refractive power of the air–cornea interface and the transparency of the cornea and the other media through which the light passes within the eyeball. The lens, the refractive power of which· can be increased by contraction of the ciliary muscles, produces the variations in total refractive (dioptric) power of the eye needed if sharp images of both near and distant objects are to be formed on the retina. While the anatomic pathway connecting afferent fibres from the retina to the efferent fibres to the ciliary muscles is known, the exact way in which a blurred image causes the appropriate change in efferent nerve output is a mystery. Then, while it is known that each point on the cerebral visual cortex (occipital lobe) receives impulses from corresponding points in *both* retinas, it is not known how the cortex can initiate and control eye movements so that the corresponding retinal points are at corresponding positions of the image of the visual field, or how both eyes can remain fixed on one object in the field when the head moves, or, conversely, how they 'track' a moving object across a stationary field, with the head held stationary or moving. It is easy to appreciate how complex are the processes involved in one aspect of the visual process.

In the conversion of light waves into nerve impulses, the process begins with a photochemical reaction. A chemical substance is changed when light falls on it. This change alters the permeability of the receptor cell and thus initiates nerve impulses, the frequency being related to both the intensity of the light and its wavelength—for there is evidence to show that our appreciation of different colours may be due to different receptors containing light-sensitive materials responsive to different wavelength of light.

Within the retinal neural layer, considerable processing of the impulses from the receptors occurs, and the axons of the retinal ganglion cells, which make up the fibres of the optic nerves and tracts, respond in various ways to a patch of light on the retina. Thus, some are stimulated by light on their receptor field (for there is considerable convergence between receptors and ganglion cells), while others are inhibited, but these may be stimulated by illuminating an adjacent portion of the retina. Again, the links between retinal receptors and optic nerve fibres are the site of complex anatomical arrangements of neurons the precise mode of action of which we do not understand.

Retinal receptors are of two general kinds—the highly light-sensitive rods, many of which can influence a single ganglion cell, and the relatively insensitive but perhaps colour-specific cones, which show much less convergence onto the ganglion cells. Therefore, cones are able to signal much more detail of the visual field, but need a brighter light to do this. It is not surprising to find that the foveal region of the retina contains only cones or that a faint point of light seen at night 'in the corner of the eye' disappears when one looks directly at it—i.e. when its retinal image falls upon the fovea.

The retina of each eye may be thought of as divided vertically into nasal and temporal (medial and lateral) halves, on each of which fall, respectively, the images of the temporal and the nasal visual fields. Thus, corresponding points on the two retinal fields fall in the nasal half of one retina and the temporal half of the other retina. The cross-over of the two nasal halves of the optic nerves in the optic chiasma ensure that, in the optic tracts, the corresponding ganglion cell axons from both retinas can approach each other and jointly relay information to other neurons in the brain. The decussation at the optic chiasma means that the left optic tract conveys fibres from the temporal half of the left retina and from the nasal half of the right retina, on both of which have formed images of the right-hand half of the visual field. Similarly, the right optic tract conveys information about the left half of the visual field (*Figure 5.7*).

Fibres leave the optic tracts and enter the midbrain to make connections with the nuclei that control the ciliary muscles—those of the pupillary opening (to control

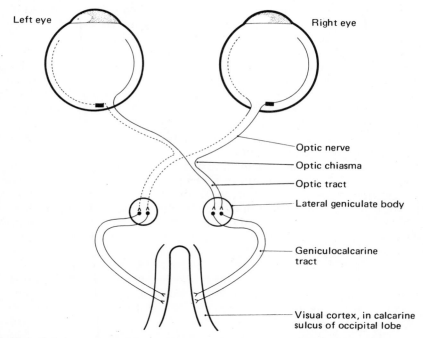

Figure 5.7 The right (temporal) half of the retina of the right eye and the right (nasal) half of the retina of the left eye both 'see' the left half of the field of vision. Owing to the crossing over of optic nerve fibres from the two nasal halves of the retinas, each lateral geniculate body and visual cortex receives *all* the impulses generated by the opposite half-field of vision

the amount of light entering the eyes) and those that control the external ocular muscles, ensuring that the images in each retina are brought to corresponding points (the accommodation-convergence reflex). The main body of optic tract fibres end on the cells of the lateral geniculate body, the axons of which pass to the primary visual cortex of the occipital lobe of the cortex.

The manner in which material becomes processed in the primary visual cortex has been extensively studied since the early 1960s. Each point (= a column of cells) on the cortex relates to a point on the retina (with the exception that the foveas are bilaterally related to both cortices), but firing of neurons in cortical points is triggered by edges between light and dark, or between shades or colours. The edge may have to be variously orientated or moving to evoke the cortical response. It is becoming possible, but beyond the scope of this book, to explain, on the basis of synaptic excitation and inhibition of the many neurons between retinal receptors and cortical cell columns, how the information has become processed in this way. But, of course, the primary visual cortex is not the end of the road. The results of its processing are passed on into the 'visual association' area. This is the region in which we begin to 'make sense' of the retinal images of the visual field, or the region in which conscious perception of the field occurs. Now, also, current visual information has to be compared with antecedent information, stored in the memory and stored also with its particular meaning. You distinguish, for instance, between a 2 m-long black and tawny striped cat and a 30 cm-long one with black and brown stripes, and both from a 2 m-long horned animal, seen to be browsing from the trees. While the last of these may be good to eat, the first will eat you if given a chance, while the small cat will treat you with a haughty indifference. Further abstractions can be learned and stored in the association cortex. A 4 in-long, two-dimensional picture of a tiger is instantly recognized, provided that you have already learned that the 'real' world can thus be represented. Finally, the shapes 'TIGER' or 'tiger' or even 'ταιγερ' may be seen to represent the dangerous beast found in forest or deep reed-bed. The visual association cortex has then to receive two main inputs. One is from the primary visual cortex and ultimately from the eyes, and the other is from the cerebral memory stores; so that, by contrasting and comparing the two, one can interpret what one is actually seeing at any one time. Presumably, it will eventually be possible to understand all these activities in terms of transmission, inhibition and conduction of nerve impulses in neurons, and the roles of the various chemical transmitters. Some people are devising electronic models of some of the simplest cortical functions, but there is no guarantee that these models will be at all like the real thing. In dreams and in hallucinations the material reaching the association area and of which we are aware will be more or less distorted, so that one 'sees' things which are not producing any retinal stimulation or input to the primary visual cortex. Disturbance of the blood supply to and thus the metabolism of the visual cortex, such as occurs in migraine, produces black patches in the visual field which may be surrounded by a jagged brilliant or flashing outline. (In one of the authors' attacks of migraine flashes occur at a frequency of 8–10 Hz, near that of the EEG's alpha rhythm.)

Hearing

Compression—expansion waves, travelling through the air at frequencies between 50 and 20 000 c/s are conducted through the tympanic membrane and the middle-ear bones to the fluid-filled inner ear. The intensity with which the waves enter the inner ear can be modified by two muscles—the tensor tympani, which alters the responsiveness of the eardrum to the incoming waves, and the stapedius, which regulates the movement of the stapes's footplate, movement of which transmits the vibrations into the inner ear. Again details of the function of the inner ear will not be given here. It is sufficient to say that different portions of the cochlear basilar membrane are tuned to vibrate in resonance with different frequencies of incoming sound waves. At the base of the cochlea is found the region with the highest frequency, while low-frequency vibrations cause resonance of the basilar membrane towards the cochlear apex. When a portion of the basilar membrane vibrates, that portion emits 'microphonic' potentials. These are also resonant with the incoming sound waves. They are not propagated action potentials or nerve impulses but are thought to be concerned, like the 'generator' potential of the Pacinian corpuscle, in the production of the nerve impulses. The frequency of nerve impulses from any portion of the cochlea is determined by the size of the microphonic potential produced by the sound waves in that portion; the only way in which frequency of sound waves is coded is by the bit of cochlea that resonates with the sound waves and thus stimulates, through the microphonic potential, its sensory nerve fibres. Another recently discovered aspect of cochlear function is that the cochlear receptors can themselves be somehow 'tuned', so that their sensitivity varies, by efferent nerve fibres running from the brain to the ears. It is possible that tinnitus may be related to this tuning process.

From the cochlea the afferent fibres pass via the eighth cranial nerve to enter the medulla of the brain. The cell bodies of these fibres, which are the analogue of the posterior root ganglion cells, are found in the spiral ganglion of the cochlea. The axons of these cells terminate on cells of the dorsal and the ventral cochlea nuclei, which are close to the inferior cerebellar peduncle (*Figure 5.8*). While most fibres from these nuclei cross the mid-line and ascend in the lateral lemniscus of the opposite side of the brain-stem, a significant number enter the ipsilateral lemniscus. Some fibres terminate in one or other superior olivary nucleus, from which axons enter the lemniscus. Further synaptic relays may occur along the course of the lemniscus and all terminate at its superior end in the inferior colliculus of the midbrain. From here new fibres run to the medial geniculate body and from there to the auditory cortex, in the floor of the lateral fissure and extending onto the superior temporal gyrus. From this description, it is seen that the 'typical' sensory pathway, of three neurons, one of which crosses the mid-line, is now known not to be true of this pathway. There are 4–6 neurons on the path from receptor to cortex, many of the fibres do not cross over, and, finally, the receptors' function may be considerably modified by efferent impulses from the brain, particularly from the superior olivary nuclei. In the auditory cortex fibres for low-frequency sounds end in the anterolateral part, while those for high frequency reach the posteromedial part of the region. It would seem, then, that our appreciation of harmony and its converse, dissonance, may depend on precisely which bits of the auditory cortex are stimulated simultaneously, and not at all on the simple ratios of the different frequencies of the tones known as common chords to musicians. Some of the most 'unpleasant' dissonance must result from simultaneous stimulation of adjacent cortical areas.

The interpretation and understanding of all sounds is performed in neighbouring areas of the temporal cortex—also known as the auditory association, or Wernicke's area. This region is of particular importance in the understanding of spoken words and, presumably, in the control of one's own speech. It should be

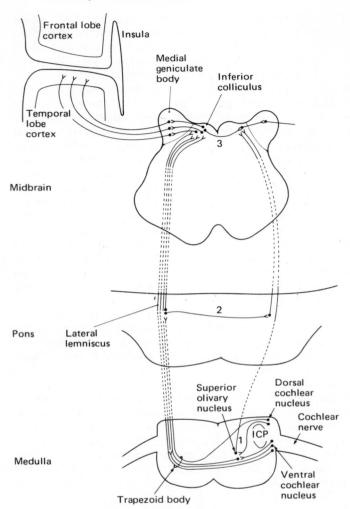

Figure 5.8 While most of the impulses from one cochlea pass to the opposite side's temporal lobe, 1, 2 and 3 on diagram illustrate the ipsilateral routes that impulses can take. ICP = inferior cerebellar peduncle

remembered, as described above, that a significant number of the afferent chains of fibres from each ear ultimately enter the ipsilateral cortex. Unilateral cortical damage does *not*, then, cause deafness restricted to the opposite ear, but some loss in both ears and some loss in the ability to judge the direction from which sound comes. This last ability depends, ultimately, on the different times at which sound waves enter the two ears. Presumably, each temporal cortex, receiving slightly asynchronous inputs from the two ears, can interpret this to determine the origin of the sound, and both temporal lobes, acting together, can also use the small differences in time of arrival of the impulses to make this determination.

Man is a social animal, and both eyes and ears are important means by which single people communicate with each other to fulfil their social natures. Defects in either system may interfere with this ability to communicate and thus disturb social contacts between people. By far the commonest visual defects are errors of refraction in the eyes' lens system, so that sharp images of the visual field cannot be formed on the retinas. These are usually corrected, more or less, by additional lenses mounted in spectacle-frames or even held in contact with the cornea. None of these are perfect, however, and none can compensate for loss of optic nerve fibres due, for instance, to the raised intra-ocular pressure of glaucoma. Nor is there any known way of preventing the errors of refraction from occurring. Although the wearing of even clear glass lenses does give a person improved visual activity, it also imparts the sensation of being withdrawn or protected from other people. Those who habitually wear spectacles are said to look naked or exposed when without them, although this may only be due to the distress felt when one cannot see one's environment clearly.

Long-sustained vigorous stimulation of the organ of Corti in the ear results in loss of hearing. This may be due to a loss of elasticity of the basilar membrane, or to actual destruction of the receptors, the hair cells, attached to the basilar membrane. (If the exposure is to particular sound frequencies, the damage may be found localized to the corresponding portion of the inner ear and the hearing loss restricted to those frequencies. If a wide range of frequencies—from machinery or 'pop' band—are applied, then deafness is correspondingly in all frequencies of sounds.) The ear can also be affected, presumably by loss of elasticity in the basilar membrane, as age advances. In this condition high-frequency loss is most severe and the loss may be replaced by tinnitus, a continuous hissing, whistling or ringing sound.

Hearing loss, too, is a powerful cause of changes in mood. One does not have to be a Beethoven to feel cut off from and suspicious of one's fellow humans as deafness develops. It becomes particularly difficult to 'sort out' a chain of sounds to which one wishes particularly to attend from a general background hubbub of noise. The deaf, then, increasingly dislike parties and prefer only tête-á-tête conversations with a single person. The increasing suspiciousness and withdrawal of a middle-aged or elderly person from social gatherings may thus be due to the development of presbyacusis and not to that of some major psychological condition.

Taste

Between the bold statement that there are but four primary taste sensations— sweet, salt, sour and bitter—and the complexity of flavours of all the foods we place in our mouths there is a considerable gap. 'Flavour' must be compounded from the primary tastes, from other oral sensations, including 'chemical heat' (as induced by chilli), temperature, texture, smell, even sight and sounds. While there is some localization of the four primary tastes (sweet at the tip of the tongue, salt at the sides, sour and bitter progressively back), it is likely that each taste bud, of which there may be 10000, containing up to 25 receptor cells, is stimulated by more than one of the primary qualities. For three of these, specific chemical groupings are involved. Thus, sweetness resides in the ketone or the aldehyde groups of sugars and saltness in negatively charged ions such as chloride or sulphate ions, while acid is dependent on hydrogen ion. Each taste bud as a whole perhaps contains one or other or combinations of the four types of receptor cell. Each one of the 250 000 receptors is innervated by several nerve fibres from different sensory neurons and each neuron innervates several receptor cells. Presumably, the vast number of variations of tastes is the results of patterns of nerve impulses of varying frequencies in many different neurons. Taste also decreases in sensitivity with age, as the number of taste buds decreases from the 10 000 found at birth. This is why older people sometimes seek more highly flavoured food than the young.

The afferent taste fibres enter the brain-stem in the seventh, ninth and tenth cranial nerves, and end in the nucleus of fasciculus solitarius of the medulla. Most authors say that the neurons of the nucleus cross the mid-line before ascending to the thalamus, although some say that they remain on the same side. The thalamic neurons, in turn, project to the lower end of the post-central gyrus and the neighbouring region of the insula. The nucleus of fasciculus solitarius also makes contact with the efferent salivatory nuclei of the seventh and ninth cranial nerves.

Smell

In contradistinction to the few (250 000) receptors and the four primary sensations of taste, there are some 50 million receptor cells in the olfactory mucous membrane on each side of the nose, and, even in man, a rich profusion of different smells is experienced and odoriferous substances can stimulate the receptors in the most minute quantities. A further distinction is that the receptor cells are themselves bipolar neurons, the specialized ends of their dendrites being the actual receptor site. The non-myelinated axons of these cells are grouped together into bundles and pass, as the olfactory nerves, through the cribriform plate of the frontal bone and enter the olfactory bulb. There, in the 2000 glomeruli, they make synaptic connections with dendrites of mitral and tufted cells. Axons of stellate cells also enter the glomeruli which, with about 25 000 bipolar cell axons and dendrites of 25 mitral and 75 tufted cells entering each one, must be the site of very considerable 'processing' of the impulses from the sensory receptor cells. The nature of this processing is not fully understood. Axons of the mitral cells partly relay in the anterior olfactory nucleus of the olfactory tract on pyramidal cells and partly run direct to the primary olfactory cortex. This is divided anatomically and perhaps functionally into three areas. The lateral olfactory area is in the uncus and the amygdaloid nucleus of the temporal lobe; the intermediate area is in the anterior perforated substance; and the medial area is on the medial aspect of the frontal lobe, beneath the anterior end of the corpus callosum. All these regions are part of the paleocortex, the first part of the cerebral hemispheres in vertebrate evolution. The main association area for smell is adjacent to the uncus in the parahippocampal gyrus. Through this there are rich connections with the neocortex, the limbic system and autonomic efferent nuclei in the brain-stem. The medial olfactory area also sends projection fibres to the brain-stem and the limbic system. This close association of olfaction and the limbic system derives from their anatomical link, in that both are found in the paleocortex. Functionally, also, smell may be the important sensory stimulus which evokes the behavioural responses characteristic of limbic system activity in lower animals. Be that as it may, in man the development of the neocortex and of auditory, visual and tactile senses has completely overshadowed this older association between the sense of smell, emotion and physical response.

Chapter 6

Initiation and control of voluntary movement

Introduction

From a strictly neurophysiological point of view, all motor activity in the CNS must be the consequence of sensory activity, of nerve impulses coming into the CNS. This may be immediate and almost reflex in nature, as when afferent impulses cause a perception of discomfort and a movement is made which alleviates this unwanted sensation. The movement may be modified by material retained in a memory store—that a vigorous scratching in response to an itch may not always be 'good manners'. On the other hand, movements may be totally determined by the memory store, itself built up by previous sensory inputs, and by perceptions and abstract thoughts arising from the inputs. Thus, one reaches for the cigarette packet because one remembers that the inhaled nicotine has a pleasant effect. When considering the control of voluntary movement, it is helpful to remember that all movements start from and finish in postures and that one could almost think of movements as adjustments of an underlying postural state. Disturbance of the mechanism that maintains posture then may cause as severe a disturbance of movement as any abnormality in those parts of the brain primarily concerned in movement.

The motor cortex

The main output centre in the cerebral cortex for voluntary movement is the area 4 histological type of cortex, found in the central sulcus and the precentral gyrus of the frontal lobe neocortex and generally called the motor cortex. It is specifically characterized by the giant pyramidal Betz cells, although these are the origin of 3 per cent only of all the axons leaving the region in the corticobulbar and corticospinal paths. Stimulation of discrete areas of the motor cortex results in discrete movements of specific parts of the body. This point should be emphasized. Stimulation of the motor cortex rarely causes contraction of individual muscles, usually contraction of a related group of muscles and relaxation of their antagonists, etc., to bring about the recognizable movements. Those parts of the body with a great repertory of movement, such as the hand, have a larger area of representation on the motor cortex than those parts with but few movements. In fact, the size

119

of an area of motor cortex will vary with the number of motor units (anterior horn cells, their axons, and their innervated muscle fibres) serving its regional muscles. On the motor cortex an analogue of the body can be drawn, as in *Figure 6.1*, showing the relative sizes and disposition of the body in the motor cortex. Finally, it should be realized that the left cerebral hemisphere controls the right half of the body and vice versa, just as in the main somatosensory system.

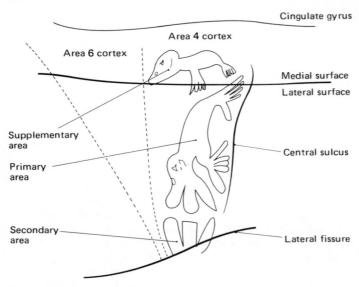

Figure 6.1 Motor areas of cortex

There is a secondary motor area in the dorsal wall of the lateral fissure and a supplementary area on the medial surface of each hemisphere, but these are not known to be of any clinical importance in man (*see Figure 6.1* for their location).

Movements can also be caused by stimulation of the histological area 6, lying in front of the precentral gyrus. These partly disappear in experimental animal preparations in which area 4 has been destroyed, which indicates that area 6 projects to the motor cortex. They are, in any case, more generalized and directional in nature, such as turning the head, twisting the trunk, or large-scale limb movements. Area 6 may, however, be associated with learned motor activities of a complex progressive nature, such as writing.

The neurological inputs to area 4 are from area 6 (as has just been described), the somataesthetic cortex and various thalamic nuclei. These may be the immediate inputs, already programmed to produce the required or appropriate outputs (voluntary movements) from the motor system, but how, in neurological terms, the appropriate response is selected from the enormous repertoire of possible move-ments is just not known. An 'ideomotor' region, located perhaps in the parietal lobe, has been postulated in which the physiological activity occurs which must accompany the concept that 'such and such a movement is required'. This region receives inputs from all the sensory association areas, from memory stores and perhaps from the regions concerned more with emotional expression in the paleocortex and the limbic system, and then activates the motor cortex via further processing in the area 6 cortex. In stating this, it should be stressed that these views are imprecise and speculative. This has to be, since exact knowledge is wanting in this subject, but it can be seen how disturbed input into such a region, as conceivably may occur in schizophrenia, could then result in the disturbances of movement which can accompany this illness.

The corticospinal pathway

About one million axons leave each cerebral hemisphere in the corticospinal and the corticobulbar tracts (*Figure 6.2*). Either directly or through interneurons these

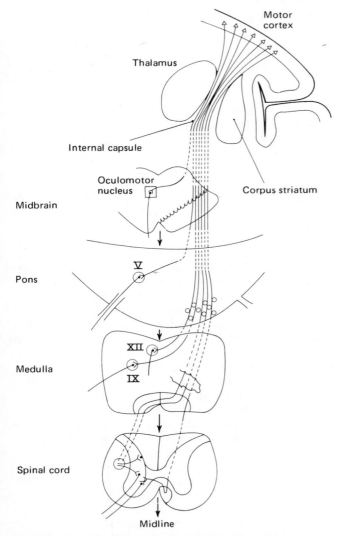

Figure 6.2 V = 5th cranial nerve nucleus; IX = 9th cranial nerve nucleus; XII = 12th cranial nerve nucleus

make contact with anterior horn cells or their analogues in the brain-stem motor nuclei. In most, perhaps in all, cases corticospinal axons cross the midline before terminating, the most important site of the crossing-over being in the decussation of the pyramids in the medulla. In the cases where corticospinal fibres stimulate anterior horn cells to activity and thus to produce muscle contraction, it is thought that they make direct synaptic contact with the anterior horn cells. Thus, for prime mover muscles there are but two neurons between motor cortex and muscle fibre, and it is scarcely surprising that these are labelled upper motor neuron and lower motor neuron, respectively. Underlying this apparent simplicity, however, the motor system is much more complex. Each anterior horn cell, or lower motor neuron, receives synaptic connections from many other sites, including both local interneurons and other long descending pathways from the brain. Some of these will be excitatory and some inhibitory. Furthermore, the motor cortex and premotor areas send axons to other regions of the brain which are concerned in the control of voluntary movement. What is known of the nature and function, so far as movement is concerned, of both these cortical efferent fibres and those descending to the lower motor neurons will be described in the following sections.

Disease or disruption of the upper motor neuron

Theoretically, damage to these cells may occur at any site from the cerebral motor cortex down to the point of the termination of their axons at anterior horn cells. In practice, however, only two conditions need concern us.

A patch of scar tissue resulting from injury or infective or neoplastic lesions may set up a focus from which epileptic activity originates. If such a focus were to lie in the motor cortex, then the seizures it caused would always start in the part of the body controlled by the affected part of the cortex, and then spread progressively to adjacent and further parts of the body. By observing the original site and spread of activity in such fits, it is sometimes possible to locate and even to remove the lesion.

The other condition is thrombotic occlusion of or haemorrhage from one of the arteries supplying the corpus striatum. The region that is most drastically affected is the internal capsule, through which the corticospinal fibres run on their way from the motor cortex into the brain-stem and the spinal cord. The results of such a lesion can be divided into two aspects. First is the loss of voluntary control of movement of parts of the body. This will be typically of the arm, leg, face and tongue of the site *opposite* to the lesion. Second, the paralysis is not flaccid, however, most of the muscles being affected by an increase in tone, and a characteristic posture is assumed. The loss of voluntary movement is ascribed to the disruption of the corticospinal fibres, while the abnormal posture is thought to result from loss of fibres running from the motor cortex to the cerebellum, the basal nuclei or other brain-stem nuclei concerned in the control of the activity in lower motor neurons.

The neocerebellum

The cerebellum can be divided physiologically into three components, although the cellular architecture of all three is similar, which suggests that its functions are performed in the same manner. The archicerebellum, concerned with postural control, and the paleocerebellum, concerned with the control of spinal reflexes, need not concern us here. They are, in man, in any case overshadowed in size and importance by the neocerebellum. The cytoarchitecture of cerebellar cortex is remarkable for the regularity of its 'wiring diagram', a situation which might lead to an understanding, in quasi-electronic terms, of how neuron systems process information coming to them in discrete nerve impulses. The cerebellar cortex receives two afferent inputs. One is via the mossy fibres and the other via climbing fibres. The former come from both spinocerebellar pathways and pontine nuclei, and the latter from the inferior olive, itself on the spinocerebellar pathway (*Figure 6.3*). Thus, the neocerebellar cortex might be said to receive information both about the 'orders' given to the motor system by the cerebral cortex and about the response actually performed by the muscles, bones and joints of the body.

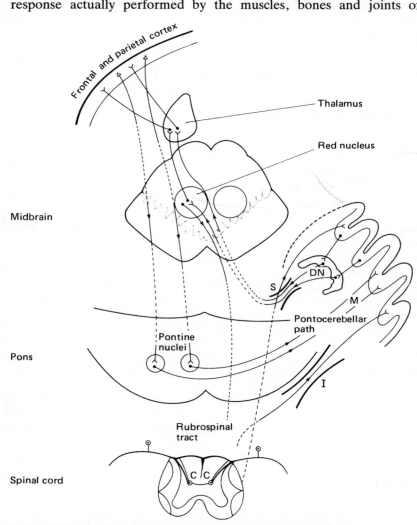

Figure 6.3 Connections of the neocerebellum: C, Clark's column of cells; S,M,I, superior, middle and inferior cerebellar peduncles; DN, dentate nucleus

Presumably, the cerebellar cortex compares command signal with result achieved, and, via its efferent pathways, adjusts and controls the output of the motor cortex, until 'command' and 'result' are accurately matched. The efferent path from the neocerebellum is via the dentate nucleus and the ventral lateral nucleus of the thalamus back to the motor cortex. It should be noted that through the corticopontine and pontocerebellar path one cerebral cortex innervates the opposite cerebellar lobe. On this return route also the axons from the dentate nucleus cross the midline en route to the thalamus and the motor cortex. It is clearly beyond the scope of this book to describe the structural and functional details of how the assembly of neurons and their interconnections may achieve this overall process, but it is sufficient to point out that the more florid symptoms and signs of cerebellar dysfunction are due to a lack of this control function of voluntary movement—the automatic adjustment and control of a movement *while it is taking place*, so that its 'aim' is accurately achieved.

This failure of 'aim' gives rise to the most important signs of cerebellar dysfunction. A finger reaching out to a given point moves slowly and in a jerky manner (asynergy). It frequently overshoots the mark, or deviates out to one side (past pointing). The defects may combine to produce a coarse tremor which becomes more intense as the finger approaches the desired point (intention tremor). Rapid alternating movements are performed slowly and clumsily (dysdiadochokinesia). Finally, there may be a reduction in basal muscle tone and the muscles tend to tire easily.

The basal nuclei of the cerebral hemispheres

These are the substantia nigra, the corpus striatum, the subthalamic nucleus and the ventral anterior and ventral lateral nuclei of the thalamus. Two 'circuits' of neurons have been described (*Figure 6.4*). One is from the motor and premotor cortex to the substantia nigra, thence to the corpus striatum, the thalamus and back to the cortex, with a two-way link between the globus pallidus and the subthalamic nucleus. The other is from the cortex to the caudate nucleus and putamen, thence to the globus pallidus (but also to the substantia nigra) and so back to the cortex via the thalamus (ventral anterior and lateral nuclei). In addition to these circuits, the basal nuclei, via the red nucleus and the brain-stem reticular formation, control activity in the rubrospinal and the reticulospinal pathways, which are two of the descending fibre systems which can influence anterior horn cell activity.

Unlike the neocerebellar cortex, we know very little about the physiological functions of these masses of neurons. The clinical condition of Parkinsonism, due to a malfunction of the dopaminergic axons of the substantia nigra, is one secure clue, but the only one we have to this system. Cells of the globus pallidus are peculiarly sensitive to prolonged exposure to carbon monoxide and this may also result in the Parkinsonian state, while the putamen and the caudate nucleus have been found to be damaged by exposure to high plasma copper concentration or some product of streptococcal infection. These conditions are associated with choreiform and athetoid movements. It might appear as though one of the two circuits outlined above, or its offshoot via rubrospinal or reticulospinal pathways, controls the tremor and rigidity of Parkinson's disease and the other circuit controls the production of irregular and non-purposive movements. It is just possible that both systems, operating together, provide a continuous background of activity in

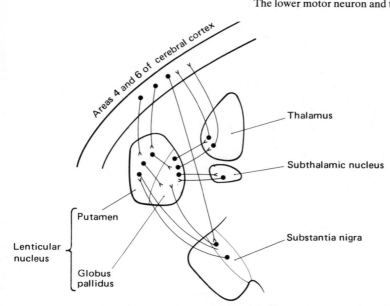

Figure 6.4 Two circuits can be traced out: 1, cortex ⟶ substantia nigra ⟶ lenticular nucleus ⟶ thalamus ⟶ cortex; and 2, cortex ⟶ putamen ⟶ globus pallidus ⟶ thalamus ⟶ cortex

both upper and lower motor neurons upon which the specific commands of some 'ideomotor' region play when initiating voluntary movements. As in so much of neurophysiology, this is but a speculative statement, pointing, perhaps, to the way investigation of the subject might proceed, particularly when coupled with the known sites of different disease processes.

The lower motor neuron and the 'motor unit'

Each anterior horn (AH) cell, through its axon leaving the spinal cord by the anterior root, or the brain-stem analogues with axons in various cranial nerves (all except 1, 2 and 8), supplies, by terminal branchings of the axon, anything from 5 to 1000 skeletal muscle fibres, and a single action potential along a single axon causes all the innervated muscle fibres to make one twitch contraction. The AH cell, its axon and the muscle fibres it innervates are therefore known as a motor unit. They function as a single entity. Once the AH cell is activated, all of its muscle fibres must respond. The number of motor units in a muscle, or the number per unit mass of that muscle, determines the fineness of control of the force that, by calling into action a varying number of AH cells, can be exerted by that muscle. Thus, the external ocular muscles, or the lumbrical muscles of the hand, have only a few muscle fibres for each motor axon, and great delicacy of control is possible, whereas in the components of quadriceps femoris or gluteus maximus many hundred muscle fibres are supplied by branches of the axon of each AH cell (*Figure 6.5a*).

Grading of contraction of muscles and the prevention of fatigue in them is accomplished in the following manner. An AH cell excited to produce a single

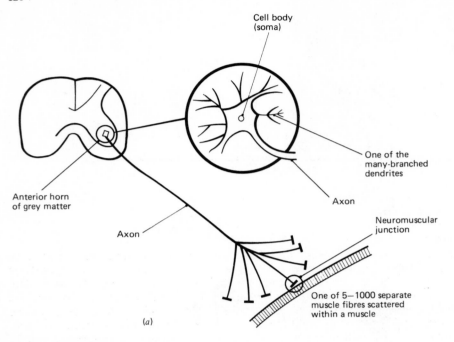

Cell body (soma)

One of the many-branched dendrites

Axon

Anterior horn of grey matter

Axon

Neuromuscular junction

One of 5–1000 separate muscle fibres scattered within a muscle

(a)

1. Twitch response to a single stimulus

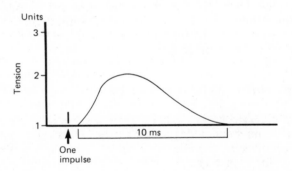

Units

Tension

3

2

1

10 ms

One impulse

2. Responses to successive stimuli

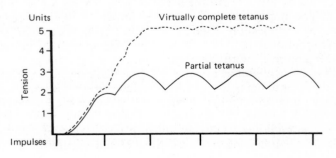

Units

Tension

5

4

3

2

1

Virtually complete tetanus

Partial tetanus

Impulses

(b)

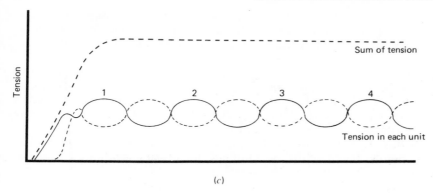

(c)

Figure 6.5 (a) Anatomy; (b) contractions in a single unit; (c) partial tetanus in two units, contracting synchronously

action potential causes a brief contraction of its associated muscle fibres, known as a twitch (*Figure 6.5b*). If the excitation of the AH cell is continuous, it responds by producing a train of impulses, which follow one another down its axon. The frequency of these impulses will depend on the level of this excitation. However, the twitch contractions produced in the muscle fibres will begin to merge as the impulse frequency rises; the total tension developed by the muscle fibres will also rise, since the activation of the muscle fibres caused by one nerve impulse will be still persisting when the next one arrives. The muscle fibres are now said to be in a state of partial tetanus (*see Figure 6.5c*), alternately partially contracted and partially relaxed, in time with the nerve impulses emitted by the AH cell. If two neighbouring motor units (or two groups of motor units) could be synchronized to be exactly 'out of phase' with each other, one contracting always as the other was relaxing, then a smoothly sustained but low-level contraction would be achieved in the muscle, without causing fatigue in any unit by having it contract more forcibly (*Figure 6.5c*). This is believed to happen in a pool of AH cells all serving the same movement or tonic function. The situation is further complicated by the fact that, in a sustained contraction—such as forms the basis of muscle tone or the body's posture—many motor units are not involved at all, while others are producing partial tetanic contraction in the reciprocal manner already described. It is found that when such an AH pool or its muscle fibres are studied electrically, while some units are active and others resting, the actual sites of activity will shift from one to another of the motor units, so that the active ones can be rested and, after a period of rest, can again resume activity. Although such electrical recordings have not been performed simultaneously with studies of the metabolic basis of muscular fatigue, it is well known that postural activity of skeletal muscle can continue virtually indefinitely in a patient with an abnormal or exaggerated postural state without any development of fatigue.

With a still higher degree of activation of AH cells and consequent higher frequency of impulse production, the individual contractions of the muscle fibres can no longer be recorded and the muscle sustains a steady high level of tension. This is the state known as complete tetanus. It may be approached when a person makes a 'maximal voluntary effort', but this can be sustained for only a very short period before fatigue occurs and the contraction strength weakens. Anecdotes of people's response under acute stress or the influence, for example, of ergot-induced hallucinations, describe levels of physical strength unattainable by normal voluntary efforts, so it may well be that even when maximal these do not cause complete tetanus of the muscle fibres.

Motor units can be affected by various disease states or by physical damage to their axons. The inevitable result of death of an AH cell or severance of its axon is paralysis of the innervated muscle fibres, and their subsequent degeneration if axonal continuity cannot be re-established. Trauma may interrupt axons at any point from their origin in the spinal cord to their terminations in muscles, and a knowledge of the origin and route taken by axons supplying any muscle would enable one to predict the effects of disruption or the possible cause of a muscular paralysis. One infectious disease that commonly, on a world-wide basis, causes death of AH cells is poliomyelitis. In many cases only some cells in the 'pool' of motor neurons serving a particular muscle group may be affected, while others may survive with full function maintained. When the muscle is studied, two characteristic consequences of the motor neuron loss are seen. The maximal voluntary power of the muscle is reduced, and at any level of effort it will develop fatigue earlier than normal. Fewer motor units are available both for maximal voluntary effort and to share out the active periods in milder contractions, so rest periods are shorter. The presence of denervated muscle fibres adjacent to normally innervated ones results in sprouts developing from the surviving axons, which re-innervate these denervated fibres. The development of macromotor units occurs. There will be recovery of maximal strength and a reduction in fatigue, but with loss of fine control of movement.

Tremor

Since various neurological and other conditions can all give rise to tremor that interferes with voluntary movement, a description of the different types of tremor should be given.

Physiological or idiopathic tremor is a fine tremor, present unchanged throughout life, and unassociated with any neurological, endocrine or physiological disturbance. It is presumably due to some inherent fault in 'wiring up' the control systems during early life.

Tremor is present in acute anxiety or the outpouring of adrenaline from the adrenal gland. It can also be produced by artificial administration of the hormone into the circulation. To what extent this adrenaline can then penetrate the blood–brain barrier and directly disturb the voluntary movement control mechanisms is unknown. The tremor of emotional states is as likely to be due to a direct cerebral action, and not to depend upon circulating catecholamines. There are adequate links between the limbic system and the motor control system to allow the former to affect the latter and disturb its normal smoothing action on voluntary movements.

Hypersecretion of the thyroid gland also produces tremor. The thyroid hormones certainly affect the function of neurons, although whether this is in some specific manner or just part of their general metabolic regulatory function is uncertain. Be that as it may, a fine tremor, most obvious in the outstretched hand, is one of the signs of thyrotoxicosis.

The intention tremor of cerebellar disease has already been described. It is most clearly distinguished from equally coarse tremor of Parkinsonism, in which condition the tremor is most apparent at rest and frequently disappears when the person voluntarily moves the affected part. Parkinsonian tremor is often seen in the resting hand, producing a simultaneous adduction of thumb and flexion of fingers, imitating manual pill rolling. In Parkinsonism the tremor is often associated with rigidity or raised muscular tone, in which case, when the physician attempts to move the patient's limb, it can be felt to 'give' in a series of regular jerks. This phenomenon is known as cogwheel rigidity.

Drug-induced tremors may be caused by compounds that incidentally block some aspect of the motor control system. Thus, Parkinsonian tremor can be produced by blockers of dopaminergic transmission, including the major neuroleptic compounds. It may be seen as a coarse, flapping tremor, associated with mask-like facies and slow, slurred speech. Other drugs can produce a tremor like the rapid, fine physiological tremor. Tremor may also be part of a drug-withdrawal syndrome, typically of alcohol or opiates. Here it may be a consequence of the anxiety experienced as part of the removal of sedative materials from the patient, or it may be that the control system, released from the damping effect of the drug, fails in its own regulating procedure.

Chapter 7

Higher functions of the nervous system

Frank J. Vingoe
Department of Psychology, University Hospital of Wales and
Department of Psychological Medicine, Welsh National School of Medicine, Cardiff

Introduction

The term 'higher functions' refers to those cognitive activities that are most developed in man, although the chimpanzee, the dolphin and other organisms may also be shown to engage in higher functions. Cognitive activity includes those processes involved in learning (i.e. the registration, processing and subsequent storage of information). Attentional processes are clearly important here in the registration and encoding of material to be stored. Processing may include thinking and reasoning (i.e. the comparison and forming of relationships between ideas and images).

While many think of our higher functions as being regulated by the neocortex, it has become quite clear that subcortical mechanisms are quite important. Whereas the specific neurophysiology may not be known, the role of the limbic circuit (system) in memory cannot be disputed (*see* next section). In addition, while the hypothalamus controls many emotional activities, such as aggressivity and sexual behaviour, there is general agreement that interactions occur between emotional activities and the so-called higher functions. While one tends to speak of a certain area of the brain in connection with a particular function, the presence of the vast number of interconnections (neural or association pathways) between different brain areas reminds us that the particular area under discussion does not function in a vacuum. Lesions in these association pathways produce a disconnection between various areas. In general, the larger the lesion or degree of disconnection, the greater the degree of dysfunction. Lesions of association pathways may be termed disconnection syndromes.

It will have become clear to the reader that the hard physiological facts of the conversion of the specific energies impinging on the receptors into nervous impulses become gradually transformed into less specific generalizations as one approaches the subject of explaining the mechanisms of perceptual integration in the CNS. The reader will also have noted that from these generalizations there appears an ever-increasing clarity of knowledge as we move down the motor system, until we can specify not only exactly how a motor unit is activated, but also the effects of its activation on the muscle cells it innervates.

In the present chapter we are going to discuss the specificity of function concept as related to the right and left hemispheres and the various lobes of each hemisphere. In addition to the psychological aspects, some of the more physiologic-al aspects of brain functioning will be considered.

The afferent neural impulses from the peripheral cutaneous and deep receptors pass through the spinal cord or brain-stem, ascending through tracts, and arrive at the primary receptive area of the cortex in the postcentral gyrus (sensory cortex), where they are perceived as sensations. From the primary receptor area these neural impulses pass to the adjacent association area. The association areas, which make up a large part of the cerebral cortex, are of great importance in the higher functions of thinking, reasoning and problem solving and, in general, in perceptual integration. It is in these areas that we interpret sensory stimuli. There is an association area associated with each lobe of the cortex. Therefore, one may speak of a frontal, temporal (auditory association), parietal and occipital (visual associa-tion) area. Electrical stimulation studies show that the area in man most implicated in somataesthetic sensitivity is an area in the postcentral cortex, which includes a part of the parietal lobe posteriorly. This is the so-called somataesthetic cortex or somatic association area (*see Figure 5.6* and Chapter 5 for a discussion of sensory functions of the brain).

We shall go on now to discuss in some detail some of the major functions of the brain and relate them to the various areas which are primarily responsible for a particular function, although, as pointed out by Critchley, it is better to speak of 'specialization of function' rather than 'localization', since the concept of 'regional equipotentiality' is generally accepted and some adjacent cerebral areas may overlap in terms of their specialization. The first major function we shall consider is that of memory, the disturbance of which is implicated in many neuropathological and psychopathological conditions.

Memory functioning

Memory refers to that capacity which enables one to store information and to make use of it at a later time. Memory enables information to be available for use in (1) behavioural tasks or (2) cognitive functioning.

One may need to keep a telephone number in mind only long enough to dial it if one does not plan to use it again. This would involve only the processes involved in immediate or short-term memory. On the other hand, should there be a future need for the number, and one is unable to write it down or to know in what directory to find it, one would need to memorize it (i.e. to ensure that it goes into long-term storage).

In thinking, reasoning or imagining, one needs to manipulate various 'bits' of information already in storage in order to solve a mental problem or to arrive at some creative response. These cognitive tasks also implicate long-term memory processes. New sensory information may also be used. The reader can see that cognitive activity may very well include the use of information from long-term storage and incoming sensory information simultaneously. It should also become clear that there is a great deal of overlap involved in perceptual, learning, short-time memory (STM) and long-term memory (LTM) processes.

What are the stages involved in the memory process? They include the following: (1) registration of the material to be used immediately and/or to be stored for future use; (2) encoding of the material in preparation for storage; (3) storage of the material; and (4) retrieval of the material from storage. Therefore, it is apparent that memory problems involve a defect in one or more of the above stages

(Vingoe, 1981). Clearly, as suggested later in the chapter, a problem of arousal (i.e. a lack of alertness or a relative inability to concentrate) may result in a memory deficit.

The assessment of memory deficits may involve asking the patient to retrieve material from long-term storage or to learn new material. Many memory problems involve a difficulty in learning new material (e.g. Korsakoff's syndrome). Learning is usually defined as a change (increase) in performance based on experience. Only through the performance of some task can one demonstrate that learning has occurred. If there is a fault in one or more of the stages involved in memory processing, then this would be demonstrated through a faulty performance. In other words, learning is inferred from task performance, which, in turn, is a function of memory processing.

Brain lesions in certain areas, such as the hypothalamus, or lesions which disconnect one specific brain area from another, may interfere with one or more of the stages in memory processing. Thus, a lesion in the brain-stem reticular formation (BSRF) may very well lead to a decreased alertness and even coma and total amnesia.

STM refers to the holding or retention of information for brief periods of time before either: (1) forgetting this information, i.e. not encoding it; or (2) encoding and storing it. In order for information to pass from STM to LTM, it needs to be practised or rehearsed, and may need some form of encoding. While STM is considered to have a limited capacity, LTM has unlimited capacity. Anxiety tends to interfere with STM and the extent to which material is passed along to long-term storage. Anxiety and other interference factors may thus result in a failure of consolidation. An example of a STM or immediate memory task would be the frequently used digit-span (DS) test, in which the patient is asked to repeat a series of numbers which are read to him at one-second intervals. A lower DS score has been found for those who exhibit a high anxiety state compared with controls. While the STM system is labile, the LTM system has been found to be quite stable once consolidation has occurred.

People who have been assessed as mentally backward typically have difficulty in STM tasks. Talland (1971) indicated that the difficulty this group of people had in new learning implied a failure to process and organize information. However, if the mentally backward and a group of matched controls learn material to the same degree, they retain the material equally well.

Memory disorders

What are some of the major memory disorders? There are four main disorders of memory:

(1) A disorder of STM, which is sometimes subdivided into (a) disorder of immediate memory (e.g. poor performance on the digit span test) and (b) disorder in recent memory (e.g. an inability or high degree of difficulty in remembering information presented, say, ten minutes earlier).
(2) A deficit in long-term or remote memory (e.g. forgetting well-known facts that were learned many years ago).
(3) Retrograde amnesia, which refers to a complete or near-complete forgetting of the events which occurred prior to an accident or illness, such as encephalitis. Retrograde amnesia may involve a relatively short period, say of a few hours, to a very extensive period of many years.

(4) Post-traumatic amnesia, also usually associated with an accident or illness, refers to the complete, or near-complete, forgetting which occurs immediately after the accident or illness. For example, during a period of unconsciousness, the patient is not able to register any (or at least very little) information from his environment. While he is concussed, and for some time after a concussion, a patient's memory is quite unreliable and he is very vague in reporting what happened.

Anterograde amnesia refers to an inability in retaining new information beyond the time involved in an immediate memory task (i.e. beyond a minute or two). Thus, one may refer to anterograde amnesia as a deficit in learning new material.

One may find deficits in STM or LTM because of widespread or diffuse brain lesions or atrophy. However, in patients with specific brain lesions the memory problem may be restricted to processing a specific type of information, such as spatial, as in remembering a geometric design; or verbal, as in remembering specific words or a paragraph of meaningful material. The deficit may also be related to the mode of presentation of the material to be remembered, such as the visual or the auditory mode. In general, it can be concluded that lesions of the left hemisphere result in memory deficits involving auditory and verbal presentation, while lesions of the right hemisphere result in deficits involving visual and praxic activities.

Korsakoff's (amnesic) syndrome

The amnesic syndrome is considered by many to be the major disorder of memory. In this syndrome the pathology is firmly based on the memory disorganization. The amnesic syndrome involves great difficulty in recalling and/or ordering past events, as well as anterograde amnesia. There is a very severe deficit in learning new material. This involves disorder 1(b) above. On the other hand, immediate memory (1a above) is intact. In addition to the defects involved in Korsakoff's syndrome (i.e. retrograde and anterograde amnesia, indicated above), two more specific aspects are frequently included as defining the disorder. These are a disorientation, not only appearing as a confusion of sequence related to past events, but also a disorientation in the present; and confabulation, in which the patient attempts to fill in gaps in his memory by manufacturing reasonable substitutions. While Korsakoff's syndrome involves extensive memory deficits, there is generally a relative preservation of the premorbid intelligence level. For example, a patient with Korsakoff's syndrome who held a responsible professional position had become a heavy drinker and maintained the habit for 7–8 years. She developed peripheral neuropathy (muscle wasting and weakness in all extremities), and the typical retrograde and anterograde amnesia. While she obtained a Wechsler verbal intelligance quotient of 126, her performance quotient was significantly lower at 112. However, her Wechsler memory quotient at 80 was barely in the Dull Normal range. Whereas she was well-oriented when tested (after a period of 'drying-out'), she showed a high degree of confabulation which, in fact, was still present 6 months later upon reassessment.

Originally, the term 'Korsakoff's syndrome' was restricted to that disorder related to chronic alcoholism leading to neuropathy and severe memory defect. It is clear that the syndrome may also occur in patients with diabetes mellitus or tuberculosis, and in various other diseases.

Memory difficulties in dementia

Clearly, with the diffuse cortical and subcortical atrophy found in demented states, extensive memory difficulties are evident. In Alzheimer's disease, a presenile dementia, a severe global amnesia is frequently obvious. Corsellis has also found evidence of hippocampal lesions in patients who exhibited presenile dementia. A very frequent finding in early dementia is a deficit in the ability to learn new material. Patients are frequently unable to learn the new associations required on the paired-associate subtest of the Wechsler Memory Scale. In cases of senile dementia memory difficulties include a retrograde amnesia, and, in severe cases, a great confusion over the chronology of past events, evidence of confabulation and an apparent unawareness of having a memory problem. A more extensive discussion of the dementias may be found in Chapter 12.

Physiological bases for memory disorders

What neural structures are essential in memory processes? Brierley (1977) concludes that the hippocampal formations, the mamillary bodies and perhaps specific thalamic nuclei in the diencephalon are necessary for normal memorization to take place. All of these structures are included in the limbic circuit, or circuit of Papez, and are intimately associated with the ascending reticular formation (*see Figure 7.2*, page 141). In addition to the memorization process, the limbic circuit is considered to be quite important to the retrieval process. Thus, the limbic circuit is implicated in the processing of information on either the input or the output side, but not in the storage of information. Brierley has shown that both retrograde and anterograde amnesias are associated with either bilateral hippocampal or other bilateral diencephalic lesions.

We turn now to a short section on language and speech before discussing the concept of cerebral dominance.

Language and speech

Language and speech can be considered as man's greatest assets. For this reason disturbances of functioning in these areas have been studied extensively. It has been found helpful to divide deficits in language or speech functioning into the expressive or motor aspect, and the receptive or sensory aspect. As one would expect, the cortical areas subserving these two aspects are near the motor and sensory areas of the cerebral cortex, respectively. Speech and language functions have been associated with the dominant hemisphere, and lesions in specific areas of the cortex may result in aphasia or, more accurately, dysphasia, deficits in the expressive or receptive functions of speech. Pierre Paul Broca in 1861 indicated that expressive or motor aphasia was associated with lesions of the posterior –inferior area (third frontal convolution) of the left frontal lobe. However, contradictory evidence has been found. For example, while complete removal of Broca's area in man may result in some aphasia, it may be only transitory. Psychosurgical treatment which has damaged Broca's area, at least to some extent, has not resulted in any reports of aphasia. Pribram, after reviewing the evidence, has concluded that a non-damaged Broca's area is not a necessary condition for normal speech, although damage in this site may lead to some disruption in communication.

In 1886 Carl Wernicke discovered that receptive aphasia was produced by damage to the posterior–superior areas of the temporal lobe. Therefore, this particular region of the cortex is usually referred to as Wernicke's area. However, as indicated by Pribram (1971), damage in this area has resulted in a disorder which varies from a nominal aphasia (a deficit in naming) to more severe disorders which interfere with the total linguistic process. Thus, while agreement exists that a communication disorder is produced by damage to the left posterior–superior temporal area (Wernicke's area), Pribram notes that the degree to which the disorder is more expressive (motor) or receptive (sensory) depends upon the degree to which the lesion extends in an anterior or a posterior direction, respectively. Further, should the lesion extend more posteriorly, then the probability is that the language disturbance is more severe and complicated. While the specific location of the lesion may vary, an expressive (motor) disorder of speech is frequently referred to as Broca's aphasia, while a receptive (sensory) disorder is still labelled as Wernicke's aphasia.

We turn now to a consideration of the concept of cerebral dominance.

Cerebral dominance

If one makes a superficial examination of the physical contours or convolutions of the human brain and compares the right and left hemispheres, one would tend to conclude that they are structurally the same. Further, if electroencephalographic (EEG) recordings were made from a normal adult in a relatively relaxed state, one would more often than not find that the EEG readings from each hemisphere were very similar. However, if one concluded that the right and left hemispheres were functionally alike, evidence from more than a century ago would prove one wrong. I refer to Broca's findings regarding the motor speech centre and Wernicke's findings on the receptive (sensory) speech centre, both of which are located in the left hemisphere for the right-handed individual. However, when both left-handed (sinistrals) and right-handed (dextrals) are considered, the situation is not so clear-cut. Hardyck and Petrinovich have suggested that 8–10 per cent of the population are left-handed. These people might be expected to have their speech centres in the right hemisphere.

It should first be noted that a number of authors suggest that the evidence does not warrant the idea of using a rigid dichotomy dividing people into strictly right- or left-handed. Rather, it is best to consider handedness as a continuous variable along a continuum from those who are strongly left-handed, through those who are ambidextrous, to those who are strongly right-handed. Contrary to what might be thought regarding all left-handed people (that they have their language functions subserved by the right hemisphere), it has been found that over 50 per cent of this group have language lateralized in the left hemisphere.

In addition, it has been suggested that some sinistrals have bilateral representation for their linguistic abilities. Following from this, it is more probable that those who are not firmly right-handed may become aphasic after damage to either the right or the left hemisphere. However, the apparent disadvantage may be accompanied by a welcome advantage, in that recovery of language deficits is more probable and more rapid for non-right-handers (Searle, 1977).

While there is evidence that speech *production* is controlled via the left hemisphere, there is support for the idea of some speech *comprehension* being subserved by the right hemisphere even in right-handed patients. Evidence from studying patients who had hemispherectomies carried out early in life suggests that our cerebral hemispheres are initially equipotential in reference to the development of linguistic skills.

Studies of split-brain patients (that is, those patients who have had their corpus callosum surgically cut in order to control their epilepsy) has resulted in much information on lateralization of function. These studies following callosal section have been mainly carried out by Sperry, Gazzaniga, Bogan, and their colleagues in America. It has been found, for example, that the right hemisphere specializes in non-verbal perceptual abilities. It is more able in dealing with form relationships and perceptual organization than is the left hemisphere.

Gazzaniga and Dimond would agree that it is no longer appropriate to consider cerebral dominance as unilateral. We should now seriously speak and think of hemispheric differentiation. It seems clear that the right hemisphere is dominant for musical ability, and for visuo-spatial, non-verbal tasks. Many authors now agree that the right hemisphere is dominant for certain functions, while the left is dominant for others. Pribram (1971) favours the view that one hemisphere exerts an inhibitory control over the other when considering a strongly lateralized function such as speech expression. Gazzaniga also argues for an inhibitory mechanism in the left hemisphere which acts to limit the level of cognitive ability and decision-making capacity of the right hemisphere. However, while accepting that certain cerebral centres specialize in particular cognitive functions, Gazzaniga also believes that there is some overlapping in specialization. Dimond and Gazzaniga agree that it is the functional integration of the two hemispheres and the brain as a whole that is of the utmost importance.

While we tend to think that we carry out our cognitive activities entirely during our waking hours, the next section, on the functions and physiology of sleep, will suggest otherwise.

Sleep

Functions of sleep

For thousands of years man has thought that the main function of sleep was to restore the fatigued organism's *milieu interieur*. While cases of so-called 'healthy insomnia' have been reported from time to time, sleep seems to be necessary for both physical and psychological health.

Physically, when one wishes to go to sleep, one attempts to decrease the number of afferent impulses coming from the immediate environment by lying down and closing one's eyes. In so doing, the muscles of the body tend to relax and, in general, somatic activity is greatly reduced. There is thus a much lowered degree of responsivity to sensory stimulation, so that a much higher intensity or more prolonged stimulation is necessary to arouse the person. In a general way, one can gauge the depth of sleep, which varies considerably during the night, by the intensity of the stimulus required to awake the sleeper. However, as shown by

Oswald, one is usually much more responsive to emotionally important and meaningful stimuli. Eventually, the level of arousal is so low that the individual becomes unaware of most types of stimulation, and even if shown to be aware at some level (for example, through the appearance of a K-complex* on the polygraph record) may be amnesic for what occurred. Supporting the idea that sleep is a state which provides a rest from the cares of waking life, autonomic variables such as heart rate and respiration rate, etc., become significantly lower.

Cognitive activity in the form of dreams and other imaginative processes take place during sleep, particularly during rapid eye movement (REM) sleep. A number of authors suggest that dreaming may provide a sort of emotional release and, in fact, may be instrumental in helping the individual solve, or to go some way towards solving, the problems encountered during the wake state. There is also evidence that during the hypnagogic state (that state between waking and going into the first stage of sleep) conditions are optimal for the occurrence of creative ideas.

Sleep studies carried out under different pharmacological and clinical conditions have led to the finding of a negative relationship (correlation) between the amount of catecholamines (particularly noradrenaline) available at brain synapses and REM sleep time. On the basis of these findings, E. Hartmann has hypothesized that there may be a feedback mechanism present which enables sleep, especially REM sleep, to restore certain norepinephrine-containing systems.

Physiology of sleep

As suggested above, another, and more accurate, way of assessing the depth of sleep, is through polygraphic recording of EEG waves, a general discussion of which may be found in Chapter 11. In addition to measuring EEG, the sleep researcher measures eye movements and muscle activity during sleep, since both eye movements and muscle activity show definite changes during paradoxical or dreaming sleep.

Sleep researchers have divided sleep into four main stages (stages 1–4). However, there are two types of stage 1 sleep: (a) initial stage 1, described below; and (b) *emergent stage 1* or *paradoxical* or *rapid eye movement (REM) sleep*. E. Hartmann has also referred to REM sleep as desynchronized or dreaming (D) sleep.

The characteristics of the EEG during the wake state and during the various stages of sleep are outlined below.

Wake state. During the wake state the EEG activity found mainly varies from alpha (8–13 Hz), a state of relaxed wakefulness, to beta activity (above 13 Hz), during which the person may be engaged in thinking or active problem solving.

Initial stage 1. During this stage there is a gradual disappearance of alpha rhythm and the emergence of low-amplitude fast beta waves. Muscle tone remains at the medium to high level, as during the wake state. Some slow eye movements may occur.

Stage 2. It is during this stage that the individual can be said to have lost contact with the external environment, in contrast to initial stage 1, during which there is some waxing and waning of one's contact. Sleep spindle activity (waves of

---

*An EEG wave form indicative of an inner or outer stimulation, occurring typically during stage 2 sleep.

12–14 Hz) is evident from a wide area of the cortex. K-complexes, which are high-amplitude, biphasic waves, occur in this stage apparently in response to some internal or external stimulation. Muscle activity may be somewhat less here than in initial stage 1.

Stage 3. About 50 per cent of EEG activity may consist of delta waves (i.e. EEG waves of less than 4 Hz and of more than 100 µV in amplitude). Some sleep spindles and K-complexes may still be evident. There is no obvious change in muscle activity from the previous stage.

Stage 4. This stage is said to occur when more than half of the EEG record is made up of delta activity below 2 Hz. There is still some evidence of muscle activity.

REM (emergent stage 1 or paradoxical) sleep. Rapid, conjugate eye movements occur, and there is a loss of muscle tone. The EEG pattern during REM sleep is similar to that in initial stage 1 (i.e. low-amplitude fast beta waves). This stage has been referred to as paradoxical, because the cortex is quite active (more like the wake state). It is particularly active in the occipital area, and the blood flow

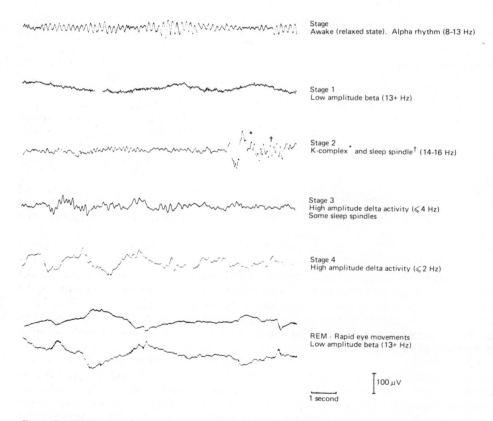

Stage
Awake (relaxed state). Alpha rhythm (8-13 Hz)

Stage 1
Low amplitude beta (13+ Hz)

Stage 2
K-complex* and sleep spindle† (14-16 Hz)

Stage 3
High amplitude delta activity (⩽4 Hz)
Some sleep spindles

Stage 4
High amplitude delta activity (⩽2 Hz)

REM - Rapid eye movements
Low amplitude beta (13+ Hz)

100 µV

1 second

Figure 7.1 EEG waves characteristic of various sleep stages. (Modified from Figures 13, 15, 16, 17, 18 and 19 in *Concept of Sleep* by kind permission of Roche, London)

through the cerebral cortex is about the same as that found during the wake state. Thus, EEG and blood flow data indicate an active cortex, not particularly suggesting sleep in the usual sense. (*See Figure 7.1* for the EEG waves characteristic of the different stages of sleep.) Autonomic variables such as heart rate and respiration rate show a greater variability as compared with non-REM (NREM) sleep, which suggests that there is a changing emotional state. There is also a quite frequent occurrence of penile erection in the male which occurs just prior to and during most of each REM period. However, it was the finding that there is, on average, about a 70–80 per cent report of dream activity associated with REM periods which caused the greatest excitement among sleep researchers. Interestingly, while the cortex is active during REM sleep, there is a loss of muscle tone and it is exceedingly difficult to awaken the individual. While initially the sleeper goes through stages 1–4 before going into REm sleep, later it is not unusual for the sleeper to go into a REM period from stage 3 or even, on occasion from stage 2. Thus, while during a typical night's sleep in a young adult there are from three to five REM periods, which have a tendency to increase in length as the night progresses, stage 4 or even stages 3 and 4 together may be omitted in certain REM cycles. A REM cycle is usually defined as the period from the onset of one REM period to the onset of the following one.

In the neonate about 50 per cent of total sleep time is taken up by REM sleep, while in the elderly this REM time reduces to less than 25 per cent. However, while the neonate may sleep about 16 hours, the average elderly person may sleep only 6 hours. In attempting to account for the large percentage of REM sleep in the neonate, it has been suggested that REM sleep facilitates the maturation of the nervous system in the very young.

Earlier research suggested that sleep deprivation could induce a psychotic-like state. However, more recent research by L.C. Johnson and his colleagues has made this suggestion less tenable, although the evidence is that *prolonged* sleep loss typically results in visual and, to a lesser degree, auditory hallucinations.

The barbiturates and other drugs used to induce sleep somewhat paradoxically also result in a much reduced, or even the complete suppression of, REM sleep during the time the drug is active. In studies in which REM-deprived subjects have been compared with those deprived of stage 4 sleep, it has been found that there is a rebound effect for each type of deprivation. In view of the high probability that REM sleep is important in regulating other body functions, and its lack results in increased anxiety and instability, the loss of REM sleep resulting from the use of many of the drugs now used to treat insomnia is to be deplored. The problem has been that loss of REM through the use of these drugs may lead to further larger doses of the drugs being prescribed. This obviously exacerbates the condition of the patient and must be avoided. However, a recent article (*Lancet*, **i**, 1981, 1256) reported on the use of a sleep-inducing nonapeptide in man. It has been found to maintain the typically REM to total sleep ratio, but increase both REM and total sleep time in insomniacs.

The normal cycle of sleep and wakefulness depends upon the integrity of the ascending reticular activating system (ARAS). Moruzzi and Magoun reported as early as 1949 that electrical stimulation of the reticular formation resulted in cortical activation as measured by the EEG. Later on, Michel Jouvet found that a small group of nuclei in the middle of the brain-stem below the reticular activating system (RAS) in the pons, the raphe nuclei, in secreting the monoamine serotonin dampens down or inhibits the alertness governed by the reticular formation, thus inducing NREM sleep.

REM sleep was postulated by Jouvet as being due to the secretion of noradrenaline from the group of neurons in the dorsal pons, called the locus coeruleus. If this area is destroyed, REM sleep no longer occurs. The noradrenaline partly releases the RAS from the serotoninergic inhibition, allowing the fast, desynchronized cortical EEG and the eye movements of REM sleep to occur, but the noradrenaline also blocks sensory input to the cortex and dampens muscular tone and activity.

Morgane and his colleagues have studied the induction of synchronized cortical activity by electrical stimulation, and correlate this with ablation studies. 'Sleep' and 'waking' centres have been found in the hypothalamus along the median forebrain bundle. Synchronization of cortical activity is produced by electrical stimulation of the preoptic basal forebrain zone, just in front of the optic chiasma. Similar results have been produced by stimulation of the region with acetylcholine. Stimulation of other subcortical regions has been shown to have similar effects. Electrical stimulation of the projection pathway from the midbrain reticular formation through the thalamus to the cortex has the effect of desynchronizing EEG activity and promoting arousal. Thus, it may be seen that a number of centres from the hypothalamus down into the lower brain-stem may be implicated in the regulation of both sleep and wakefulness.

A discussion of various sleep disorders and their treatment may be found in Vingoe (1981).

The emotions and their expression

In this section the discussion will be limited to considering the emotions in a general sense. Aggression, anxiety and sexuality are discussed in later chapters.

While it is difficult to define emotion, it is generally agreed there is a subjective aspect involving 'feelings' and a behavioural aspect seen in changes in facial expression and posture, etc. Most people think of emotions as feelings and as involving organismic changes which may be expressed in 'feeling high, buoyant or elated' or 'feeling low, blue or depressed' (Vingoe, 1981). An emotion or mood state may occur either as a result of sensory stimulation or by a cognitive stimulus such as a thought or visual image.

Both the limbic system and the autonomic nervous system (together with the endocrine glands) are implicated in the emotions and their expression. We start by discussing the limbic system, or the so-called emotional circuit of the brain.

The limbic system

A section of the limbic system consists of archicortex or rhinencephalon. In organisms lower down on the phlyogenetic scale the rhinencephalon is mostly concerned with olfaction, or the sense of smell.

While physiologists and others may not be in full agreement as to the particular structures to be included in the limbic system, they are in agreement that the limbic system is of the greatest importance in the mediation and expression of emotion. The limbic system includes the cingulate and subcallosal gyri on the medial surface of the cerebral hemispheres, and the hippocampus, parahippocampal gyrus and associated structures in each temporal lobe. In addition, it includes subcortical nuclei, notably the amygdaloid nucleus (already seen as the terminal of the lateral olfactory tract) and, finally, thalamic and hypothalamic nuclei (*see Figure 7.2*).

The hippocampus receives axons from many cortical areas, particularly the sensory association regions, including the amygdaloid nucleus, via the parahippocampal gyrus. The cingulate gyrus also receives afferents from many neocortical regions, and passes fibres to the hippocampus. From the hippocampus, axons pass in the fornix to the hypothalamus, particularly to the mamillary body. From the mamillary body fibres run in the mamillothalamic tract to the anterior and intralaminar nuclei of the thalamus, which, in turn, innervate the cingulate gyrus.

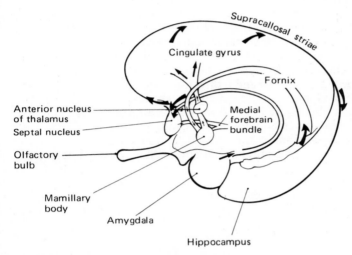

Figure 7.2 Neural connections of the limbic system

There is thus a Papez circuit (—cingulate gyrus—hippocampus—mamillary body—thalamus—cingulate gyrus) into which other cortical regions feed information, particularly those regions concerned with perception. Information may also enter the circuit from the non-specific multineuron path from the spinal cord, which we have already seen terminates in the intralaminar nucleus of the thalamus.

The main output of the limbic system is through the median forebrain bundle, which is a multisynaptic system running through the hypothalamus into the brain-stem reticular formation, and the autonomic nervous system nuclei. From the hypothalamus, the limbic system may also affect the secretions of the pituitary. The importance of this output route is considered further in the chapter on anxiety, while the autonomic nervous system is discussed below.

The main function of the limbic system is that of its involvement in emotion. Lesions which have been made in the hippocampus and the adjacent amygdala (certainly always lesions made in the amygdala) of experimental animals have led to a response of passivity–docility. From this it has been concluded that the intact amygdala usually facilitates the expression of emotion and, in particular, anger. That the amygdaloid nucleus is particularly implicated in anger and aggression has been supported by stimulation experiments in animals and ablation studies in man. On the other hand, electrical stimulation of a different part of the amygdaloid nucleus has led to fear-like behaviour. It seems highly likely that the amygdala serves different emotional functions. In addition, the limbic system is quite important in memory processing, as indicated in an earlier section of this chapter.

A number of limbic structures have been termed 'pleasure centres', in that, when electrically stimulated in experimental animals, they have been found to be rewarding to the animal. In these experiments the animal, through pressing a lever or bar, is able to administer an electric shock via electrodes implanted in his brain. Provided that the electrodes are in a pleasure centre, the animal may administer as many as 11 000 shocks to himself in an hour. Many animals have shown that they prefer to work for these small shocks than to work for food. There are also so-called 'punishment centres' in which the experimental animal wishes to stop the electrical stimulation. Punishment centres are not so widely distributed. They have been found in the dorsal midbrain and in certain hypothalamic and thalamic areas. (For more details on this subject see the chapter on anxiety.)

The lateral hypothalamus seems to be the area which the animal will stimulate itself at the highest rate. This certainly supports the concept of the hypothalamus as a centre of vast importance in emotional and motivational behaviour, in addition to its role in water balance, food intake and the regulation of body temperature. The role of the hypothalamus in the regulation of body temperature and in food intake (appetite and satiety) will be discussed later in this chapter.

Before going on to a discussion of the autonomic nervous system and the endocrine glands, a word of caution may not be amiss. Most of our information regarding the limbic system has been obtained in animal studies, which are, at times, notoriously difficult to interpret. Therefore, it is well to be quite cautious in generalizing the results of these animal studies to man, and to apply equal caution in dealing with the information obtained from that brain damage and those diseases which involve the limbic system in the human being.

The autonomic nervous system and the endocrine glands

The autonomic nervous system (ANS), with its sympathetic and parasympathetic branches, together with the endocrine glands serve a homeostatic function in that they control the composition of the internal environment. While some of the endocrine glands and their hormones are touched upon in this section, the more specific interactions between the CNS, endocrine secretions and behaviour are described in Chapter 8. The effectors of the ANS innervate the various internal organs such as the heart, lungs, etc., glands such as the adrenals, and smooth muscle. The two branches of the ANS tend to work together in integrating their actions, although at first glance they might appear to be antagonistic. When the organism is under stress and needs to be ready to engage in fight or flight, the sympathetic branch goes into action, in that the organism becomes aroused not only autonomically, but centrally as well. When the sympathetic branch is most dominant, more energy is made available through the increased secretion of adrenaline from the adrenal medulla, which leads to the release of glucose from the liver and fat from adipose tissue. Under sympathetic activation there is an increase in heart rate, blood pressure and respiration rate. On the other hand, peristalsis and other digestive processes come to a standstill. The sympathetic system is frequently referred to as adrenergic, in that the neurotransmitter substance at the postganglionic effector junction is the catecholamine noradrenaline.

In some contrast to the sympathetic branch, the parasympathetic is more dominant during states of quiescence, and is involved in the conservation of energy resources rather than the opposite. Thus, there is a decrease in heart rate, blood pressure and respiration rate, and digestive processes tend to be facilitated. The parasympathetic branch is also referred to as cholinergic, in that the neurotransmitter substance is acetylcholine. While the sympathetic system acts in a rather diffuse manner, which results in changes throughout the body, the action of the parasympathetic system is much more specific.

The ANS can be considered as a complex system of negative feedback control loops and servo mechanisms which serve a homeostatic function, in which a small input produces a large output. In servo mechanisms the output may be of a completely different form from the input; thus, it is not merely amplification. Negative feedback refers to an action which results in the inhibition or dampening down of an ongoing process. For example, should the thyroid gland produce an overabundance of thyroxine, this thyroxine suppresses the thyroid-stimulating hormone (TSH) production via blood circulation to the pituitary. The TSH stimulated the thyroid to produce thyroxine in the first place. Study of the preservation of the 'constant internal environment' of the living cells of the body has been a primary concern for physiology throughout its existence as a scientific discipline since the 1850s, when Claude Bernard began his research career. In this study the role of the ANS and the secretions of the endocrine glands have frequently been observed as the mechanisms through which the internal environment is controlled. In more recent years, however, attention has turned somewhat from study of Bernard's internal environment, that of the pericellular fluids, to the intracellular environment—the medium in which the intracellular organelles such as ribosomes, mitochondria, endoplasmic reticulum and transmitter granules and vesicles all exist. It is to be expected that, in the future, some aspects of nerve cell function of great importance to psychiatrists will be found to depend on studies of how nerve cells control their own internal chemical and physical states. The homeostatic mechanisms of the ANS are largely mediated through centres in the medulla, although the hypothalamus is concerned with body temperature regulation. Many endocrine glands are completely independent of the nervous system, but the pituitary gland, and through it the thyroid, the adrenal cortex and the gonads, are all dependent upon the hypothalamus.

Many of the responses of the ANS to physical activity are initiated by regions in the hypothalamus and the midbrain tegmentum which have received the name 'alerting reaction centres'. It is interesting to note that these are very similar to the 'punishing' centres already mentioned. The alerting reaction centres, it should also be noted, are on the outflow path from the limbic system. The physiological reactions associated with fear and anger are also those of physical activity, and it is not too fanciful to suggest that this is a necessary relationship when one considers the human species 'in the wild'. These reactions lead to a state of readiness for fight or flight, and include an increase in rate and force of the heart beat, constriction of arterioles in the splanchnic region, skin and kidneys and of all veins, and the mobilization of glucose from the liver and of fatty acids from fat depots. If vigorous physical activity follows, the muscle blood vessels dilate and the glucose and fatty acids are used as sources of metabolic energy in the exercising muscle, and the arterial blood pressure is little affected. If, however, the stimulation of the alerting reaction is *not* followed by exercise, a large rise of arterial blood pressure will occur, the work of the heart will be considerably increased to no purpose, and a hyperlipidaemia will ensue. If this occurs frequently enough, there is a much higher probability of the development of a cardiovascular disorder. The response of the cardiovascular system to the alerting reaction centres is mediated by the sympathetic nervous system, either directly through the noradrenergic postgang-lionic fibre activity or through the liberation of adrenaline from the medulla of the adrenal gland into the blood stream. Adrenaline causes the mobilization of liver glucose. However, it is uncertain whether it is the circulating adrenaline or noradrenergic sympathetic nerve stimulation that causes fat liberation from adipose tissue. A further discussion of this area may be found in Chapter 14, on anxiety. The next section discusses the regulation of body temperature.

The regulation of body temperature

It is necessary that our body temperature be maintained within certain narrowly defined limits. Fortunately, since man is homoiothermic, we are not affected as much as cold-blooded (poikilothermic) animals by the varying temperature of our external environment. This may, however, be less true for the increasing percentage of elderly people in the population, who are at greater risk for hypothermia than the rest of us.

When the body temperature is changed, receptors in the skin and anterior nuclei of the hypothalamus are stimulated. Hypothalamic mechanisms adjust for those significant changes in body temperature. That is, the homeostatic regulation of body temperature is carried out by centres in the hypothalamus. Thermal receptors in the hypothalamus also continuously assess the temperature of the blood flowing through it and, if the blood is higher or lower in temperature than normal, send neural impulses to the skin and other structures in order to initiate behaviour that will correct for the 'deviant' temperature.

There is a region in the anterior hypothalamus which serves to prevent hyperthermia. High-temperature blood leads to the inhibition of neural impulses via the sympathetic nervous system to the skin blood vessels, which results in their vasodilation, leading to a greater flow of blood just under the skin and a greater heat loss from the skin into the surrounding air. The sweating rate is caused to increase by sympathetic *stimulation* of sweat glands and the sweat evaporates. Thus, if there is a lesion in the anterior hypothalamus, hyperthermia may well result.

A region in the posterior hypothalamus serves to prevent hypothermia. In this case, neural impulses from cold cutaneous receptors and cool blood bathing the hypothalamus result in the transmission of impulses via the sympathetic nervous system to the skin, causing vasoconstriction which reduces heat loss. In addition, increased metabolism in muscles, and perhaps elsewhere, produces more heat, A lowered sweating rate and shivering are produced which act to increase body temperature. Clearly, then, damage in the posterior hypothalamus may result in hypothermia (i.e. a poikilothermic person who is unable to maintain a constant body temperature).

Temperature is associated with our metabolic rate, typically being higher when we are fully awake and active, and lower when we are asleep. Various studies have established that our temperature follows a 24 hour or diurnal cycle, as does our pulse rate. Our temperature is at its lowest some time during the early hours when we are asleep, and reaches its peak some time during the afternoon or early evening. While both muscular activity and food intake partially affect the 24 hour rhythm, this is probably determined by some biological 'clock' within the CNS. The location and mode of action of this clock are not yet known. It affects not only temperature regulation, but also many endocrine secretions.

Appetite and satiety

The importance of the hypothalamus in appetite and satiety has already been mentioned. Two hypothalamic areas, the ventromedial and the lateral hypothalamic areas, work as a 'stop' emotional mechanism and a 'go' motivational mechanism, respectively (Pribram, 1971). It has been found that the destruction of the ventromedial nucleus, close to the midline, results in hyperphagia. Therefore, it has been concluded that the main function of this site is to inhibit eating, and it has come to be referred to as the *satiety centre*. If an animal is electrically stimulated in this area while eating, the eating behaviour becomes inhibited. It might also be mentioned in passing that bilateral destruction of the ventromedial nucleus results in aggressive or even rage behaviour (*see* Chapter 14).

The lateral hypothalamic area has been referred to as the *feeding centre*, in that stimulation induces eating behaviour. Destruction of this site produces inhibition in eating behaviour, which may lead to starvation and death unless special feeding methods are instigated. Since changes in the degree of glucose utilization seem to correlate with the frequencies of unit discharges from satiety and feeding centre cells, it has been postulated that glucose-sensitive cells are active in the hypothalamus. When blood glucose level is low, impulses from the hypothalamus to the brain-stem result in responses associated with eating behaviour such as chewing, swallowing and stomach contractions. On the other hand, when the glucose level increases, electrical indications of increased activity are found in the satiety centre. More recent research by R.M. Gold has indicated that only when lesions extend beyond the ventromedial nucleus do they produce obesity. Gold has shown that excessive eating is produced by electrical or chemical stimulation, blockage or damage to the ventral ascending non-adrenergic bundle or its terminals*.

The reader should not conclude from the above discussion that only organic factors are implicated in disorders of food intake. It is clear that psychological factors are also important in such conditions as obesity. Two other disorders involving appetite will now be briefly discussed: first, anorexia nervosa and, secondly, the rare Kleine–Levin syndrome.

The symptoms of *anorexia nervosa* include primary or secondary amenorrhoea, loss of appetite and weight loss, which cannot be attributed to any physical or psychiatric disorder. Anorexia nervosa is primarily an adolescent problem, mostly restricted to females, and results in mortality in about 10 per cent of those afflicted. A.H. Crisp has reported its incidence as 1 in 150 girls between 10 and 18 years of age. It would seem to have psychological aetiology and to involve faulty perceptual functioning. Therefore, cognitive aspects are quite important. Successful treatment may involve both behavioural and psychotherapeutic methods.

The so-called *Kleine–Levin syndrome* is most frequently found in adolescent males, and is frequently attributed to hypothalamic dysfunction, in that it involves sleep, appetitive and sexual symptomatology. The two major symptoms include chronic attacks of hypersomnia, during which the patient spends long periods (even days) asleep, and periods of megaphagia (extreme hunger). There may also be evidence of hypersexuality. The afflicted person may spend most of his time either eating or sleeping. During an attack there may be cognitive confusion, heightened motor activity, irritability and hypersexuality. Between attacks the patient is

---

*Since this chapter was written, we have noted the work of Margules, which implicates an opioid receptor in these mechanisms.

physically and psychologically normal. Not only is the patient normal between attacks, but also the progress is good, remission of the disorder occurring after a few years.

Chapter 8

Neuroendocrinology

In this chapter two areas are going to be considered. First is the detailed manners in which the CNS is involved in controlling the secretion of hormones by the endocrine glands, and second is the way in which many hormones affect the function of brain cells and thus behaviour. In this latter area it is important to remember that hormones, reaching nerve cells via their blood supply, may enter the cells and affect nuclear mechanisms and so enzyme synthesis, etc. This is the mode of operation of steroid hormones. Polypeptide hormones, however, act as do some transmitters, on nucleotide cyclase activity or on the Ca^{2+} mechanism of enzyme activation. These actions may 'modulate' the target neurons' response to the transmitters released at synaptic terminals, enhancing or diminishing such responses. In these mechanisms, then, such hormones will be acting in a manner analogous to those transmitters also thought to act through the nucleotide cyclase or Ca^{2+} mechanisms, although the effects of the blood-borne hormone will be very much more prolonged than those of the neurotransmitter.

Substances recognized as hormones in the body may affect CNS function in various ways. Thus, a substance may simultaneously be a hormone in, for example, the gut, and also a neurotransmitter. A hormone, by regulating some metabolic function, may incidentally affect behaviour simply as a side-effect of its regulatory role, and disturbances in behaviour will accompany the metabolic disturbances that result when its secretion rate is altered. Finally, some neurons may be among the specific target cells of hormones, and thus behaviour as well as specific physiological processes in other organs may be affected by the hormone.

Most of the experimental studies on the way hormones may affect behaviour have been performed on laboratory rodents. One must beware the too-liberal extrapolation of these to the human species, in which the determination of behaviour is so much more complex. However, many endocrine disturbances affect behaviour, each in its characteristic manner and it may sometimes be possible to link the change in behaviour to a change in metabolic activity. In other instances psychological disturbance may produce hormonal changes and these then may feed back upon the CNS and produce further mental changes. Finally, profound changes in behaviour, particularly in sexual orientation, may occur in man without any evidence of any endocrine abnormality at all. We are not going to attempt in this chapter to give a complete survey of all the neuroendocrinological interconnections, but, as above, to indicate some of the principles of the subject and our present understanding of some of its growing points.

The hypothalamus and endocrine glands

The hypothalamus is intimately concerned with the functions of both the anterior and posterior lobes of the pituitary gland and, through the anterior pituitary, those of the adrenal cortex, the thyroid gland and the gonads. The posterior pituitary gland produces two hormones, antidiuretic hormone (ADH) and oxytocin. Each is an octopeptide and the two differ in only one constituent amino acid. They are secreted by axon terminals in the posterior pituitary gland, the cells of origin of which are in the supraoptic and paraventricular nuclei of the hypothalamus. It is these cells which form the secretions (ADH in supraoptic nucleus, oxytocin in paraventricular nucleus), which then pass down the axons to the terminals. Both hormones are only released from the terminals when, in response to the appropriate receptor stimulation, nerve impulses pass down the axons. Osmoreceptors exist within the supraoptic nucleus which are stimulated by a rise in solute concentration of the blood. The resultant secretion of ADH results in water retention by the kidneys and consequent dilution of blood solutes. These supraoptic nucleus cells are also thought to be inhibited by a stimulation of the volume receptors in the great veins and atria of the heart, so a rise in circulating blood volume would cause an increase in water excretion by the kidneys. Although ADH has this very precise action on body water and solute concentration, it has also recently been suggested that it has an equally specific action on the incorporation of new material into the memory store. This action, unlike the antidiuretic and vasopressor actions, survives removal of the glycinamide residue from the natural molecule, thus supporting the suggestion that this effect on memory retention is a specific one on the relevant part of the CNS. The reflex mechanism of oxytocin release is thought to begin in the stimulation of cutaneous receptors around the nipple caused by an infant's suckling, since one important action of this hormone is the contraction of the myoepithelial cells of the ducts of the lactating breast.

Six hormones are produced by the two types of secretory cells of the anterior pituitary gland. They are: follicle-stimulating hormone (FSH), luteinizing hormone (LH), prolactin, thyroid-stimulating hormone (TSH), adrenocorticotrophic hormone (ACTH) and growth hormone. Production of each of these is stimulated by a specific 'releasing factor' and of two production is stopped by a 'release-inhibiting factor'. These factors are produced by hypothalamic neurons and are released into blood vessels in the median eminence, whence they pass in the pituitary portal vein, down the pituitary stalk and into the sinusoids bathing anterior pituitary cells (*Figure 8.1*). Release of the factors from their axon terminals is dependent upon nerve impulses passing down the axons from the cell bodies, exactly as in the case of release of posterior pituitary hormones. The hypothalamic cells that produce these factors are themselves sensitive to the blood concentrations of the products of target hormones. Thus, the neurons that produce TSH releasing factor (TSH-RF) are inhibited by an elevated blood thyroxine level and stimulated when the level of this hormone is low, which forms an example of negative feedback control. Similar actions exist for controlling activity in the adrenal cortex and the testis. The cyclical activity of the ovaries is determined by a more complex system of both positive and negative feedback control.

The chemical identity of some of these factors is known in some cases. TSH-RF is a tripeptide, LH-RF is a peptide containing 10 amino acids, while somatostatin or growth hormone release-inhibiting factor contains 14 amino acids with a disulphide bridge between cysteine molecules at the third and fourteenth positions. LH

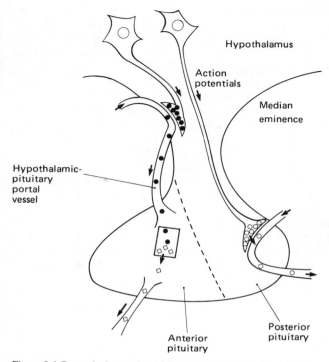

Figure 8.1 Control of secretion of the pituitary gland. The posterior lobe (neurolypoplysis) secretes directly from nerve terminals into blood vessels (○). Axon terminals of hypothalamic neurons secrete releasing (or release inhibiting) factors (●) into blood vessels which carry these to anterior lobe cells which then release their hormones (□) into the blood

release-inhibiting factor turns out to be dopamine. All these have been found in other sites than in the hypothalamic neurons that release them into the pituitary portal blood supply and they have been shown to affect neuronal activity when artificially applied, but only TSH-RF and dopamine have been shown to be released by nerve impulses, and even this release does not mimic synaptic activity, in terms of postsynaptic membrane ionic conductance or potential changes. However, some animal studies with LH-RF shows that, when applied to the right part of the hypothalamus of an ovariectomized, oestrogen-primed female, this substance can induce mating behaviour patterns. Similarly, somatostatin, when injected into cerebral ventricles in animals, causes decreased motor activity, loss of slow wave and REM sleep and raised appetite. The hypothalamic neurons producing these pituitary regulating factors are themselves the targets of other activity in the CNS and may be synaptically excited or inhibited. For instance, 'stress', presumably operating through the limbic system on the hypothalamus, can interfere with the homeostatic mechanism. Thus, a person having to make up his mind that his present working conditions are intolerable and that he must resign his job and seek a new post showed an increasing blood level of glucocorticoids until he gave in his notice, when the level promptly returned to normal. The disturbing factors that alter thyroid gland activity are not known. In fact, one could regard thyroxine as a hormone in search of a role. Although variations in thyroid secretions affect metabolic rates of all cells, there has never been more than a faint suggestion that general levels of metabolism (which might be of importance in the regulation of body temperature or of body fat-store size) are regulated through the thyroid hormones. Alterations of thyroxine levels produce their characteristic mental changes, the hyperthyroid person being almost always overactive, irritable, easily distractable and labile in mood. The thyroid-deficient adult shows lack of initiative and spontaneity, cannot concentrate, and becomes indifferent and apathetic to his state. Extreme passivity and mental retardation are important and, if untreated, irreversible effects of congenital hypothyroidism. Through what metabolic mechanism all these changes are produced is not known.

The hypothalamic neurons whose axon terminals liberate the releasing or release-inhibiting factors are, as suggested above, themselves subject to excitatory and inhibitory influences. Some will arrive in their blood supply, while others will be neurotransmitters released at synaptic terminals impinging on these neurons.

The effects of target gland hormones on some of the releasing-factor cells has already been described, as has the role of dopamine as LH release-inhibiting factor. Work on the roles of neurotransmitters is proceeding and conflicting statements appear in current literature. *Table 8.1* perhaps best summarizes the present state of

TABLE 8.1

Neurotransmitter \ Hormone	GH	Prolactin	ACTH	TSH	FSH	LH
5-HT	+	+	+	+	+	+
Dopamine	+ or −	−		−	−	−
Acetylcholine			+			
Catechol α receptor	+		+			
Catechol β receptor	−					

knowledge (1980). The effects on pituitary hormones themselves are shown, but it must be presumed that these are mediated via the hypothalamic release or release-inhibiting factors. Gaps in the table indicate actions that have not yet been sought for or demonstrated. However, it is clear that activity in other cerebral regions (for instance, limbic and other cortical sites), as well as in the other hypothalamic sites, may, through the actions indicated, have an effect on the control of the pituitary gland by the hypothalamus. Thus, 'mental stress', acting through either 5-HT, acetylcholine or noradrenergic alpha receptors, can stimulate ACTH production. It is further to be expected that any disturbance of normal cerebral function that may become manifest as a 'mental illness' may also affect endocrine secretions. Treatments that are aimed at modifying the actions of neuotransmitters and primary disturbances of transmitter function will be certain to have similar effects.

Endocrine disorder and psychological disturbance

Endocrine diseases have a wide range of effects on mental state which are often non-specific. In other words, according to many secondary interactions, hormonal upset may give any one of several patterns of disturbance in psychological functioning. The observed changes may mimic or induce organic states (acute or chronic brain syndrome), mood (depression, euphoria, anxiety), neurotic symptoms (instability, immature behaviour, unpredictable behaviour, etc.), cognitive abnormality (loss of concentration and interest, inefficient thinking, the acute or chronic brain syndromes mentioned above) and vegetative changes (libido, appetite, sleep, energy, etc.). The type of factor in the individual determining which kind of dysfunction he or she manifests depends on factors such as social isolation or support, perceptual impairments (deafness, loss of sight), interpersonal. The following is a brief and incomplete summary of some of the interfaces between psychiatric conditions and the endocrines. This is an important and expanding area, and the reader is advised to undertake further reading.

Stress and arousal

During stressful situations one effect is on the hypothalamic–pituitary–adrenal axis which liberates cortisol under these conditions. The 'cortisol response' varies in magnitude between individuals but is fairly constant for each person. Novel or threatening circumstances are effective stimuli. Acute stress, as in examinations, can produce surprisingly high levels in some individuals.

Psychologically arousing conditions, pleasant or unpleasant, lead to the liberation of catecholamines, the amounts produced again being characteristic of the person and more or less proportional to the level of arousal produced.

The chapter on anxiety deals in part with this area.

Psychiatric illness associated with hormonal dysfunction

Two examples of the hormonal disruption accompanying psychiatric illness have been chosen—affective illness and anorexia nervosa.

In depressive affective illness cortisol is secreted not only in more frequent larger bursts, but also throughout the day without the normal diurnal variation. In normal individuals the secretion of cortisol is partly inhibited by dexamethasone, a synthetic steroid given in small doses of 1–2 mg at 2300–2400 hours. From 40 to 67 per cent of depressives of endogenous type do not suppress to dexamethasone, and return to normal responses on recovering only if they are not going to suffer an early relapse.

Thyroid-stimulating hormone is liberated by thyrotrophin-releasing hormone, but in about a third of depressed patients (? unipolar only) the response of TSH to TRH is blunted. What is more, it is accompanied by a paradoxical (abnormal) liberation of growth hormone.

GH responses to hypoglycaemia and production of luteinizing hormone are both reduced in postmenopausal women.

Depressives as a group produce normal amounts of prolactin but the diurnal pattern is disrupted.

Finally, bipolar patients may have a disturbance in their renin–aldosterone system. It is characterized by high renin activity, a blunted response of renin to posture and inappropriate rates of secretion of aldosterone.

These data indicate marked disruption in the hypothalamic–pituitary and other mechanisms in the body.

Anorexia nervosa is a puzzling condition in which there is weight loss, delusions of body size and pathological feelings about eating. The neuroendocrine abnormalities associated with it include reduction in gonadotrophin levels and in oestrogens in females and testosterone in males. In females the cycloid gonadotrophin pattern of the menstrual cycle is lost. The amounts of oestradiol present fall and there is a relative rise in the biologically less active compound oestrone. The normal response of GH to hypoglycaemia or to dopamine agonists is reduced, yet there is a normal response of GH to arginine infusion. TRH induces secretion of GH, a phenomenon not seen in normal subjects. Plasma cortisol is secreted in larger amounts than normal, sometimes with loss of diurnal variation as in depressives, but cortisol metabolism is also changed and has a short half-life in the body.

The endocrine diseases and the psychiatric syndromes they evoke

As mentioned above, the type of psychiatric syndrome produced by any one hormonal disease is dependent on host characteristics and the interaction of this with severity of the endocrine disturbance.

Thyroid gland

(1) The individual with hyperthyroidism is overactive, anxious and unstable. The usual misdiagnosis is that of an anxiety state, but some develop depressive affective disorder, paranoid state, hysterical symptoms, panic attacks and depersonalization. Acute brain syndrome occurs sometimes in thyrotoxic cases.
(2) Cretinism is mental subnormality resulting from failure of function of thyroid activity.
(3) Psychological abnormalities are almost the rule in hypothyroidism and are often the features which present and lead to the diagnosis. At the forefront is usually some degree of cognitive impairment—loss of interest, drive, concentration and initiative, together with deterioration in recent memory. Affective changes do occur but perhaps less often than in hyperthyroidism. As hypothyroidism becomes more severe, there is progressive apathy and indifference, and there may be clouding of consciousness, depressive and paranoid features and hallucinations. Ultimately the condition may progress to coma.

Parathyroidism

Hyperparathyroidism induces alterations in mood and both overactivity and underactivity of the parathyroid gland may produce organic syndromes.

Anterior pituitary

At least half of the patients with Cushing's disease have psychiatric symptoms and 15–20 per cent become psychotic. Symptoms vary between loss of energy, amenorrhoea and loss of libido, deterioration in memory, mood change (depression, anxiety and, particularly, hypomania), general emotional lability, auditory hallucinations and paranoid delusions. There may be periods of excitement or withdrawal, apathy and stupor. A wide range of psychiatric symptoms may accompany the treatment of patients with ACTH and glucocorticoids, but unlike Cushing's disease mania symptoms is one of the syndromes.

Addison's disease

The usual findings in Addison's disease are depression, anergia, apathy, loss of initiative, instability and decreased libido. Alternatively, there is a mild chronic brain syndrome, and in Addisonian crises, delusion and stupor.

Diabetes mellitus

Excluding the effects on consciousness of an excess of hypoglycaemic drugs and the delirium which results from uncontrolled diabetes, the main psychiatric problem is that of a tendency to affective disorders. Depression occurring in undiagnosed illness often clears with adequate treatment.

Hyperinsulinism

Insulinomas produce weakness, hunger, disturbance of consciousness and anxiety, leading on to coma in some patients. If severe enough or untreated, the individual may develop neurological damage, including chronic brain syndrome.

Premenstrual tension

Despite the claims of imbalance in female sex hormones, there seems to be more to this syndrome than that. It is accompanied to a varying extent by anger, depression, instability, drowsiness, swelling of breast and abdomen and sometimes peripherally. The symptoms can be severe but are accepted (or ignored by male doctors) because of their brevity.

Acromegaly

Patients with acromegaly rarely have severe psychiatric disturbances, perhaps some degree of memory disturbance, changes in libido and mild depression or elation. It is claimed that acromegalic individuals are passive in nature.

Panhypopituitrism

Even more than in Cushing's disease, panhypopituitrism is the source of much psychopathology. The great majority of patients show some abnormality such as loss of libido, excess need for warmth and rest, sluggishness, loss of initiative, depression or apathy and instability. The acute brain syndrome proceeding to coma is not infrequent.

Diabetes insipidus

The characteristic psychiatric accompaniments of diabetes insipidus are loss of energy and libido, lability of mood, apathy and instability.

An important effect of psychological activity on the hypothalamus and pituitary is seen in the descriptions of aggression and anxiety (*see* Chapters 13 and 14), in which, in particular, the roles of ACTH and of testosterone are described.

Sex and gender differentiation

One way in which endocrine secretions have been thought by some to impinge on personality is in those aspects which are sexually determined. In man, as well as in other mammals, many aspects of behaviour, which can be studied objectively, as well as the more subjective and introspective attributes of personality, are dimorphic, and separate along lines that conform with the dimorphic sexual structures and functions. It is becoming the practice to refer to the anatomical and physiological differences as sexual, and to use the adjectives 'male' and 'female' in referring to them. The behavioural and personality differences are described as 'genderal' and the adjectives 'masculine' and 'feminine' are used when referring to these. Since a large part of our sense of personal identity is related to matters of gender, and in so many ways our sense of gender and the behaviour appropriate to masculine and feminine persons determine our daily lives, it is essential to consider how the self-identity and the behaviour arose, and the extent to which they are determined by genetic and endocrine factors.

While much speculation surrounds this topic, various errors of endocrine function provide some objective evidence so far as the human species is concerned. One defect concerns the adrenal cortex gland. A stage in the production of glucocorticoid is defective and the gland produces large amounts of its immediate precursor, which is androgenic. A genetically female infant with this state, the adrenogenital syndrome, is born with partly male external genitalia and may be incorrectly assumed to be a boy. Synthetic progesterone-like hormones, prescribed to prevent spontaneous abortion, may have the same effect, for they have been given at the time, 6–12 weeks from conception, when the external genitalia begin to differentiate into the male and female types. In another condition there may be a complete or partial failure of tissues of a male fetus to respond to testicular androgens. At birth such an infant has the external genitalia of a female and will be reared as such. These wrongly assigned infants usually develop happily in the assigned gender, despite the discordance between genetic sex and assigned gender, the chromosome arrangement XX or XY having no effect on the personality.

The evidence concerning the role of the hormones in determining behaviour comes from animal experiments, and also from the observations of, among others, Dr John Money of the Johns Hopkins Hospital's gender identity clinic, and also from anthropologists' observations of different human cultures. However, many of these latter observations are negative ones, which shows that human behaviour may not be determined by the gonadal hormones.

In most mammals the adult male is potentially always ready to be aroused into sexual behaviour, but in the female arousal occurs periodically, and the times of arousal are linked to periodic activity in the ovaries. In fact, the whole mechanism, hypothalamus–pituitary–ovaries, is periodic in the female, regular cycles of ovulation and receptivity alternating with periods of sexual and reproductive quiescence. It has been found that such periodicity can be induced in males of some species by a brief exposure of the hypothalamus to oestrogens. In rats this is soon after birth, even though in female rats the periodicity does not appear for some months. Not only do the injected males develop rhythmic activity in their hypothalami, but also their whole behaviour pattern alters. They respond to other male rats as do normal females and indulge in specifically female activities such as nest-building. In these oestrogen-treated males, then, we have a switching over of both physiological function and behaviour to that appropriate to the females of the species.

There is as yet no evidence that the same can occur in man, except for the possibility that androgen-exposed female fetuses may later show behaviour at the 'tomboyish' end of the scale of feminine behaviour. What evidence there is can be interpreted in the opposite sense. Unlike the laboratory rat, a person can tell us what sex he is and what gender role he wishes to assume, and we can observe the degree to which his behaviour fits one or other of the masculine or feminine roles we have come to accept as belonging with the male or female sex. In a small number of people there is a partial or complete discordance between the bodily sex and the sense of gender identity and even the observed gender role adopted by a person. Such people have been labelled transvestite (where the gender identity sense and the adopted role is confused or mixed and in whom the presenting symptom is a compulsive and episodic desire to adopt the clothes and appearance of the other gender) and transsexual, where the sense of gender identity is completely discordant with the sex. Transsexuals occur among both men and women. On the genetic level there is usually no doubt but that their karyotypes are 46XX if their bodies are female or 46XY if male. Equally, their gonads are quite normal, producing the appropriate sex hormones and gametes. Many transsexual men have been fathers; and some transsexual women, mothers. Thus, no known genetic or hormonal cause produces their strong sense of an inappropriate gender identity, which frequently stems from early childhood, and the transsexual will talk of resenting being forced into a role which 'he' felt did not fit in with what 'he' thought 'himself' to be, but which was nevertheless the one appropriate for the person's anatomy and physiology. Left to themselves the transsexuals will adopt all aspects of social gender role that is appropriate to the sense of gender identity, and not to the objective facts of the anatomical and physiological sex. Thus, in these people at least, it is clear that gender is in no way determined by either the karyotype or the sex hormones.

Similar evidence comes from a study of different human societies. We know, from a study of our modern Western European and North American society, which attributes belong to men and which to women. That is, we have a clear idea of the gender dimorphism that goes with our sexual dimorphism, and this extends from superficial markers such as clothes or hair styles to emotional expressions such as weeping. But even our own society, if we look back to the eighteenth century, has changed considerably in its gender roles, and the period since the middle 1960s has seen the start of another change. Furthermore, a look at other human societies shows that they differentiate genders differently from ours. One New Guinea tribe, the Tchambuli, has an almost reversed pattern from the familiar western society, and others have virtually no differentiation at all, men and women both playing, on the social level, the same roles in respect to such important matters as crop and food production, the rearing of children and communal activity. The minimal allowance possible is made for the different reproductive roles of the males and females. These studies, like the individual ones on transsexual people, and those of cases of malassignment of sex at birth, serve to indicate that gender role and gender identity are not necessarily dependent upon either genetic or endocrine factors.

The development of these must, then, be due to environmental factors, to teaching, example, learning or mimicry of behaviour. The little boy knows he is one because he wears trousers or because his father takes him out to look at trains, while the little girl identifies her female anatomy with pretty dresses or helping mother in the house. In this most important area of personal identity, the endocrine glands have little part to play in either the normal or the unusual cases of discordant identity.

Some other hormonal/behavioural interactions

ACTH

Receptors to this hormone are present in CNS tissue as well as in the adrenal cortex. One study confirming the specificity of these receptors was performed on those in the periaqueductal grey matter. ACTH and β-endorphin are both naturally occurring ligands to the opiate receptors of this region, but the ACTH receptors are not stereospecific to opiates, nor are they naloxone-sensitive, but the β-endorphin receptors possess both properties. The two ligands have opposite effects both on the adenyl cyclase activity and on behaviour. In man the possible effects of ACTH cannot be separated from those of the glucocorticoids. Apathy results from their absence and hypomania is part of the Cushing's syndrome state. In rodents ACTH and glucocorticoids both decrease aggressive and increase submissive behaviour.

Sex steroids and pheromones

Hormones may be directly involved in pheromone production or, in animals, release behavioural/neurological activities that cause pheromone production. Pheromones are then involved in aggression, marking territory and sexual activity. Synchronicity of oestrus occurs in some colonies of females of a species and this may be due to pheromone production. About the only indication that pheromones have any role in human behaviour is certain accounts that all-female human communities may develop a synchronization in their menstrual cycle.

Melanocycle-stimulating hormone (MSH) and melatonin

The former is a polypeptide, found as part of the ACTH molecule. It is secreted from the pars intermedia of the pituitary. Melatonin comes from the pineal gland and is a tryptophan derivative, N-acetyl 5-methoxytryptamine. Both substances act on melanocytes, the black pigment cells of human skin. MSH causes pigment formation, and melatonin causes the retraction of pigment granules and thus a paling of skin where this property is present (but probably not in man). Melatonin production is stimulated when the sympathetic nerve supply to the pineal gland is reflexly stimulated by light entering the eyes. Both substances have effects on behaviour that are quite apart from their actions on pigment cells. Thus, MSH is required for the normal reflex responses to fear-producing situations. Melatonin is stated to induce sleep, but without affecting the normal ratio of REM sleep. In this it seems to be unique among hypnogogues. Its metabolism is affected, but in opposite ways, by chlorpromazine and by hallucinogens such as LSD. This has led to some speculation that melatonin may be involved in schizophrenia.

Chapter 9

Psychopharmacology

General points

With one or two notable exceptions, the compounds used in psychopharmacology have as their target organ the brain, and to reach the central nervous system they first have to gain entry to the blood stream. Possible means of administration of drugs are by oral, intramuscular, intravenous, subcutaneous, percutaneous, buccal or rectal routes, and the drugs used in psychiatry are largely confined to the first two routes. This means that psychopharmacological agents given orally have to pass across gastric and jejunal mucosa and intestinal capillaries, and, when drugs are given by intramuscular injection, across the walls of skeletal muscular capillaries.

There are several ways by which substances cross mucosal and capillary walls. Cell membranes consist of lipids interleaved between two monomolecular protein layers, and they can most easily be traversed by substances which dissolve in the lipid component. Most psychopharmacological agents have this property of high lipid solubility and therefore can easily pass across intestinal mucosa or capillary walls.

Routes of administration of drugs

Oral

Oral administration of drugs has the advantages of convenience, flexibility and comfort. It has the disadvantage of requiring repeated acts of will on the part of the patient, and is therefore subject to a whole range of uncertainties and vicissitudes, from the effects of the latest medical programme on the media to plain human forgetfulness.

Assuming that the patient takes the drug, whether there is food in the stomach will decide how quickly it passes on into the jejunum and to what extent gastric absorption will occur. Food reduces drug absorption by the gastric mucosa and delays movement on into the jejunum.

A further factor determines the pattern of intestinal absorption. Many drugs are either weak acids or weak bases. In solution they exist in both ionized and non-ionized forms, with an equilibrium between the two. Weak acids are ionized to

157

a greater extent in an alkaline medium and weak bases in an acid solution. Since the non-ionized form is the more lipid-soluble and therefore more easily absorbed when ionization is reduced to a minimum, absorption will be faster. Many psychotropic drugs are weak bases, so that it follows that a smaller proportion will be ionized in the jejunum and a larger proportion in the acid environment of the stomach. This means that absorption of psychotropic drugs tends to be slow from the stomach but rapid once they have passed on into the jejunum.

The way in which a drug is prepared will determine its ease of absorption. Those in aqueous solution are immediately available, but various ways have been used for delaying uptake to produce a smoother, more continuous pattern of absorption. Methods of slowing absorption include incorporating the drug in a fatty or waxy matrix which disintegrates slowly. Drugs have also been made up in substances which form a surface gel when put in an aqueous medium. The gel disperses slowly, after which the next layer of the matrix forms a gel, and so on, until the final part of the tablet disintegrates. The surface gel prevents rapid absorption and early disintegration of the tablet. These and other formulations which delay absorption are of particular use where a peak concentration due to rapid absorption can give rise to side-effects. In some cases, however, the use of slow-release preparations is of questionable benefit to the patient, and extravagant claims on their behalf should not be accepted uncritically.

A theoretical disadvantage of delayed-release oral preparations is the possibility of their traversing the gut before all the drug has been absorbed, and this can be a serious disadvantage, particularly if the degree of absorption is variable from day to day, depending on rate of gastrointestinal transit.

Intramuscular

The intramuscular route has some clear advantages. An injection given into a muscle is usually absorbed in 10–30 minutes, so this is of particular value when speed is of importance. It also makes it possible for the clinician to observe the effect of a known dose over a given time and, if used intelligently, can allow careful matching of doses to needs, and a shortening of the time needed to control distressing feelings or uncontrolled behaviour. It must be remembered, however, that absorption from a muscle will only be rapid and predictable if the whole dose is injected intramuscularly (and not partly subcutaneously in fat depots, etc.) and that muscle blood flow (and therefore rate of absorption) will be increased considerably by emotional arousal and by activity of the muscle.

It must not be assumed that a drug given intramuscularly *necessarily* reaches the brain in adequate levels faster than if given orally, unless this has been demonstrated.

Finally, there is a corpus of knowledge and experience concerned with the use of preparations which for several reasons gain only slow entrance to the systemic circulation from an intramuscular injection site and whose effects continue for weeks. The main use of these compounds has been in the depot neuroleptic compounds, principally for the maintenance treatment of schizophrenia.

Intravenous

The intravenous administration of drugs is a somewhat marginal activity in psychiatry—e.g. for rapid sedation. We are familiar with the rapidly acting anaesthetics and muscle relaxants used for electroconvulsive therapy, and a few centres use the intravenous route for a tricyclic drug (usually clomipramine). Perhaps the future will see an expansion of the use of this route with the advent of antidepressant and other drugs with a low incidence of toxic effects on the heart and with fewer autonomic problems.

Metabolism of drugs

Because of the high lipid-solubility of many psychotropic drugs, they are not readily excreted from the body in their unchanged form. They may pass out with the glomerular filtrate, but pass back across the tubular membrane with equal facility. To dispose of them needs some modification to their structure, which will render them less lipid-soluble (and often more water-soluble). This is largely carried out by the liver, and one of the main processes is by one particular enzyme system. This is in the microsomal fraction of hepatic cells which contain the cytochrome P450 enzyme system, which catalyses a whole series of oxidative mechanisms on many foreign substances, including the majority of psychotropic drugs. The activity of this process tends to be fairly constant in one subject from one time to another, and it has a range of up to a twofold difference between individuals. It is one of the factors determining the pattern of response and sensitivity to drugs in any one person.

The behaviour of this enzyme system is influenced by a number of extraneous circumstances. In the presence of two substances, each a substrate for the enzyme, the rate of metabolism of both will be reduced. This is because the two substrates compete for the available enzyme. The enzymic modification of both compounds is thus impeded, and their metabolism is reduced. Such an interference would be most obvious at the outset when two drugs are given together. This is the process of enzyme inhibition, but another mechanism, enzyme induction, may modify the pattern further.

A drug which is lipid-soluble and which is a substrate for the drug-metabolizing system may induce the production of more enzyme; this is a property which some compounds have to varying degrees and others do not. Thus, after days or weeks of administration of, for instance, orphenadrine, chlorpromazine, a barbiturate, etc., new enzyme will be produced in the liver, and the rate of destruction of the compound in question and of other substances using the same enzyme system will gradually rise. The extent to which this mechanism of enzyme induction can occur is not known. However, enzyme induction is most obvious in those with initially low levels of activity of the enzyme and it can lead to at least a doubling of activity. It takes several days to weeks to develop, and subsides over several days to a week after discontinuation of the drug. The phenomena of competition for enzyme and of enzyme induction are arguments either against polypharmacy or for an active awareness of how different drugs may modify their own metabolism and that of concurrently given substances. It is particularly difficult to allow for the fact that competition for enzyme (enzyme inhibition) and enzyme induction work in opposite ways and to different time schedules, and to differing extents with different drugs. The assessment of the combined and continuing effect of two drugs on each other at the onset of treatment, during treatment and also after withdrawal of one of them is a problem.

Perhaps it should be stressed at this point, however, that while these interactions are important, and we should be aware of them in clinical practice, the effect of the sum total of interindividual differences in the management of drugs by different people far outweighs them, and leads, for instance, to tenfold, twentyfold or even larger differences in plasma levels of drugs. To what extent these large differences in plasma levels mirror changes in the availability of the drug at their target sites is a task for future research. More also needs to be known about differences in individuals' responses to drugs, and about specific and non-specific induction of hepatic enzymes by food contaminants (e.g. insecticides), alcohol, nicotine, contraceptive steroids and many other extraneous substances.

After their metabolic modification in the liver, some drugs are conjugated and are excreted as relatively lipid-insoluble glycuronates, acetates or sulphates. In fact, many drugs are 'inactivated' and are then excreted in these forms.

Specific interactions between drugs and between drugs and foodstuffs, etc., are discussed below in the appropriate section on different types of psychotropic drugs.

'First pass' metabolism

Because of the efficiency of the liver in metabolizing drugs, there is what is known as a 'first pass' effect. By this is meant that drugs which are given orally, and thus have to pass through the liver to reach the systemic circulation, may be modified there before reaching the general circulation, so that, for instance with chlorpromazine, only a proportion of the parent compound reaches the brain in unaltered form. In some individuals this proportion (of unaltered drug) may be quite small, and instead of a preponderance of the parent compound, the brain is exposed to a spectrum of derivatives, some therapeutically active, some inactive, and each person may have a pattern of metabolites idiosyncratic to the individual. It is even thought that in some, perhaps rather exceptional, patients endowed with particularly active hepatic enzyme systems, it may be difficult to achieve adequate therapeutic levels of some drugs by the oral route, and the clinician may be puzzled by the failure of these patients to respond. (Of course, the most likely cause of lack of response is failure to take the drug.) The situation is enhanced for some substances (e.g. the phenothiazines) where there is an enterohepatic circulation when some of the drug is excreted by the liver in the bile, and is then reabsorbed and repeatedly exposed to the hepatic cells and their transformations.

This 'first pass' effect can be avoided by giving the drug parenterally, when it will be distributed more equally to the tissues, including the brain, and a much smaller proportion will be modified initially by the liver.

The existence of the 'first pass' effect accounts for the much greater activity of phenothiazines given parenterally, for the considerable efficacy of depot neuroleptics and for the 'escape' from control sometimes seen when disturbed patients are transferred from intramuscular to oral therapy at too low a level of oral dosage.

Protein binding

Some drugs circulate in the blood in part bound to plasma proteins, mostly albumin, and the moiety in association with the protein cannot cross the blood –brain barrier. This may result in one of two processes. If the transport, metabolism, etc., of the drug is rapid, the 'bound' fractions can be thought of as a reservoir; if the converse is true, the low levels of free drug may limit entry to tissues, especially the brain. It is mostly lipid-soluble compounds such as warfarin (90 per cent bound), or lipid-soluble organic bases which are bound (the latter to another site on the protein molecule). In general the drug–protein complexes dissociate rapidly.

Plasma proteins are not the only sites for association between protein and drugs, and any drug bound in plasma is likely also to be similarly in association with proteins in the interstitial spaces, in the cell membrane and even intracellularly. Highly lipid-soluble drugs may be sequestered in fat depots which can constitute up to 50 per cent of the body mass in fat individuals.

The importance of binding is that with a highly bound drug such as chlorpromazine (90 per cent) or phenytoin (70–95 per cent) toxicity may result from displacement from new protein–drug complexes by other drugs, leading to much higher 'free' concentrations.

Of the drugs stored in fat depots, two examples are disulfiram and thiopentone, 70 per cent of the latter being in fatty tissues within 3 hours of its administration.

Drug interaction

Drugs may interact with one another in synergism or antagonism, or they may produce unusual interactions with other substances in the body or in the diet.

Within the gut itself, drug interactions are quite unusual. One of the noteworthy exceptions are antacids and chlorpromazine. Antacids can absorb chlorpromazine so that less of the phenothiazine is available for absorption. A number of psychopharmacological agents have anticholinergic properties which are perhaps theoretically advantageous in that gut motility is reduced so that more complete absorption might occur. In practice, absorption of psychotherapeutic agents tends to be rapid in any event, so this is unlikely to be of importance. What could be of greater significance is where two or more drugs with anticholinergic effects act together to slow the gut down to a dangerous extent, to the point of causing severe constipation or even paralytic ileus in some patients.

Inside the body two important aspects of drug interaction in the form of competition for enzyme and enzyme induction have already been discussed above, and it should be stressed again that the algebraic sum of the two actions would be difficult to predict in any one individual.

Monoamine oxidase inhibitors probably act in the body to modulate the level of amines in the brain. They also have a protective function in the gut mucosa and liver preventing sympathomimetic compounds in food from gaining access to the circulation. Monoamine oxidase inhibitors remove this protection so that tyramine and probably other sympathomimetic substances enter the circulation to give serious rises in blood pressure. Directly acting sympathomimetic substances such as noradrenaline are relatively safe, probably because catecholamines have the enzyme catecholamine o-methyl transferase, which deals with circulating amines. It is the indirectly acting compounds that enter aminergic cells and release amines which have most potential danger. Indirectly acting sympathomimetic drugs and naturally occurring compounds in food, particularly in fermented or badly stored protein foods, are equally risky.

Monoamine oxidase inhibitors have what are probably non-specific effects on a variety of enzyme systems. They may interfere with the metabolism of pethidine and barbiturates in some individuals. It seems that they block other enzymes as well as the monoamine oxidases.

There may be an as yet imperfectly understood interaction between MAOI drugs and anti-Parkinsonian compounds.

Tricyclic antidepressants block the presynaptic re-uptake mechanism for amines. Among other things, this re-uptake mechanism is the means by which aminergic transmission in the synapse is terminated so that the effect of exogenous noradrenaline or adrenaline (e.g. in a local anaesthetic) will be increased.

The presynaptic amine re-uptake site for noradrenaline and adrenaline is the entry point for some antihypertensive drugs (e.g. guanethidine) and also for indirectly acting sympathomimetic compounds. Both of these types of compound will be inactivated or partly antagonized by tricyclic drugs.

Neuroleptic drugs

One of the major advances in psychiatry has been the introduction of neuroleptic drugs, otherwise known as ataractics or major tranquillizers. The centre of the stage has been held by the phenothiazines (*see Figure 9.1*) and in particular by chlorpromazine, which can be taken as a 'specimen case'. Their most striking properties have been seen in the treatment of psychotic and excited states and in the way they modify behaviour in animals. Their therapeutic actions of quietening without sedation and their antipsychotic activity have important applications in psychiatric illness.

Bernthsen synthesized the phenothiazines in 1883 but it was not until the 1940s that they came to be used in medicine, first as putative antihelminthics and then for their antihistaminic properties. Laborit, a French surgeon, tried promazine in an attempt to enhance the actions of anaesthetic agents. In the search for more powerful drugs, Charpentier synthesized a group of new phenothiazine compounds, one of which, chlorpromazine, Laborit suggested, could be used in psychiatry. This advice was followed rapidly by reports from Sigwald and Bouttier in 1951 and Delay and Deniker in 1952 of the antipsychotic effect of chlorpromazine and its benefit in excited states.

It soon became apparent that phenothiazines and, for that matter, other antipsychotic drugs had a wide range of activities on many central and peripheral systems, a property which incidentally earned chlorpromazine the trade name of 'Largactil'. This ability to interfere with and modify the function of many physiological and biochemical processes leads to a present confusion. Here are drugs which, among other things, are likely to modulate the activity of every monoaminergic synapse in the brain and whose action includes modification of the function of the brain-stem reticular function. These observations must be assessed with parallel observations on the profound changes in complex behaviour and function, as seen in animals and man (including the remarkable antipsychotic properties of these drugs). Immediately a gap becomes apparent between knowledge of the activities of these drugs at molecular and cellular levels, and what occurs in the whole animal or human. This difficulty in correlating specific local effects with generalized responses, including those involving higher integrated function and behaviour, makes for confusion in the description of the actions of neuroleptic drugs. There is a plethora of knowledge but as yet it is not possible to systematize the findings adequately.

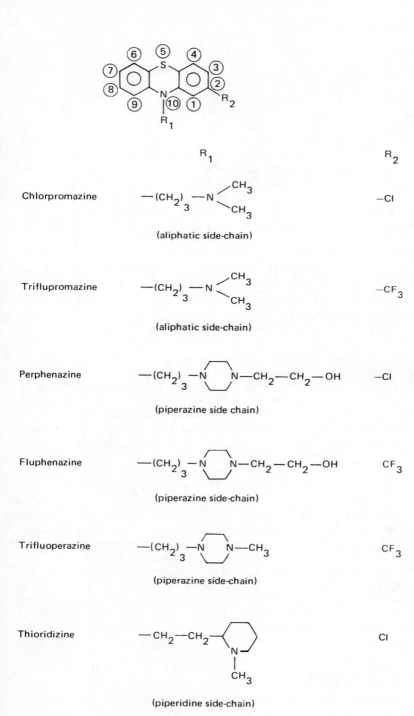

Figure 9.1 The parent phenothiazine structure and six compounds

The neuroleptic syndrome

With the introduction of the major tranquillizers came early descriptions of their global effects on patients. Shortly after taking these drugs patients tended to feel sleepy, but this passed off after a few days, so that there was little or no impairment of consciousness at the usual doses used. In the established 'neuroleptic syndrome' the patients had little spontaneous speech, showed little initiative and did not express demands, preoccupations or preferences. The effects of external stimuli were damped down, so that it was necessary to repeat questions, to which they replied with apparent indifference after a short delay. Topics which would be expected to evoke enthusiasm or pleasure had little effect, and they appeared immersed in a pleasant indifference, separated from the environment by an invisible curtain. These observations went hand in hand with similar observations on the drugs' remarkable effects on disturbed states, particularly in mania and schizophrenia.

As stated above, as yet the following account of the pharmacology of phenothiazines cannot claim to provide a full explanation of their therapeutic or other actions.

Pharmacology of chlorpromazine

PERIPHERAL

Chlorpromazine has a powerful peripheral antiadrenaline activity in the form of alpha-adrenergic blockade. This property is partly responsible for its effect in lowering blood pressure, including postural hypotension, and in causing failure of ejaculation. Its effect on the blood pressure is only partly peripheral and its overall action on the cardiovascular system is discussed below. Chlorpromazine is also a peripheral 5-HT blocking agent and is weakly antihistaminic and weakly anticholinergic. Although it has never been used as such, chlorpromazine is a powerful local anaesthetic.

CENTRAL

Chlorpromazine acts in the brain, tending to block transmission across noradrenergic, dopaminergic and serotoninergic synapses. From this property alone its effects would be considerable, because the ascending aminergic systems are distributed widely to many brain structures (see Figures 4.17, 4.20 and 4.21).

Phenothiazines vary in the strength of their anticholinergic activity, from the weak (chlorpromazine) to others (e.g. Thioridazine) where this property is well developed. Excluding aminergic pathways, the degree to which anticholinergic activity, or activities at synapses with other characteristics, enters in the overall effect of phenothiazines on the brain is not known. Some authorities attribute the main effects of phenothiazines to their aminergic blocking properties.

DOPAMINERGIC SYNAPSES

The effect of phenothiazines and other antipsychotic drugs on dopaminergic synapses have been a focus of considerable interest for two reasons.

First, these drugs are most powerful blockers of catecholaminergic synapses, and this action on dopaminergic neurons in the basal nuclei is responsible for the well-known extrapyramidal side-effects attributed to postsynaptic blockade of the dopaminergic receptor. This blockade of dopaminergic receptors allows unbalanced activity of the opposing cholinergic mechanism in the basal nuclei and the development of extrapyramidal symptoms. The relative freedom of some neuroleptics from extrapyramidal side-effects has been explained by their high anticholinergic activity. This limits the otherwise unbalanced cholinergic activity and prevents Parkinsonian side-effects.

The second and perhaps more important area of interest in the effects of neuroleptics on dopaminergic systems comes from the school of thought which equates this action with the antipsychotic action of these drugs (*see also* section on haloperidol, page 172). It is suggested by the proponents of this hypothesis that dopaminergic blockade is the means by which neuroleptics exert their antipsychotic effect (but *see* later discussion).

That neuroleptics are useful drugs for the treatment of schizophrenia and excited states is now well established, and it was noticed that most of the effective drugs of this type also produced Parkinsonian side-effects, presumably, as stated above, by blocking dopamine receptors in the basal nuclei. It has been found, for instance, that *in vitro* measures of blockade of dopaminergic receptors closely paralleled the empirically found and well-established chemical dosages of these drugs, and there is the tantalizing way in which the molecular conformations of chlorpromazine and dopamine can be superimposed (*Figure 16.5*).

The importance of dopaminergic blockade was studied further using flupenthixol. This is in two isomeric forms, one of which acts on dopaminergic receptors and one of which does not. The 'normal' drug, as marketed, consists of a mixture of the two. When the isomers were given separately to schizophrenics, the one lacking the ability to blockade dopaminergic receptors was no more active than placebo in suppressing symptoms. The active, dopamine receptor blocking compound was significantly better than both its 'twin' and placebo. These two isomers shared many other pharmacological activities, and since it was argued that other properties were unlikely to be involved, it was suggested that this experiment may demonstrate the importance of blockade of dopaminergic transmission in the antipsychotic activity.

The site of this was unlikely to be the basal nuclei, because the antipsychotic properties of drugs did not parallel their ability to evoke Parkinsonian side-effects. Another site has been proposed, the dopaminergic mesolimbic system (*Figure 4.19*), within which antipsychotic drugs may be acting. This does not necessarily imply that the functional disorder underlying psychotic symptoms is within this system. It may be that antipsychotic drugs in schizophrenia could be reducing mesolimbic dopaminergic activity to balance loss of activity in an as yet unknown opposing system.

Dopaminergic synaptic blockade is also responsible for the effect on prolactin and luteinizing hormone. A dopaminergic pathway, the tuberoinfundibulum tract, normally inhibits the release of prolactin, and when this pathway is blocked by phenothiazines, prolactin is released. This is one of the effects of phenothiazines in the endocrine system.

In the brain-stem medulla is a 'chemoreceptor trigger zone' which is connected to the vomiting centre in the dorsal part of the lateral reticular formation. The chemoreceptor centre contains dopaminergic receptors stimulated by apomorphine, and this effect of apomorphine is antagonized by chlorpromazine, a property which seems to be common to the neuroleptic drugs. A 'useful' antiemetic property in man (e.g. Thioridazine) is not implied.

TEMPERATURE CONTROL

Control of temperature is a complex and imperfectly understood process which involves at least cholinergic, serotoninergic and noradrenergic neurons, and which depends largely on posterior hypothalamic and anterior hypothalamic/preoptic centres. Chlorpromazine can lower a raised temperature, and also can lead to hypothermia in temperate environments. In general, it impairs temperature regulation, so that under particularly unfavourable conditions control of temperature can be lost, causing either hypothermia or hyperpyrexia.

RETICULAR FORMATION

The reticular formation is a poorly defined network of fibres containing more than 50 nuclear masses distributed throughout the tegmentum of the brain-stem, which has important ascending and descending projections. Destruction of parts of the reticular formation in the midbrain leads to profound somnolence, and stimulation of this region in intact animals leads to EEG desynchronization and behavioural alerting. The reticular formation receives collaterals from the main sensory pathways which maintain the thalamocortical pathways responsible for wakefulness via ascending projections.

It is possible to monitor conduction of impulses in the reticular formation while observing EEG or behavioural arousal, and to assess the effects of input via a sensory pathway. It was found that barbiturates and phenothiazines had quite different effects on this system.

Barbiturates blocked behavioural and cortical arousal by a direct depressant action on the reticular formation itself, since it could be shown that they reduced conduction of an evoked impulse within this system. By contrast, chlorpromazine gave only a negligible increase in the arousal threshold to direct stimulation of the reticular formation, but instead blocked responsiveness to incoming sensory stimuli. Thus, chlorpromazine selectively reduced the influence of afferent stimuli entering the reticular formation via collaterals from the sensory pathways which would have had an alerting effect. There have been other explanations for this effect. It has been suggested that reticular formation activity was increased by chlorpromazine, but that this stimulated a 'gating' effect, the blocking of a proportion of the impulses passing through the reticular formation. In this latter suggested explanation the input to the reticular formation may be increased but the drug enhances a filtering mechanism in the region which reduces the 'throughflow' of inessential information. In man, moderate doses leave intellectual functioning intact, but vigilance and distance attention are reduced, possibly as a result of the effect of chlorpromazine on the reticular formation.

MOTOR ACTIVITY

Chlorpromazine decreases muscle tone, in part possibly by modification of brain-stem or basal ganglion control mechanism, and in part by decreasing activity of the alpha efferent system. There is no neuromuscular blockade.

THE CARDIOVASCULAR SYSTEM

Chlorpromazine has a complex effect on the cardiovascular system. Peripherally, its antagonism of adrenergic receptors results in loss of vasomotor tone and a tendency for blood pressure to fall. Centrally, chlorpromazine depresses the vasomotor control mechanisms in hypothalamic and bulbospinal regions of the brain, and this contributes to the tendency of chlorpromazine to lower blood pressure and produce postural hypotension.

REDUCTION OF SHAM RAGE

Some but not all animal species respond with 'sham rage' if transected above the thalamus. By this is meant that quite trivial stimuli provoke signs of aggression; in the cat spitting, piloerection and clawing. When this reaction is found, it appears to be dependent not on the severed connections to the neocortex, but on interruption of pathways from the limbic cortex and the amygdala. Chlorpromazine blocks the 'sham rage' reaction.

GENERAL EFFECTS

Effects on animal behaviour

Once again we must remind ourselves that we are examining drugs with widespread effects in the nervous system. In general, animals given chlorpromazine have reduced motor activity, respond less than normally to external stimuli and have little interest in their environment. Motor power and co-ordination are unchanged and there is no tendency to sleep excessively. Cats show increased sociability and reduced hostility, and similarly in a number of species which ordinarily would be aggressive or defensive, the drug has a 'taming' effect. This is one of the more remarkable and interesting properties of neuroleptics.

Learning

Animals can be trained to make a conditioned response in the presence of a stimulus (e.g. a warning noise) to avoid an unpleasant experience, such as an electric shock. If the animal fails to take the necessary avoiding action and receives the unpleasant stimulus, it may jump or flinch. This is the unconditioned response. The effects of various drugs on the type of behaviour has been studied. Barbiturates, for instance, depress both the conditioned avoidance and also the unconditioned response. In moderate dosage, chlorpromazine has no effect on the unconditioned response, but the conditioned behaviour is impaired, so that the animal fails to take avoiding action and therefore receives more shocks.

In the 'training' of conditioned reflexes, chlorpromazine tends to delay acquisition, but when given to animals with established conditioned reflexes, it does not delay extinction.

Another type of circumstance has been used to study the effect of chlorpromazine in complex behaviour in animals—that of conflicting drive conditions or 'experimental neuroses'. Here a 'normal behaviour'—e.g. catching mice by cats; going to a source of food in rats, etc.—is coupled with 'punishment', say in the form of an electric shock. The normal reaction to this is a reduction in the frequency of the activity in question; when given chlorpromazine, the cat will continue to pounce or the rat will persist in eating in the presence of a noxious stimulus. It is as though the animal ignores the warning of impending punishment, while at the same time, at smallish doses, it is still able to make the unconditioned response—e.g. escaping once the 'punishment' has been given.

Obviously the presence of these types of effect by chlorpromazine and other neuroleptics on conditioned avoidance responses and 'experimental neuroses' is a basis for hypotheses about their mode of action in psychiatric disorders.

STRUCTURE–ACTIVITY RELATIONSHIPS

Figure 9.1 shows the parent phenothiazine structure with the sites at positions 2 and 10 at which substitutions have been made in modified phenothiazine molecules. Basically the molecule consists of two benzene rings joined by sulphur and nitrogen bridges to make a three-ring structure. Some of the substitutions and the resultant molecules are listed in *Table 9.1*. Closely related are thioxanthene neuroleptics (*Figure 9.2*).

TABLE 9.1. Chlorpromazine: additional properties, side-effects and toxic effects

Autonomic	Postural hypotension	dry mouth
		difficulty in accommodation
		blurred vision
		constipation
	Anticholinergic side-effects	tachycardia (reflex from BP and atropine-like actions)
		retention of urine
		paralytic ileus
Cardiac	Direct depressant action on heart muscle	
	EEG: flat T waves, lengthened QT interval	
	Arrhythmias	
	Cardiac arrest	
CNS/muscles	Drowsiness—transient early effect	
	Parkinsonian: sometimes dyskenesias irreversible	
	Seizures in epileptic subjects; in normals limbic epileptic activity at high doses	
	Poikilothermia; hyperpyrexia; hypothermia	
	Toxic confusional state	
	Muscle weakness (early Parkinsonism?)	
	Unmasking myasthenia gravis; worsening myaesthenia gravis	
Liver	Choleostatic jaundice	
Bone marrow	Eosinophilia	
	Agranulocytosis, thrombocytopenia, pancytopenia (three serious toxic effects)	
Eyes	Pigmentary retinopathy (thioridazine above 600 mg/day)	
	Pigmentation lens and cornea	
Skin	Photosensitivity with deposit of pigment in skin, cornea, lens	
	Urticaria	
	Maculopapular or petechial rashes	
	Contact dermatitis (nursing staff)	
	Oedema	
Endocrine	Galactorrhoea	
	Menstruation: irregular, scanty, absent	
	May block ovulation	via prolactin
	Loss of libido	
	Impotence	
	? Decreases growth hormone	
	Peripheral oedema: perhaps secondary to inhibition of ADH	
	Reduction in production of ACTH	
Metabolic	Gain in weight	
	Increase in cholesterol in plasma	
Shock	Chlorpromazine protects in part against traumatic and haemorrhage shock	
Tolerance	Is non-addictive	
	Abrupt discontinuation may or may not lead to exacerbation psychosis, muscle discomfort, difficulty in sleeping	

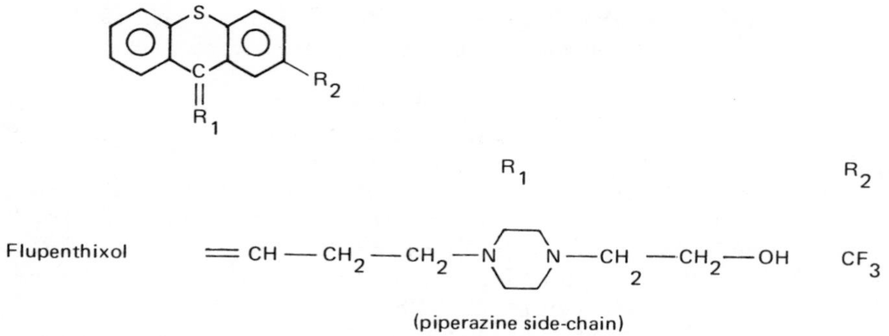

Flupenthixol R_1: $= CH - CH_2 - CH_2 - N$ (piperazine) $N - CH_2 - CH_2 - OH$ R_2: CF_3

(piperazine side-chain)

Figure 9.2 The thioxanthine structure and one derivative

One variant on the phenothiazines theme has a two-carbon chain between the nitrogen at the 10 position and the terminal nitrogen, and some antihistamine and sedative drugs (e.g. promethazine) are of this type. In general, it is the molecules with three carbon atoms between the two nitrogen atoms from the 10 position which have been most useful in psychiatry.

Taking the parent component promazine, substituting a Cl atom on position 2 (chlorpromazine) gives enhanced depression of motor activity and greater effect on conditioned avoidance in animals coupled with a more powerful antipsychotic action. Replacing the Cl atom with CF_3 (trifluopromazine) further improves the antipsychotic properties and heightens the antiemetic action but increases the likelihood of inducing extrapyramidal side-effects. The three-carbon chain between the nitrogen atoms from position 10 is associated with peripheral adrenergic blockade activity. The three main types of side-chain at position 10 are the aliphatic (as in chlorpromazine), piperidine and the piperazine.

Piperazine and piperidine side-chains have greater antipsychotic and antiemetic actions and a greater tendency to Parkinsonian side-effects than have the aliphatic groups and, in particular, the piperazine compounds contain some of the most powerful antipsychotic drugs.

Finally, substitution of carbon for nitrogen at position 10 gives thioxanthine compounds. For instance, the thioxanthine analogue of chlorpromazine has high antiemetic and anti-Parkinsonian activity and is less sedative.

ABSORPTION, METABOLISM AND EXCRETION

Chlorpromazine is rapidly absorbed from the gut and following intramuscular injection. An oral dose gives peak concentrations in plasma in anything from ½ to 3 hours, depending on food intake, which has a very variable effect. Some antacids delay absorption, probably owing to binding of the drug to the gel formed by these preparations. Anticholinergic drugs can both delay absorption and decrease the amount of drug reaching the circulation; there is an intestinal microsomal oxidase which with gastrointestinal slowing has longer to act to initiate degradation of the drug. This may be a factor in poor response to treatment—a reduction in intestinal absorption. Certainly it has been shown that in patients suffering from schizophrenia, whose absorption of the drug was reduced and whose response was poor, clinical improvement sometimes followed changing over to the intramuscular route.

In steady state conditions the intramuscular route also gives much higher plasma levels than the orally given drug. From 90 to 95 per cent of the compound is in bound form to proteins, mostly albumin in plasma, and brain levels may reach 4–5 times those in plasma.

Plasma levels vary widely between individuals, which indicates large differences in metabolism. A very large number of metabolites of chlorpromazine have been identified, some of which are therapeutically active. When taken by mouth, the metabolism is somewhat different from that of parenteral administration, because, as discussed above, oral therapy is accompanied by the 'first pass' effect, the result of the dose passing initially through the liver and being converted to a larger proportion of metabolites, many of which take part in an enterohepatic circulation—excretion in the bile and reabsorption in the gut. With parenteral administration of drugs a larger proportion of unchanged drug reaches the brain and other parts of the body than when it is taken orally.

Chlorpromazine induces the microsomal enzyme catalysing hydroxylation (as described above), thereby accelerating its own metabolism. Thus, some individuals on fixed doses may have progressively decreasing free drug levels in plasma with time. This is seen from the increase of plasma levels of chlorpromazine, which reach a peak after 2 weeks' treatment. In the third week plasma levels decline to new lower levels. The fact that chlorpromazine induces the microsomal enzyme in the liver is further supported by the gradual increase in one of the metabolic products of this route, the glycuronated compounds, which achieve a late peak at 3 weeks.

Phenothiazines remain in the body for many months after they have been withdrawn.

Chlorpromazine is non-addictive, and there are no appreciable effects on even abrupt withdrawal. It has a wide therapeutic index and is remarkably safe in most circumstances, even in overdosage.

The distribution volume of chlorpromazine is about seven times that of body water, which indicates a high degree of localization in tissues. Much of this is drug bound intracellularly to the membranes of microsomes and mitochondria, with much less binding to nuclei and soluble cell constituents.

Chlorpromazine and its metabolites also bind to red cells, possibly with the parent substance at the cell surface and some of its metabolites within the cells themselves, and red cells could be of importance in carrying the drug and its active metabolites to the brain.

The main site of metabolism of chlorpromazine is the hepatic microsomal P450 cytochrome enzyme. Much of the drug is initially hydroxylated at positions 3 and 7, and then conjugated to glycuronic acid (to give 30 per cent of the urinary metabolites in chronic dosage). A smaller but significant amount is converted to the sulphoxide.

TABLE 9.2. Chlorpromazine: drug interaction

Alcohol: additive effect on CNS
Amphetamines: antagonism
Guanethidine: antagonism
Antihypertensive drugs: antagonism
Hypoglycaemic agents: antagonism (possibly an effect on puerperal use of glucose)
Phenytoin: increased depression of CNS

Tricyclic antidepressants: hepatic enzyme { induction / competition

Morphine } potentiation
Pethidine }

Following a single dose, the main products are sulphoxide and demethylated compounds, but with time the pattern mentioned above of predominance of glycuronated derivatives establishes itself, probably as a result of hepatic enzyme induction. It has been suggested that this might be part of the basis of tolerance to the early side-effects experienced by some patients—the gradual replacement of more biologically active metabolites by the inactive polar derivates.

SIDE- AND TOXIC EFFECTS

The side-effects of chlorpromazine are mainly extensions of its pharmacological actions.

CNS
Some patients may complain of drowsiness in the early days of treatment, especially with dimethylamino and piperidine compounds.

Extrapyramidal side-effects
An early manifestation of *akinesia* may be weakness, especially in muscles used repeatedly. The condition may progress on to the Parkinsonism, with tremor, rigidity, festinant gait, mask-like face and excess salivation.

Akathisia occurs mostly with the piperazine phenothiazines, and consists of uncontrolled restlessness, sometimes associated with seborrhoea.

Dystonic reactions occur mostly with the trifluomethyl compounds, and take the form of inco-ordination of movement, retrocollis, torticollis, facial grimacing and distortion, protrusion of the tongue, dysarthria, oculogyric crises and opisthotonus.

Finally, there are the tardive dyskinesias involving repeated inco-ordinated movements which may or may not be irreversible.

Autonomic nervous system
In summary, the effects of chlorpromazine on the autonomic nervous system are complex and have been described above in various sections. Chlorpromazine has alpha-adrenergic blockade activity, has some cholinergic-blocking actions and probably also acts in part like tricyclic antidepressants in blocking amine re-uptake mechanisms at the presynaptic membrane. It also blocks 5-HT receptors.

The anticholinergic activity results in blurred vision, reduction in gastric secretion, constipation and urinary retention. The alpha-adrenergic blockade is responsible for chlorpromazine's ability to block or reverse the pressor effects of noradrenaline, reduce baroreceptor reflexes, and the effects of sympathomimetic drugs on the iris and nictitating membrane, the lowering of the lethal dose of adrenaline, and it may be responsible for inhibition of ejaculation.

Tables of side-effects and interactions have been given on pages 168 and 170.

Uses of phenothiazines

The most outstanding uses of phenothiazines have been in the treatment of schizophrenia and in the control of the symptoms of mania, particularly in the more seriously disturbed patients. They have been helpful for acute or chronic confusional states and in very disturbed depressed patients, and have also had a place in the management of severe anxiety and poor impulse control. They are not used widely in the management of alcoholism now, except perhaps for the treatment of alcoholic hallucinosis.

Phenothiazines have been employed for the treatment of a number of conditions which give rise to nausea and vomiting, such as radiation sickness, chemotherapy of malignancy, uraemia, carcinomatosis, during therapy with morphia, etc.

Table 9.3 lists some of the neuroleptics with their approximate equivalent doses. The number of compounds presents a bewildering choice to the clinician and this could result in some confusion when deciding on the most appropriate. However, this should rarely be a problem.

In general, all of the compounds substituted in the 2 position are antipsychotic but some are less potent (weight for weight) than others. Examples are chlorpromazine and thioridazine, drugs which will require a larger dose to achieve the same effect than, say, trifluperazine or flufenazine. With matched doses the low-potency and high-potency drugs should produce similar antipsychotic actions. This is not to say that for other reasons one neuroleptic is not better than another in a particular patient, and different drugs and formulations have their special uses.

In choosing neuroleptics it is better to select three or four drugs and use them continuously to develop expertise in their use, rather than jump from one to another. Similarly, if one neuroleptic is being given at optimum dosage and is ineffective, another is unlikely to do better. Polypharmacy with neuroleptics is not justified and only confuses the picture.

Of course, it may not be possible to achieve optimum levels with one drug. For instance, a patient may become hypotensive with chlorpromazine but tolerate haloperidol.

Cardiac problems may dictate the choice of drug. Arrhythmias occur more commonly with low-potency drugs such as thioridazine, a drug which also causes irreversible retinopathy at doses over 600 mg/day. On the other hand, its high anticholinergic activity minimizes Parkinsonian side-effects.

For the agitated patient the low-potency drugs are preferred because they tend to be calming. On the other hand, the apathetic thought-disordered individual will do better with the more activating high-potency compounds such as fluphenazine, or haloperidol (*see* below).

As already stated, individuals susceptible to alpha-adrenergic blockade and therefore liable to hypotensive crises might have haloperidol, trifluoperazine or flufenazine instead of chlorpromazine.

To these drugs the clinician must add a long-acting neuroleptic for maintenance therapy, mostly in chronic schizophrenia. These include long-acting intramuscular preparations of flufenazine, flupenthixol and fluspiriline (*see Table 9.4*).

These suggestions may not cover all eventualities but should provide a basis to suit most purposes in which mixing of neuroleptics will be unnecessary.

Butyrophenones

There are now quite a number of butyrophenones and related diphenylbutyl piperidines of possible use as neuroleptics (*Figure 9.3*). The first one of interest in the series was haloperidol, a butyrophenone synthesized by Janssen and introduced in 1958. On first examination it would seem to have different characteristics from those of the phenothiazine neuroleptics, but, as Janssen and Van Bever have pointed out, neuroleptics tend to be tertiary (rarely secondary) amines containing at least one aromatic ring linked to the basic amine portion (−N<) of the molecule by an intermediate chain of general formula

$$Ar-\alpha-\beta-CH_2-CH_2-N<$$

With the butyrophenones the aromatic moiety (Ar) is 4-fluorophenyl, α is a keto function and β stands for a methylene group, to give:

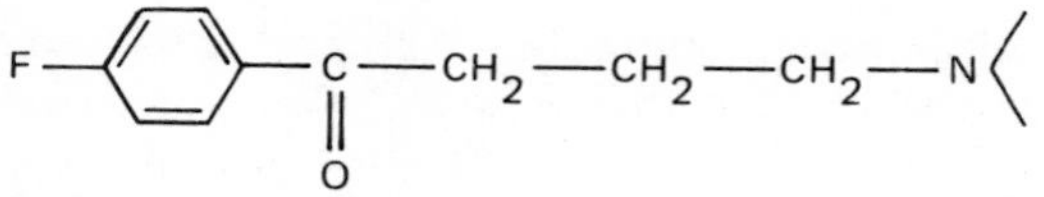

$$F-\underset{O}{\underset{\|}{\overset{}{\bigcirc}}}-\overset{}{\underset{\|}{C}}-CH_2-CH_2-CH_2-N\big\langle$$

When the keto group is replaced by a 4-fluorophenyl methine group (4-F–C_6H_4–CH=), this gives the general formula of the diphenylbutylpiperidines (e.g. pimozide).

In animals this group of drugs given in low doses decreases operant behaviour, reduces exploration of the environment and suppresses conditioned avoidance behaviour (e.g. pressing a lever to avoid an aversive stimulus such as electric shock). The animals tend to give fewer and slower responses to a whole range of

Butyrophenones

Haloperidol
(Serenace, Haldol)

Droperidol
(Droleptan)

Diphenylbutylpiperidines

Pimozide
(Orap)

Penfluridol

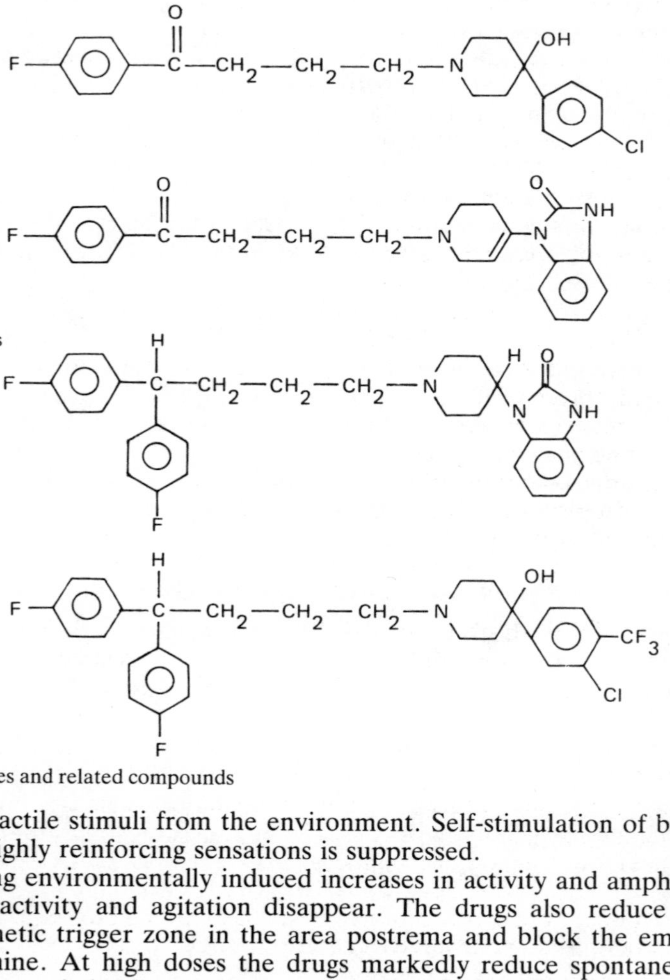

Figure 9.3 Butyrophenones and related compounds

visual, auditory or tactile stimuli from the environment. Self-stimulation of brain centres producing highly reinforcing sensations is suppressed.

Naturally occurring environmentally induced increases in activity and amphetamine-induced hyperactivity and agitation disappear. The drugs also reduce the sensitivity of the emetic trigger zone in the area postrema and block the emetic effects of apomorphine. At high doses the drugs markedly reduce spontaneous mobility and exploratory behaviour to the point eventually of catalepsy.

Taking chlorpromazine as a comparative measure, dose for dose the butyrophenones in general are much more potent than this parent neuroleptic. They tend to differ from chlorpromazine both in lacking even the initial sedative effect of this drug and in having minimal or no adrenolytic actions (so that problems from hypotension are infrequent) and little or no anticholinergic activity.

Like the phenothiazine neuroleptics, they block the dopaminergic receptors. The drugs have quite potent effects on the dopaminergic pathways, increasing firing rates, and on turnover of dopamine. The latter effect is achieved via the (hypothetical) autoreceptors. They may have other presynaptic actions, increasing the availability of dopamine in the dopaminergic synapse. The postsynaptic dopaminergic receptors can be demonstrated by binding to labelled dopamine or labelled haloperidol, and it has been suggested that the receptor might have a two-state model—the agonist form, to which dopamine binds, and the antagonist configuration, to which haloperidol and other neuroleptics will bind. A remarkably close correlation has been found between the affinity of both phenothiazine and butyrophenone neuroleptics for the ^{3}H-haloperidol binding site and their respective neuroleptic activities in animals and man. Furthermore, increases in binding to dopaminergic receptors has been shown following presynaptic lesions (cutting the nigrostriatal tract to the corpus striatum) and after chronic treatment with neuroleptics. Such manoeuvres as discontinuing chronic treatment with neuroleptics may be accompanied by increased sensitivity to dopamine agonists, which suggests the development of dopaminergic supersensitivity (but *see* arguments on these points in Chapter 16).

These findings underline the possible importance of dopaminergic receptor –neuroleptic interactions, a line of enquiry also discussed further in Chapter 16.

PHARMACOLOGICAL PROPERTIES IN HUMANS

Haloperidol can be taken as the 'parent compound' for butyrophenones, which, like chlorpromazine and the other phenothiazine compounds, produces the neuroleptic syndrome described above. Haloperidol is similar in some ways to the piperazine phenothiazines. Like these, it is a potent antipsychotic drug which calms and quietens excited patients, and which has been used successfully for both manic and schizophrenic patients and for other conditions.

ABSORPTION, METABOLISM AND EXCRETION

Haloperidol is absorbed readily from the gut and reaches a peak in plasma 2–6 hours after ingestion. Fall-off in levels thereafter is slow, with detectable amounts remaining for weeks. Excretion is via the bile and through the kidneys.

EFFECT ON CENTRAL NERVOUS SYSTEM

As stated above, the drug calms and quietens the excited or psychotic patient with minimal sedation. The EEG becomes slowed, with increased theta activity, and the seizure threshold may be lowered.

AUTONOMIC AND CARDIOVASCULAR ACTIONS

With a reduced level of adrenolytic and anticholinergic properties as compared with chlorpromazine, as would be anticipated, these actions are much less troublesome and ECG efforts have not been described. Nevertheless, there may be minor problems over blood pressure, dry mouth, difficulty in accommodation and tachycardia.

EFFECT ON ENDOCRINE SYSTEM

Like the phenothiazines, haloperidol blocks the dopaminergic pathway, which inhibits prolactin secretion, so that prolactin is produced in abnormal amounts. In other words, when this dopaminergic pathway is blocked, there is 'release' of prolactin secretion. This can lead to galactorrhoea, and menstrual and other sexual side-effects described for chlorpromazine. There is some controversy as to whether haloperidol has any marked effect on weight. Recently it has been shown that luteinizing hormone is also under the control of a dopaminergic pathway and will be influenced by dopaminergic blocking drugs.

SIDE- AND TOXIC EFFECTS

Side-effects with haloperidol are relatively uncommon, with the exception of Parkinsonian symptoms, dealt with above in the section on chlorpromazine. As stated above, anticholinergic effects are minimal, and hypotension is rarely a problem of any magnitude. The problems come down mostly to extrapyramidal effects, and those produced via prolactin. Occasionally leucopenia is seen, and rarely agranulocystosis.

Recently the possibility has been raised that haloperidol and lithium may interact together to give earlier Parkinsonian side-effects or enhanced CNS toxicity from lithium or even more serious effects in the form of brain damage. Very many patients have received these two drugs together without experiencing toxic interactions, and this useful combination should not be discontinued when and where it is indicated. It would be wise, however, to keep plasma lithium levels (12 hour) to below 1 mM and limit haloperidol to 20 mg daily where the two drugs are used together.

At our present state of knowledge, serious toxic effects and brain damage are only likely to be the outcome of toxic doses of one or other or both drugs. Haloperidol is essentially a safe drug.

Substituted benzamides

These are a new class of compounds (*Figure 9.4*), some of which have the behavioural effects of classic neuroleptics—i.e. they decrease hyperactivity induced by injection of dopamine into the nucleus accumbens, and inhibit apomorphine-induced circling, climbing behaviour and increased activity. Some block the stereotyped behaviour produced by apomorphine or amphetamines.

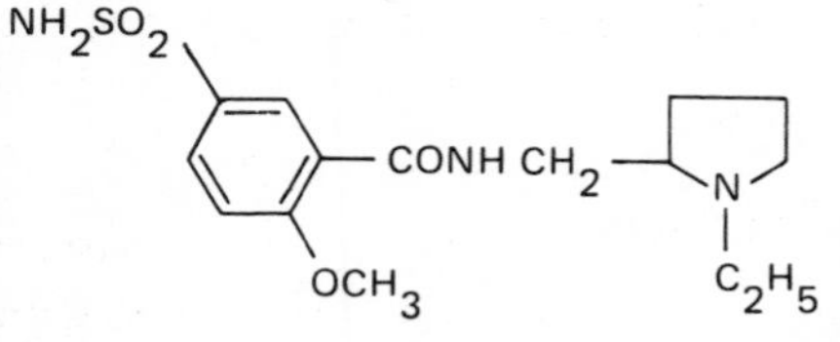

Sulpiride

Figure 9.4 Substituted benzamide

TABLE 9.3. Relationships between some of the phenothiazines and thioxanthines

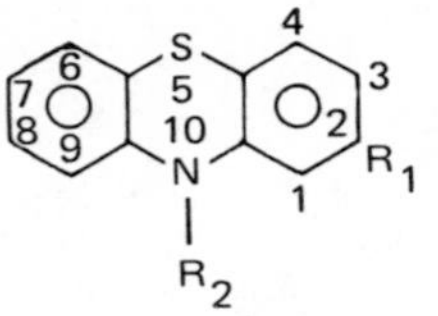

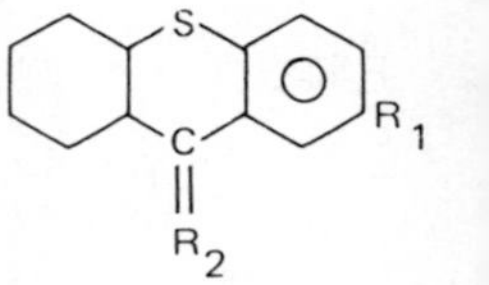

Phenothiazines

R_2		R_1	
	H	Cl	CF_3

Aliphatic

$--CH_2-CH_2 \cdot CH_2 N(CH_3)_2$

Promazine (Sparine) 300 mg	Chlorpromazine (Largactil) 100 mg	Trifluorprom (Vesprin) Canada and U 40 mg

Piperidine

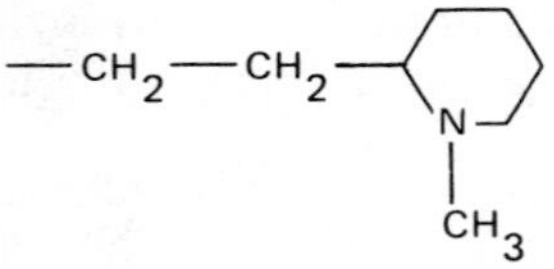

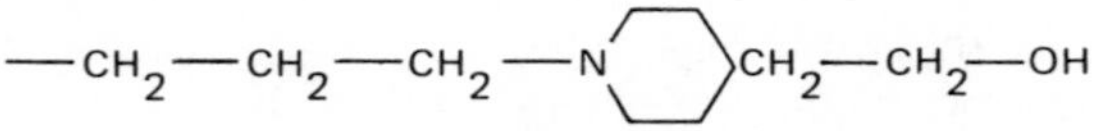

$-CH_2-CH_2-$ [piperidine ring with CH_3]

$--CH_2-CH_2-CH_2-N$ [piperidine ring] CH_2-CH_2-OH

Piperazine

$-CH_2-CH_2-CH_2-N$ [piperazine] $N-CH_3$

$-CH_2-CH_2-CH_2-N$ [piperazine] $N-CH_2-CH_2-OH$

$-CH_2-CH_2-CH_2-N$ [piperazine] $N-CH_2-CH_2-O-\overset{O}{\overset{\|}{C}}-CH_3$

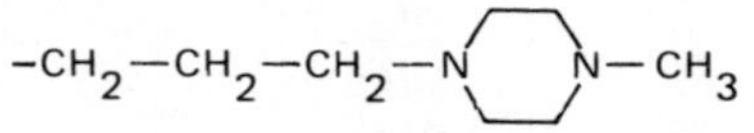	Prochlorperazine (Stemetil) 15–30 mg	Trifluorperaz (Stelazine) 5–10 mg
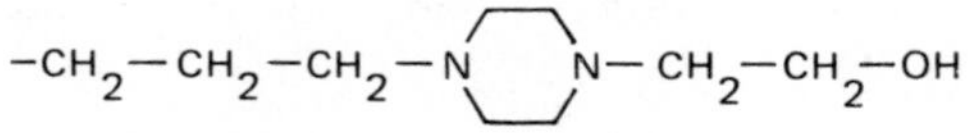	Perfenazine (Fentazine) 10 mg	Flufenazine (Modecate) Prolixin (USA 2 mg
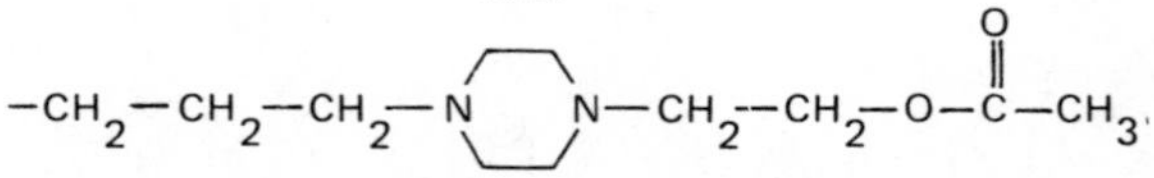	Thiopropazide (Dartalan) 10 mg	

Thioxanthines

Aliphatic

$-CH-CH_2-CH_2-N(CH_3)_2$

Chlorprothixene (Taractan) approx. 50 mg	

Piperazine

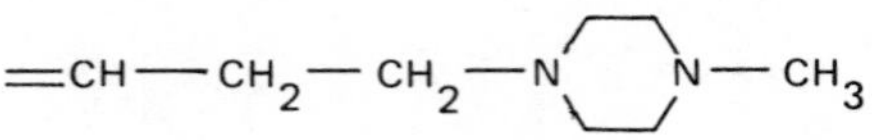

$=CH-CH_2-CH_2-N$ [piperazine] $N-CH_3$

$=CH-CH_2-CH_2-N$ [piperazine] $N-CH_2-CH_2-OH$

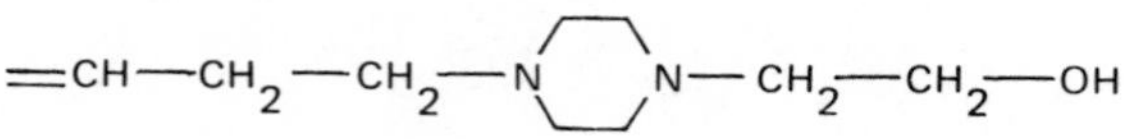	Flupenthixol (Fluanxol, Depixol) 3 mg

$SO_2N(CH_3)_2$ $S-CH_3$ $-\overset{\overset{O}{\|}}{S}-CH_3$ $-\overset{\overset{O}{\|}}{C}-CH_3$ $-\overset{\overset{O}{\|}}{C}(CH_2)_2-CH_3$ $-\overset{\overset{O}{\|}}{C}-CH_3$ $-\overset{\overset{O}{\|}}{C}-CH_2-CH_3$

Thioridazine   Mesoridazine
(Melleril)   (Serentil)
100 mg   Canada and
  USA
  50 mg

Piperacitazine
(Quide)
Canada and USA
10 mg

Butaperazine   Acetophenazine¹   Carphenazine
(Repoise)   (Tuidal)   (Proketazine)
USA   USA   USA
10 mg   20 mg   25 mg

Thiothixine
(Narvane)
5 mg

Their ability to induce catalepsy is relatively weak. Like other neuroleptics, they raise levels of prolactin, induce extrapyramidal symptoms and prevent apomorphine-induced vomiting.

They increase dopamine turnover in the brain and displace radioactively labelled butyrophenones from their binding sites, but at a lower level of affinity than other neuroleptic compounds. This activity is not in parallel with their antipsychotic activity. The difference is seen in the dopamine-sensitive adenyl cyclase system, which phenothiazines and thioxanthines block in proportion to their therapeutic behaviour, and butyrophenones in a way not closely related to their clinical efficacy. This contrasts with the substituted benzamides, which are different from all the other known dopamine antagonists, leaving dopamine-sensitive adenyl cyclase unaltered except when the drug is at very high concentration. Thus, it seems likely that substituted benzamides act on a sub-population of dopamine receptors or, alternatively, on a part of the receptor which is independent of adenyl cyclase. There is more than one type of dopamine receptor and these compounds may be effective at only one of these.

In fact, the substituted benzamide sulpiride can displace only a proportion of labelled butyrophenone binding sites, but dopamine receptors sensitive to this class of compound occur in all the main dopaminergic sites—cortical, mesolimbic, striatal. The evidence suggests that they have little, if any, activity presynaptically but are functioning at postsynaptic sites on, as stated above, a sub-population of receptors independent of adenyl cyclase.

Cholinergic and GABAergic pathways do not influence the actions of substituted benzamides, and, for instance, classical neuroleptics produce an increase in dopamine turnover which can be at least partially blocked by anticholinergic drugs. Sulpiride does not influence GABA binding sites and leaves turnover of norarenaline and 5-HT unchanged.

Reserpine

Reserpine is one of a large number of alkaloids which have been isolated from a family of climbing shrubs (*Rauwolfia serpentina*) (*Figure 9.5*). It is included here

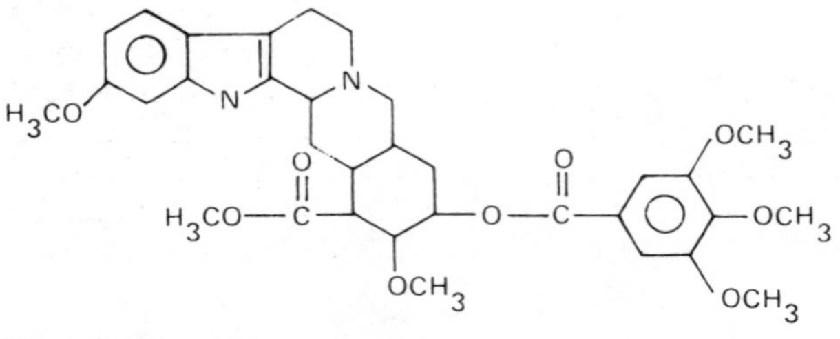

Figure 9.5 Reserpine

mainly because of its place in the history of antipsychotic and antidepressant drugs, but it is not in common use now. It was introduced into psychiatry as an antipsychotic agent by Kline in 1954, and subsequently the ability experimentally to antagonize its effects, either on animal behaviour or aminergic systems, etc., was used as a means of selecting potential antidepressants.

General pharmacology

The most obvious and well-known action of reserpine is to produce irreversible interference with the intracellular storage of biogenic amines—5-HT, noradrenaline and dopamine—in storage granules in brain neurons. Similarly, in the periphery 5-HT (and histamine) are released from platelets which can no longer store amines, and catecholamines are liberated from the heart and postganglionic adrenergic neurons. Storage of amines in the gut (5-HT) and adrenal medulla (catecholamines) are less affected than are amines in other tissues.

The actions of reserpine are complex—there is displacement of amines from the vesicular binding sites, but it also seems to influence transport (possibly interfering with the ATPase-dependent uptake mechanism in the granule membrane) and possibly also reducing release of amines. Depletion of amines in the CNS has occurred in 1 hour after administration, and is complete at 24 hours, and there is then a major disturbance in the function of aminergic neurons. Thereafter, a very small amount remains firmly bound in the tissues. In view of the early but then prolonged effects of reserpine persisting when so little remains *in situ*, it has earned the title of a 'hit and run' drug. Certainly, restoration of normality has to await the synthesis of new storage granules and their delivery down to the aminergic terminals.

The actions of reserpine are antagonized by tricyclic antidepressants and MAOI, and if the latter is given before reserpine, there may be brief 'excitement' because of the release of amines which cannot be degraded to inactive components.

Effects of reserpine

Unless there is a brief period of excitement following previous MAOI administration or very large doses of the drug are given, reserpine produces sedation, tranquillization, unreactiveness, indifference to surroundings, and nightmares. The 'taming' action of neuroleptics in animals is seen also with reserpine. With prolonged high doses there may be extrapyramidal complications, usually dystonia and/or akathisia, and susceptible individuals may develop psychotic depression. Because of loss of sympathetic tone and parasympathetic 'release', patients may experience excess salivation, nausea, diarrhoea, nasal congestion, flushing, fall in blood pressure (often with postural hypotension), bradycardia, peripheral oedema and acute peptic ulcer. Seizures occur at high doses. There are a number of hormonal effects due to disruption of the regulation of hypothalamic hormones; these include amenorrhoea, and reduced fertility in women and altered sexual function in men, due to blockade of release of gonadotrophins. There is also release of ACTH and a resultant stimulus of the adrenal cortex; possibly release of ADH, and production of prolactin. The increased production of prolactin may be responsible for a report of increased incidence of cancer of the breast in patients taking reserpine.

Uses of reserpine

Reserpine has been given for the treatment of hypertension and Raynaud's disease, but, as stated above, it has fallen into disuse in psychiatry. This has been because its actions and its neuroleptic properties are less predictable and less easily controlled than are those of phenothiazines and butyrophenones, and because of the problem of side-effects.

Benzodiazepines

Benzodiazepines are a group of compounds first synthesized in the 1930s which have come to occupy a prominent position in recent years, chiefly as hypnotic or antianxiety agents. Early animal studies of these compounds suggested that they may have muscle-relaxant, antistrychnine and spinal reflex blocking capacity, but it was their 'taming' effects which led to their trial as antianxiety agents. One of their useful properties is anticonvulsant activity. As a group, they are characterized by a remarkable lack of toxicity, even at very high doses, and inactivity at peripheral sites. Even in large quantities benzodiazepines do not induce anaesthesia.

Metabolism, absorption, etc.

The metabolism of the benzodiazepines is somewhat complicated, because with some compounds many of the metabolic products are equally as active as their parent compound. These active derivatives have their own metabolic fates, half-lives, etc. This interrelationship of benzodiazepine metabolites has been exploited in the search for short-acting compounds where active compounds near the 'end' of the degradation process have been consciously selected so that they would be without the disadvantage of giving rise to other drugs, or even a series of active substances.

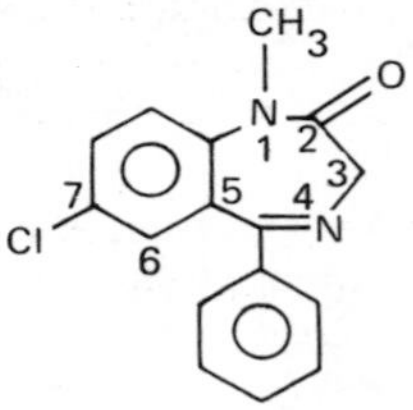

Diazepam

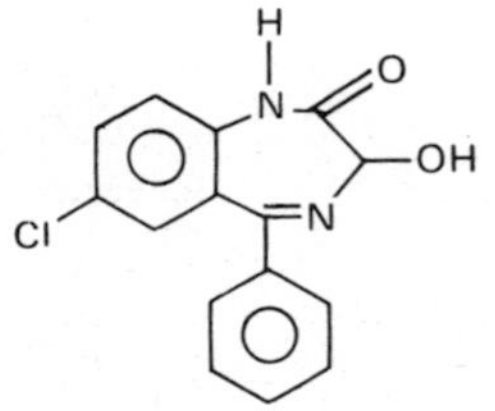

Oxazepam

Figure 9.6 Benzodiazepines

The structure of two benzodiazepines is given in *Figure 9.6*. Increased activity is given by substitution of a halogen in position 7 and having a carbonyl group at 2. The substitution at 7 is essential for activity and 7-chloro compounds are quite common. It is the relative persistence of the 7 and 2 substitutions which can result in the continuance of pharmacological activity in the metabolites of benzodiazepines. Some of the processes in the degradation of benzodiazepines involve the hepatic microsomal system, but these drugs, while they may be degraded more rapidly if there is enzyme induction, do not appear to induce the enzyme themselves to a significant extent. Benzodiazepines can modify their metabolism, however, as is shown by the changing pattern with time of the balance between a parent substance and a derivative (*see* below).

Diazepam

Diazepam has been taken in this section as a representative of the benzodiazepine group. It is readily absorbed from the gut to give peak levels in about 30 minutes, but intramuscularly the peak level takes 60 minutes to achieve. The intramuscular route also gives a much lower peak than that of the orally given drug, probably because of tissue binding at the injection site. Comparative peak plasma levels in one trial were 1600 mg/ml (intravenous, 5 minutes), 490 mg/ml (oral, 30 minutes), 270 mg/ml (intramuscular, 60 minutes). Plasma levels may differ considerably between different individuals on the same dose, and diazepam has earlier peaks and longer plasma half-lives in young children.

One route of metabolism is demethylation to desmethyl-diazepam, an active compound with a longer half-life than diazepam, which therefore tends to accumulate. With time, diazepam accumulates in plasma and then tends to decline slightly, probably because of some enzyme changes leading to increased formation of the desmethylated derivative. This has been confirmed by the fact that chronic users given a test dose produce a lot more of the desmethylated derivative than they do after a long period off the drug.

Brain concentrations of diazepam vary from region to region, in proportion to the richness of blood supply, with largish concentrations in frontal grey matter, thalamus and mesencephalon.

The therapeutic actions of diazepam and its desmethyl derivative differ somewhat, with the parent compound being most helpful for psychic tension, depressed mood and complaints centred on some autonomic disturbances (dry mouth, flushing, perspiration, giddiness), and desmethyl diazepam for gastrointestinal-related complaints.

While the main product of diazepam is desmethyl-diazepam, this is converted into oxazepam and demoxepam (still active), both of which are present in smaller amounts than is the desmethyl compound.

SIDE- AND UNWANTED EFFECTS

Benzodiazepines are remarkably safe under normal circumstances and are unlikely to be fatal in overdose. In susceptible individuals they can give rise to ataxia and mild confusion and disorientation, and may also enhance the effects of alcohol. Occasionally they give rise to paradoxical effects—release of overactivity or previously partially suppressed feelings. On long-continued high-dosage patients may become habituated to the drug and develop anxiety, apprehension and/or fits on withdrawal. These drugs can lead to lapses of attention which may make driving or the use of machinery hazardous. A few people gain weight on benzodiazepines.

PHARMACOLOGY

Central nervous system

Benzodiazepines have a variety of activities. They have important actions on conditioned conflict punishment schedules in animals, which are discussed further below. Like barbiturates, but at high doses, they block EEG arousal during stimulation of the brain-stem reticular formation, and they depress spinal reflexes. They have a significant depressant effect on the electrical discharge from the limbic system, including the septal region, the amygdala and the hippocampus. They have

TABLE 9.4. Haloperidol and related compounds

	Starting dose (daily unless otherwise stated)	Maintenance dose or other dosage regimens (daily unless otherwise stated)	Notes/uses, etc.
Haloperidol (Serenace, Haldol)	1–6 mg disturbed patients oral 6–15 mg more disturbed patients 0.5 mg b.d. anxiety states 2–10 mg i.m. hourly increasing to 30 mg hourly if required*	These doses may have to be increased according to response to 60, 80, 100 or even 200 mg	Wide uses—acute/chronic schizophrenia, mania, organic brain syndrome, alcohol withdrawal, delirium tremens, nausea and vomiting, premedication, anxiety states, Gilles de la Tourette syndrome
Trifluperidol (Triperidol)	0.5–3 mg	6–8 mg	Used—acute/chronic schizophrenia, mania
Benperidol (Anquil)	0.25 mg	0.25–1.5 mg	Suppression of antisocial sexual behaviour
Droperidol (Droleptan, Thalamonal)	2–20 mg	5–15 mg i.v. up to 10 mg i.m. 5–20 mg oral	Used—premedication and 'adjuvant to anaesthesia', mania, agitation, antiemetic. May exacerbate depression.
Pimozide (Orap)	2–4 mg	2–10 mg	Contraindicated in mania and in psychotic and other states with aggression and agitation. Useful in withdrawn apathetic schizophrenia with thought disorder. May aggravate depression. Low side-effects claimed.
Fluspiriline (Redeptin)	2 mg/week i.m.	2–8 mg/week i.m. to 10 mg i.m. in some cases	Maintenance therapy schizophrenia. Antipsychotic action lasts 5–15 days.

*See Reading list

a hypnotic action in which REM sleep is not suppressed in the usual dose range, but they diminish or abolish stage 4 sleep. Benzodiazepines increase the seizure threshold and therefore can be used as anticonvulsants. The EEG is increased in amplitude and there is an increase in fast beta activity. They have negligible effects on the cardiovascular system and on respiration, but produce a significant degree of muscle relaxation.

Effects in conditioning experiments

Benzodiazepines have opposing effects in goal-directed behaviour. In high doses and initially they depress such behaviour and at low or repeated doses they often facilitate it. Their effects are most readily elicited in conditioning experiments in schedules which demonstrate behaviour contingent on either reward or punishment. It has been suggested that in these types of behaviour the reward system is controlled largely by noradrenergic pathways and that the punishment system is at least partly mediated by serotoninergic neurons.

Some of the studies of the actions of benzodiazepines have combined punishment and reward schedules. During training the animals are given a reward (e.g. food) at infrequent and irregular intervals in response to some action (e.g. lever pressing).

This is the reward schedule, which is interspersed with another in which, following a different type of signal (e.g. a sound), the presentation of food is accompanied by a punishment (e.g. an electric shock delivered to the feet through the floor grid). With training, high rates of lever pressing will accompany the non-punished or reward routines, and low rates the punished programme. The punished schedule results in inhibition of behaviour which would have occurred in the absence of the punishment, or, after training, the warning of impending punishment. In this case the action which is inhibited is the taking of food, but it might equally have been some other kind of action and response to another reward.

Benzodiazepines have a disinhibitory effect on the punishment behaviour. In other words, despite the 'warning' of impending punishment, the previously inhibited behaviour is not blocked but returns, so that the animal, as it were, ignores the imminent threat of a noxious stimulus. This property of benzodiazepines has been equated with its antianxiety action in humans. It is by no means certain that this extrapolation to human emotions is valid, but it is of interest that the antianxiety effect of benzodiazepines in humans is not an effect which habituates with time. The punishment behaviour disinhibition also continues with repeated doses, showing no appreciable habituation.

Benzodiazepines have an additional effect—they also decrease the activity in the non-punished (reward) schedules. This is an effect, however, to which tolerance appears rapidly and, therefore, is seen only at the beginning of chronic treatment programmes.

One group has suggested that at whatever site benzodiazepines act, their ultimate effect in these experiments is via 5-HT systems in the punishment schedules, and on noradrenergic systems in the non-punishment programmes. In both instances it was proposed that the action is to decrease activity in aminergic systems: in noradrenergic pathways in non-punished responses, and in 5-HT pathways in the punished mechanisms. They also suggest that their antianxiety actions in humans are mediated by their influence on the 5-HT systems. The effect on these systems, if correct, would be indirect (*see* below).

Possible site of action of benzodiazepines
Benzodiazepines bind to postsynaptic sites at GABAergic synapses. It follows that their actions should be widespread because of the wide distribution of these synapses in the central nervous system. That they act via GABAergic pathways is supported by the observation that they produce their effect only in the presence of endogenous GABA, and the changes they produce are most obvious when the action of GABA systems is submaximal. The upper limit of potentiation of GABAergic transmission in test systems is limited and occurs at about ×10 the threshold dose of the drug.

Sites with high affinity binding for benzodiazepines have been identified in the brain. Subsequently displacement of the drug from binding compounds (e.g. triazolopyridazines and β-carboline-3-carboxylate) pointed to the presence of at least two types of benzodiazepine receptor, called BZ_1 and BZ_2. BZ_1 sites account for about 75 per cent of the cortical and 50–60 per cent of the hippocampal binding, and no brain region has less than 50 per cent BZ_1. However, there were relatively high numbers of BZ_2 receptors in the caudate nucleus, the putamen and the dentate gyrus, and in the superficial layer of the superior colliculus (in the rat). Two proteins, of 51000 and 55000 daltons, respectively, have been found which can displace benzodiazepines from binding, the first probably being associated with

BZ_1, the latter with BZ_2; and there are smaller amounts of other proteins with similar properties.

At the time of writing it seemed likely that anxiolytic and anticonvulsant activity lay in BZ_1 and sedative properties in BZ_2 receptors.

The situation is further complicated by the finding of a polypeptide of 15 000 daltons and a peptide of 3000 daltons, both of which can displace bound benzodiazepines.

Inosine, hypoxanthine and nicotinamide are endogenous compounds which bind to the benzodiazepine receptor, and concentrations of the order of 1 mM are required to displace 50 per cent of diazepam binding. It seems probable that these compounds would have a significant effect *in vivo*, although a related exogenous compound, caffeine, if taken in appreciable amounts in tea, coffee, etc., could modify GABAergic function.

Of the substances used to define the two types of receptor, one, β-carboline-3-carboxylate, was isolated from human urine. It was capable of displacing half the diazepine binding at 4–7 nM, as compared with 5 nM for the highly active benzodiazepine clorazepam. It is probably not a functional endogenous modifier of GABAergic activity. It is likely that with these various competitors at the benzodiazepine receptor sites a whole range of compounds selective for different properties will be synthesized.

USES

Benzodiazepines have their greatest use in the relief of anxiety and as hypnotics. They are also used in alcoholic withdrawal, as a preoperative medication, in labour, as an anticonvulsant in status epilepticus, and for the treatment of tetanus. They are of some benefit as muscle relaxants in upper motor neuron disease, etc.

Barbiturates

Barbiturates are derivatives of barbituric acid, which was first synthesized by von Baeyer in 1864. They are compounds which depress the activity of many systems, mostly probably by their effects on electrical stabilization of cell membranes, but they have been used for their actions on the nervous system because of its particular sensitivity to these substances.

The basic structure of barbituric acid and that of some of the barbiturates is given in *Figure 9.7*. Active compounds are made by substituting alkyl or aryl groups for both hydrogen atoms at position 5. Two alkyl groups are needed at this site for sedation, while aryl or reactive alkyl side-chains are anticonvulsant.

Speed of onset and duration of action are inversely related to lipid solubility, which is increased by substituting sulphur for oxygen at 2 (thiobarbiturates), or by attaching a methyl group to one of the nitrogens.

The barbiturates are absorbed easily from the gastrointestinal tract and from subcutaneous or intramuscular injection.

The most rapidly and brief-acting barbiturates, i.e. those with high lipid solubility, act by virtue of their quick penetration into the brain (and other tissues high in fatty material). The process is reversed equally rapidly, however, as the drug is redistributed from fatty tissues to the whole body.

The barbiturates are metabolized in the liver by the hepatic microsomal system by oxidation of the side-chains from site 5, removal of sulphur from the thiobarbiturates, and splitting off of the alkyl groups. Enzyme competition can occur for metabolism of substances passing down the same pathways, and after exposure to barbiturates there is induction of the enzymes in the system. This may cause problems with other drugs.

Most barbiturates have sedative and hypnotic actions, but some, such as phenobarbitone, have more anticonvulsant properties. It is possible, e.g. with phenobarbitone, to separate anticonvulsant from hypnotic activity by abolishing the sedation with amphetamines. The basis of this difference is not quite clear.

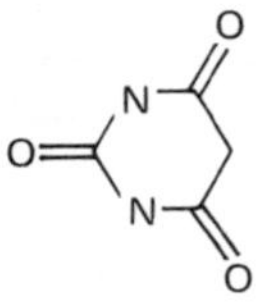

Barbituric acid

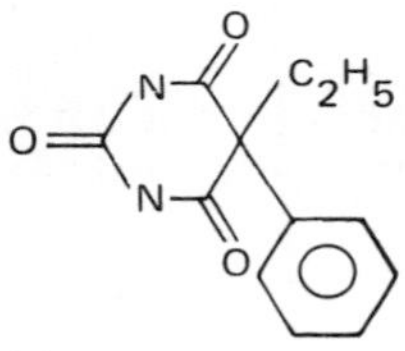

Phenobarbitone

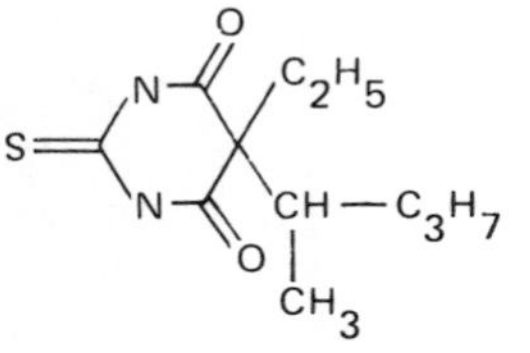

Thiopentone

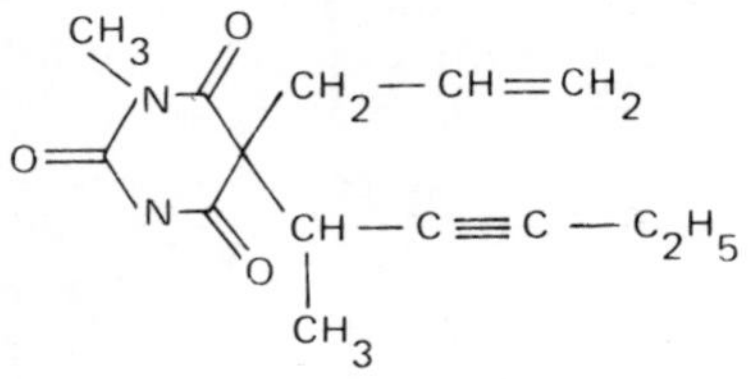

Methohexitone

Figure 9.7 Barbiturates

In general, the barbiturates depress transmission more than conduction, so that the membrane potential is unaltered, and the most obvious changes they produce are at the synapses. The regions of the brain most sensitive to barbiturates are the cortex and the reticular formation.

Initially, at low doses there may be an increase in electrical activity, possibly due to a release of the cortex from inhibitory pathways from the reticular formation; but thereafter excitatory impulses from the reticular system are diminished, leading to sedation, hypnosis and finally, with sufficient of the drug, anaesthesia. With increasing doses the drug affects first the cortex and the reticular system, then lower centres, and finally the medulla and the spinal cord.

Overall, barbiturates tend to depress excitatory and have variable effects on inhibitory synapses—e.g. they block the excitatory but not the inhibitory noradrenergic synapses in the cortex.

Part of the effect of barbiturates may be via GABAergic neurons, where release of GABA may be prolonged both postsynaptically and at presynaptic inhibitory synapses. Another possibility is that barbiturates may interfere with the 'depolarization–calcium–release of transmitter' process, preventing the entry of this cation into the cell, and thus preventing release of the transmitter.

In animals these drugs reduce activity, cause ataxia or stupor, and interfere with learning processes such as acquired conditioned reflexes. They control conflict behaviour in experimental neurons.

In man performance of tasks, especially those requiring sustained concentration and vigilance or those which are complex, is impaired. Small doses are activating and/or euphorant; higher doses lead through sedation and drowsiness, to sleep and then deep anaesthesia. Initially, there is a slight fall in blood pressure and depression of respiration, but marked autonomic and respiratory depression only occur at high doses.

Barbiturates have largely fallen out of use in psychiatry. This is because tolerance develops to them (through enzyme induction), and larger doses are needed for the same effect. More importantly, the brain habituates to their presence. A true physical dependence develops, with serious side-effects on withdrawal, such as panic, insomnia, epilepsy, etc. Other unwanted effects include toxic overdosage and drug rashes.

Tricyclic antidepressants

In the late 1950s a number of drugs with structures similar to those of the phenothiazines were being tried out for their sedative or hypnotic characteristics. One of these was imipramine, a drug which has a similar structure to promazine and differs from it only in the substitution of an ethylene bridge for the linking S atom of the phenothiazine structure. Because of their three-ring molecular conformation this group of drugs became known colloquially as the 'tricyclic' antidepressants.

It was Kuhn who noticed that this new compound, imipramine, was ineffective in quieting agitated psychiatric patients but seemed to have antidepressant qualities. Subsequently, he gave the drug to patients with a range of depressive syndromes and came to the conclusion that it was those with depression of the endogenous type who did best.

Formulae

The formulae of some of the tricyclic antidepressants are given in *Figure 9.8*. They bear a striking resemblance to the phenothiazine structure and, in fact, as mentioned previously, imipramine, the first compound of the group, was an attempt to develop the promazine structure into a more actively antipsychotic drug. The considerable and important differences between these two superficially similar groups of compounds may be in their molecular conformations. The phenothiazines have a planar structure, in contrast to the tricyclic drugs, where the

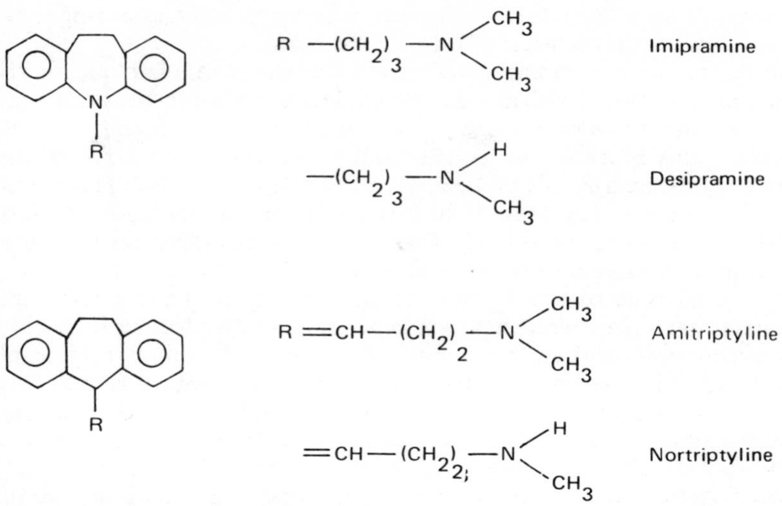

Figure 9.8 Tricyclic antidepressants

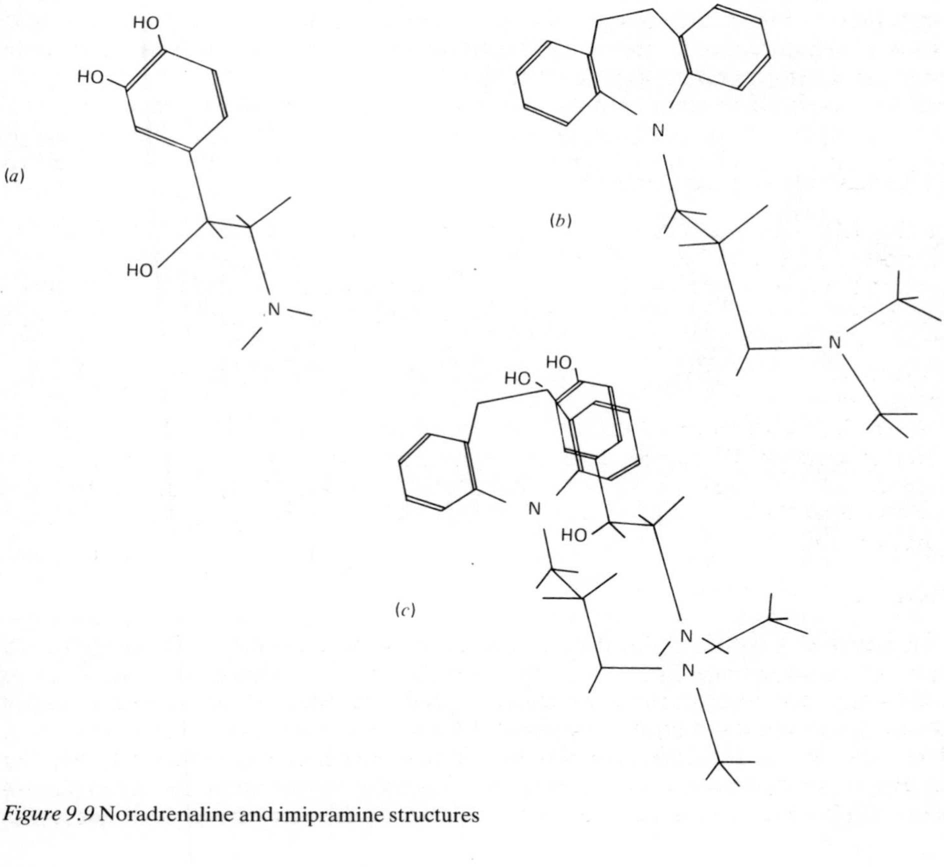

Figure 9.9 Noradrenaline and imipramine structures

substitution of the ethylene bridge gives the benzene rings a dihedral angle of 90–180° between them—a quite different form of structure.

Quite a lot of the discussion on tricyclic drugs will centre on their blockade of uptake of noradrenaline and 5-HT at the presynaptic membrane of aminergic neurons. It is assumed that this process involves a receptor site to which the drugs also bind to achieve this blockade of uptake, and there have been attempts to describe the possible characteristic of this site. One possible conformation has been suggested for noradrenaline together with a possible corresponding preferred conformation for imipramine (*Figure 9.9*). The two crucial binding sites on these molecules for the noradrenergic re-uptake receptor are the phenyl ring (or one benzene ring on the tricyclic structure) and the distal nitrogen of the side-chain, which clearly correspond. However, there are other possible conformations.

Similar attempts, not illustrated here, have been made to compare crucial binding sites on the 5-HT molecule with tricyclics which block uptake of 5-HT.

Pharmacology

The property of tricyclic antidepressants of blocking uptake of noradrenaline or 5-HT at the presynaptic membrane of aminergic neurons is one which should increase the amounts of these amines in the synaptic cleft into which they have been released. The process of uptake is a high-affinity temperature-dependent mechanism requiring metabolic energy and the activity of Na/K-stimulated ATPase, and that for noradrenaline is stereospecific for the L-isomer. The actions of tricyclic drugs on it are by competitive inhibition.

Tricyclic antidepressants tend to be one of two types—the tertiary dimethylamine compounds (imipramine, clomipramine, amitryptiline, etc.) and the secondary methylamines (desipramine, nortriptyline, protriptyline, etc.). They tend to act on both noradrenergic and 5-HT neurons but to different extents. Both types act on noradrenergic neurons, but the secondary amine drugs (nortriptyline) are the more powerful in this respect, and act predominantly on this system.

For the 5-HT pathways, on the other hand, the tertiary amine drugs (amitryptyline, etc.) are the more active. It should be emphasized, however, that even the tertiary amine drugs have more effect (in most instances) on the noradrenergic than on the serotoninergic neurons. The exception is clomipramine, which is 3–10 times more potent on 5-HT uptake than on that of noradrenaline. (However, *in vivo* it will be converted to its secondary amine product, which again tends to select noradrenergic neurons.)

None of the tricyclic drugs has much effect on the re-uptake of dopamine.

Many of the studies of the effects of tricyclic antidepressants have been after acute treatments, but there has been an increasing interest in some of the longer-term actions which may mimic their use in humans more closely than do shorter-term experiments.

It is becoming clear now that with time adaptive changes take place in aminergic systems treated with tricyclic drugs. For instance, it has been shown that there is a decrease in firing rate in 5-HT pathways (raphe), and a decrease in turnover of 5-HT. Similarly, noradrenaline turnover is reduced, and this is associated with a slowly developing reduction in activity of tyrosine hydroxylase.

Receptor activity is changed by chronic administration of tricyclic drugs. For instance, in the rat the response to a 5-HT agonist by cortical cells is reduced in acute exposures to imipramine, but is enhanced if a brief wash-out period is allowed in the chronic experiment. This suggests increased receptor responsiveness by 5-HT receptors in the type of treatment used in antidepressant therapy in humans.

What might be expected from the properties of tricyclic drugs on re-uptake of noradrenaline is their activity at low dosage to potentiate the effects of endogenous and exogenous noradrenaline at peripheral sites, as demonstrated in the cardiovascular system, etc. They block the actions of indirectly acting sympathomimetic drugs and adrenergic blocking hypotensive compounds such as guanethidine. This is a result of competition at the re-uptake receptor, preventing these drugs getting into noradrenergic neurons.

Tricyclic antidepressant drugs reverse the syndrome in rats and mice elicited by reserpine or tetrabenazine, and, indeed, this property was used to detect new antidepressant compounds. The reserpine syndrome is characterized by inertness and failure to explore the environment, extrapyramidal signs, and increased parasympathetic and decreased sympathetic activity (ptosis, meiosis, diarrhoea, bradycardia, salivation) and hypothermia. Antagonism of central and peripheral effects of reserpine is largely due to potentiation of noradrenergic pathways.

In the chapter on depression there is a further discussion of the possible modes of action of tricyclic drugs. At this point it should be pointed out that not all tricyclic drugs block presynaptic amine re-uptake (e.g. Opipramol and iprindol), although these drugs have other actions on aminergic mechanisms.

In general, tricyclic and some other antidepressants tend to decrease beta and increase (some) 5-HT and alpha postsynaptic receptor sensitivities.

Effects in man

NORMAL CONTROLS

Unlike some other drugs with antidepressant properties, the tricyclic group do not alter the mood of normal individuals appreciably. Such people given imipramine tend to feel sleepy and are quietened; they may experience a fall in blood pressure and sometimes feel light-headed. Some find the experience unpleasant, with activation of anxiety, poor performance in work tests, etc.

There are accompanying anticholinergic side-effects, as evidenced by dryness of the mouth, blurred vision and difficulty in micturition. Normal people also may complain of their tiredness and clumsiness, and after a few doses may feel that their concentration and thinking processes are impaired.

DEPRESSED PATIENTS

For reasons which are not clear most depressed patients tolerate imipramine and, indeed, other tricyclic drugs more readily. In contrast to normals, their mood is elevated, but although the process is progressive, it is slow, taking many weeks to be completed.

Patients with the bipolar type of affective illness may become manic, which may or may not be an effect of the drug on any one occasion. Some patients, thought otherwise to have unipolar illness, seem to have a 'driven', slightly overactive phase at the end of a period of treatment with tricyclic antidepressants, which some clinicians hesitate to label as 'hypomanic' and often consider to be a side-effect of the drug.

OTHER EFFECTS IN MAN

Some of the tertiary amine tricyclic antidepressants have a quite powerful hypnotic effect but are not used much for this purpose, because they tend to produce a hangover. These hypnotic antidepressant drugs tend to decrease the number of awakenings, increase stage 4 and diminish REM sleep. In contrast, secondary amine tricyclics may be activating and therefore are of use with the apathetic or retarded patient.

Tricyclic antidepressants have variable actions on the autonomic nervous system. The configuration of the side-chain gives them anticholinergic side-effects (dry mouth, blurred vision, constipation and urinary retention). Some of their actions on the autonomic nervous system are not immediately explicable. They partially inhibit autonomic ganglia to blunt cardiovascular reflexes. This is most in evidence in the common side-effect of postural hypotension.

On the whole, however, tricyclic antidepressants are not advisable where there is any cardiac pathology. They tend to produce tachycardia (possibly from potentiation of noradrenaline; possibly from an atropine-like action), produce inversion and flattening of T waves and increase the tendency to arrhythmias.

It has been suggested that a particularly harmful combination of tricyclic antidepressants, cardiac disease and stress can lead to cardiac arrest.

Absorption and metabolism

As a group, the tricyclic antidepressants are readily absorbed and rapidly distributed. As mentioned above, the tertiary amine tricycylic compounds are partly converted to their secondary amine derivative, so that amitriptyline is converted to nortriptyline, imipramine to desmethylimipramine, etc. Other routes of metabolism include oxidation and aromatic hydroxylation, the pharmacological activity being lost in hydroxylation at the 2 positions. The hydroxylated compounds are excreted as glucuronates in urine or faeces (via the bile).

There is a very wide spectrum of plasma levels at steady state and in half-lives of the drug. These drugs are metabolized by the hepatic microsomal enzymes, so that drugs which inhibit or evoke these will affect the metabolism of tricyclic compounds. Excretion of the drug is quite rapid. Since the activity of the hepatic systems is so variable in different individuals, similar doses of a tricyclic drug may give 20–40-fold differences in plasma levels.

Quite a lot of work has been done on plasma levels and their relationship to antidepressant response. Some reports have shown no relationship, while some (especially with the secondary amine tricyclic nortriptyline) suggest an inverted U-shaped plasma level–response curve—a therapeutic window with high and low levels being relatively ineffective. Some reports on tertiary amine tricyclics have given a proportional response with no upper limit, while others do not. Clearly, the situation has to be clarified further.

It is claimed that with time patients develop some tolerance to anticholinergic side-effects and postural hypotension. It is premature to claim this, in the absence of detailed information on change of level of drug in the body. Although tricyclic

TABLE 9.5. Benzodiazepines

Benzodiazepines	1	2	Structure 3 (see page 192)	4	7	*	Initial oral dose (mg)	Daily dose range (mg)	Approximate mean half-life of parent compound (hours)
Chlordiazepoxide (Librium)	–	NH CH$_3$	H$_2$	O	Cl	–	10–50	15–200	12
Diazepam (Valium)	CH$_3$	O	H$_2$	–	Cl	–	5–20	6–40	32
Medazepam (Nobrium)	CH$_3$ H$_2$		H$_2$	–	Cl	–	5–15	5–30	2
Oxazepam (Serenid)	H	O	H,OH	–	Cl	–	15–60	30–120	8
Lorazepam (Ativan)	H	O	HOH	–	Cl	Cl	1–2.5	1–7.5	12
Clonazepam (Rivotril)	H	O	H$_2$	–	NO$_2$	Cl	0.5	2–8	53
Nitrazepam (Mogadon, Remnos)	H	O	H$_2$	–	NO$_2$	–	5–10	5–20	28
Flurazepam X^a (Dalmane)		O	H$_2$	–	Cl	F	15	15–30	1
Clorazepate (Tranxene)	H	OH.OK	HCOOK	–	Cl	–	7.5–30	15–60	2
Clobazam (Frisium)	CH$_3$	O	H$_2$	O	Cl	–	20	20–60	18
Normison	CH$_3$	O	H$_2$	O	Cl	–	10–20	10–60	5–8

^{a}X $= -(CH_2)_2N(C_2H_5)_2$

drugs are not powerful invokers of the hepatic microsomal enzyme system, they have some effect, and levels in the body may fall with time. This could explain part of the 'habituation' process in regard to side-effects.

Drugs which compete with the hepatic microsomal system decrease rate of degradation of tricyclic drugs. This property has been used by giving methylphenedate continuously with imipramine, which has led to rises in steady state levels as high as 2½-fold.

There are a few reports of some side-effects on acute withdrawal from high doses, but this is not a common phenomenon, and usually patients experience no effects from sudden cessation of therapy.

Mild side-effects include those due to the anticholinergic properties, dry mouth, constipation, difficulty in accommodation, difficulty in micturition and others such as sweating (of unknown origin), weakness and fatigue (probably central) and,

TABLE 9.5. Continued

Benzodiazepines	Active metabolites (approximate half-life in hours)			
Chlordiazepoxide (Librium)	1. Desmethyl chlordiazepoxide (14)	2. Demoxepam (37)	3. n-Desmethyl-diazepam (65)	4. Oxazepam (8)
Diazepam (Valium)	1. n-Desmethyl-diazepam (65)	2. Oxazepam (8)		
Medazepam (Nobrium)	1. n-Desmethyl-diazepam (65)	2. Oxazepam (8)		
Oxazepam (Serenid)	None			
Lorazepam (Ativan)	None			
Clonazepam (Rivotril)	None			
Nitrazepam (Mogadon, Remnos)	None			
Flurazepam (Dalmane)	n-Hydroxy-ethyl flurazepam	N_1-Desalkylflurazepam (65)		
Clorazepate (Tranxene)	1. n-Desmethyl-diazepam (65)	2. Oxazepam (8)		
Clobazam (Frisium)	N-Desmethyl clobazam (42)			
Normison (Temazepam)	None			

quite commonly, headache, fine tremor and epigastric discomfort. Side- and toxic effects are most often seen in the elderly. Bipolar patients may become manic and, as mentioned above, arguably, unipolar patients may become overactive. Hallucinations, delusions and confusional states occur but are not too common in the usual dosage range.

Mild Parkinsonism may be seen, especially in the elderly, and people subject to fits may have seizures precipitated by the use of tricyclic drugs. Allergic jaundice, probably of the chlorpromazine type, is a rare complication of tricyclic therapy, as are agranulocytosis, eosinophilia, skin rashes and photosensitivity.

Tricyclic drugs may interact with MAOI, central depressive drugs, thyroid hormones, antihypertensive drugs of the guanethidine type, sympathomimetic drugs and indirectly acting sympathomimetic drugs, as discussed above.

TABLE 9.5. Continued

Benzodiazepines	Uses	Comments			
Chlordiazepoxide (Librium) Diazepam (Valium)	Anxiety, insomnia, status epilepticus, muscle relaxant, DTs, LSD reactions, abreaction, premedication	Long half-lives } Steady state	Then single daily dose is sufficient	With habituation withdrawal symptoms may occur 5–7 days after cessation of drugs	
Medazepam (Nobrium)	Night terrors } in children Somnabulism	Rarely abnormal paradoxical reactions, aggression, excitement, confusion, uncovering of depression			
Oxazepam (Serenid)	Anxiety states, phobic states, insomnia	No active metabolites }	Steady state 2 days	Fairly short half-life, 4–20 h	
Lorazepam (Ativan)	Phobic states, anxiety states, premedication				
Clonazepam (Rivotril)	Anticonvulsant				
Nitrazepam (Mogadon, Remnos)	Usually for insomnia but half-life can result in hangover effect	May give confusion in elderly because of length of half-life			
Flurazepam (Dalmane)	For insomnia and daytime sedation, anxiety states, phobic states and premedication				
Clorazepate (Tranxene)	As for diazepam	Long half-life (see diazepam and chlordiazepoxide above)			
Clobazam (Frisium)	Anxiety states	Fairly long half-life			
Normison (Temazepan)	Insomnia, anxiety states				

They are used for the treatment of depression, obsessive compulsive disorders and eneuresis.

New antidepressants

Nomifensine

The structure of this novel compound is given in *Figure 9.10*. It has been tried as an antidepressant from 1970 onwards, with promising results.

Nomifensine is absorbed rapidly from all routes of administration, gives peak plasma levels in 1–2 hours and has a half-life of about 2 hours. The drug is bound to protein in plasma, but is rapidly distributed throughout the body.

TABLE 9.6. Tricyclic antidepressants: Drug interactions

Drug	Interaction	
MAOI	Excitement, restlessness, dilated pupil, muscle twitching, hyperpyrexia, loss of conciousness	Start the two drugs together. Use only well-tried combinations—e.g. phenelzine and amitriptyline
Sympathomimetic agents noradrenaline	Enhanced precursor effects	
adrenaline (e.g. in local anaesthetics) isoprenaline	Enhanced and prolonged broncho-dilator effects	
indirectly acting sympathomimetics	Prevention of their action (tricyclics block their entry to sympathomimetic neurons)	
Hypotensive agents guanethidine bethanidine desbrisoquin vasodilators	Blockade of their effect by prevention of their entry to sympathomimetic neurons	
Analgesics/antirheumatics phenazone phenylbutazone	Effects prolonged Reduced absorption from gastrointestinal tract	
Anticoagulants bishydroxycoumarin	Enhanced effect (enzyme inhibition)	
Anticonvulsants	Tricyclics may enhance convulsant activity or induce it *de novo*	
Anticholinergics e.g. antihistamines, antiemetics	Enhanced atropine-like actions, blurred vision, dry mouth, urine retention, increased intraocular pressure, constipation, paralytic ileus	
Tranquillizers alcohol barbiturates ethchlorvynol chlorpromazine	Enhanced CNS depression Increased antidepressant effect (enzyme inhibition)	

Nomifensine   Mianserin   Viloxazine

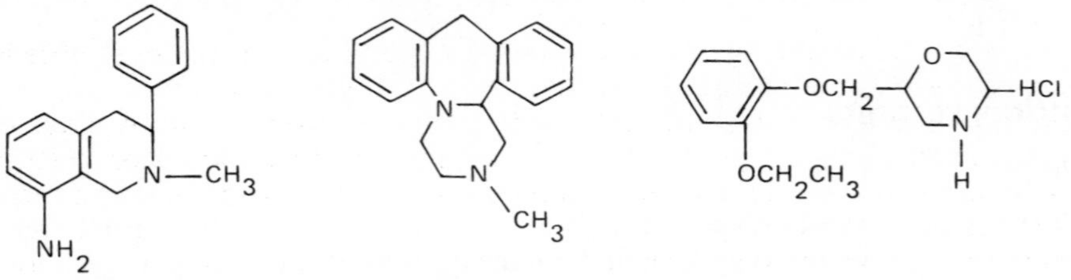

Figure 9.10 New antidepressants

TABLE 9.7. Tricyclic antidepressants

	Usual daily dose (mg)
Iminodibenzyl derivatives	
Imipramine (Tefranil, Berkomine, Dimipressin, Impramin, Praminil, Co-Caps, Imipramine)	75–300
Desimipramine (Pertofran), Norpramin, Petrofane (Desmethylimipramine)	75–300
Trimipramine (Surmontil)	50–300
Clomipramine (Anafranil)	75–200
Dibenzocycloheptadiene derivatives	
Amitriptyline (Laroxyl, Lentizol, *Limbritol, Saroten, Tritafen-DA, Elavil, *Triptafen-Forte, *Triptafen Minor, Tryptizol, Glavil, Endep)	75–300
Nortriptyline (Allegron, Aventyl), *Altilev, *Motival	50–150
Protriptyline (Concordin, Vivactyl)	15–60
Butriptyline (Evandyne)	150–300
Other tricyclics	
Doxepin, Sinequan	50–300
Dothiepin, Prothiaden	75–250
Opipramol, Insidon	150–300
Dibenzepin, Noveril	160–560
Mianserin, Bolvidon, Norval	20–120 or more
Tricyclic with 'bridge'	
Maprotiline, Ludiomil	75–150

*Formulated with other drugs.

Most of the drug or its metabolites appears in the urine within the first 2 days of administration, and there is no accumulation of the drug in the body.

Like many other antidepressants, nomifensine antagonizes the effects of reserpine in animals. It does not inhibit monoamine oxidase, but seems to act by blocking the re-uptake of noradrenaline and dopamine at the presynaptic membrane. This involvement of dopamine and nomifensine has been demonstrated *in vitro* (platelets), it antagonizes the behavioural effects of depletion of dopamine and produces stereotypes in rats similar to apomorphine and amphetamines. There is some evidence for and against a postsynaptic activation of dopamine receptors.

Release of catecholamines is probably unaffected by nomifensine. Nomifensine has little *direct* activity in 5-HT systems (although *in vivo* stimulation of dopaminergic neurons will influence serotoninergic pathways). A metabolite, 4-hydroxynomifensine, blocks re-uptake of 5-HT at the presynaptic membrane, but this substance is present in very low concentration after the administration of the parent drug.

Nomifensine has few side-effects, is considered at this time to be relatively safe in patients with cardiovascular disease and has no epileptogenic activity.

Nomifensine has both anxiolytic and antidepressant properties, but it tends to counteract inhibition and restore drive. This means that care should be used in giving it by itself to severely depressed patients who are a suicidal risk, and it is unsuitable for the agitated depressive.

Nomifensine can be given in sequence following MAOI and vice versa without problems. There are no published data on the use of MAOI and nomifensine together.

TABLE 9.8. Side-effects of tricyclic antidepressants

Early (within 24 h)	Dry mouth, difficulty with accommodation, postural hypotension, sweating, constipation, headache, difficulty in micturition
	Tertiary amine tricyclics (e.g. clomipramine, amitriptyline) tend to be sedative and cause drowsiness and ataxia
	Secondary amine tricyclics (e.g. nortriptyline) tend to be activating
	Potentiation effects alcohol and CNS depressants
	With special susceptibility (often pre-existing pathology) or drugs:
	Retention of urine, glaucoma, tachycardia*, arrhythmias*, heart block*.
	Hypertension in some patients on some antihypertensives (e.g. guanethidine).
	Epilepsy *de novo* or worsening established epilepsy
	Sudden death usually in stressed individuals (cold, exercise, emotional, etc.)
Later (2 or more weeks)	Tremor, gain weight, epilepsy, toxic hallucinosis (especially elderly), paralytic ileus, Parkinsonian tremor, akinesia, rigidity muscles.
	Disturbed sexual function.
	Hypomania
Rare effects	Allergic skin rashes, choleostatic jaundice, agranulocytosis, anxiety and agitation, insomnia
Withdrawal	Usually no effects.
	Gastrointestinal disturbances—nausea and vomiting
Overdosage	Agitation, hallucinations, hyperpyrexia, hyperreflexia progressing to coma 1–3 h. Arrhythmias and hypotension.
	Convulsions, status epilepticus

*CVS effects include tachycardia, prolonged QT interval, depressed ST segments, flattened T waves.

Mianserin

Mianserin is a tetracyclic compound (*Figure 9.10*) synthesized in 1966, which was thought of initially as useful as a potential 5-HT antagonist. That it might have antidepressant qualities was deduced from the finding that an analysis of its effects on the EEG were similar to that of amitriptyline. Since then clinical trials have supported the claim that it is an effective antidepressant.

It is readily absorbed orally, giving a plasma peak at 2–3 hours; its half-life is 6–12 hours, and a steady state is achieved after about 2 weeks. There is significant 'first pass' metabolism of the drug; the drug is bound in the plasma but widely distributed in the body. It enters the brain readily and is distributed evenly throughout the brain. Very little of the drug leaves the body in unchanged form, but there are few data on the activity of the various metabolites. The pattern of pharmacological activity is quite different from that of the tricyclic drugs and it does not inhibit monoamine oxidase. Any effects on blockade of re-uptake mechanisms of amines are so weak as to be negligible, as also is anticholinergic activity.

One action is to block presynaptic α_2-receptors and thereby increase stimulus-induced Ca^{2+}-dependent release of noradrenaline *in vitro* and *in vivo*, and turnover of noradrenaline. It is sedative and of use in alleviating anxiety.

Cardiotoxicity is much less than with tricyclic drugs. In general, it has few adverse effects—like many other antidepressants, it can activate latent epilepsy, and must be given with care to patients with unstable diabetes mellitus.

One group have suggested an inverted 'U' plasma response curve for mianserin—i.e. the existence of 'a therapeutic window' for this drug.

Recently an interaction with phenytoin (increased levels of the latter) has been suggested.

Viloxazine

Viloxazine (*Figure 9.10*) was synthesized in 1967 by ICI. It is unlike other antidepressants in structure and is related chemically to propranolol. While chemical trials have shown it to be antidepressant, the number of patients who develop nausea and/or vomiting have prevented its use on a large scale.

Like other antidepressants, viloxazine antagonizes reserpine-induced effects in animals, and its main pharmacological action seems to be that of blockade of re-uptake of noradrenaline across the presynaptic membrane. There are no effects on dopamine and minimal effects on 5-HT systems.

The main justification for retaining viloxazine as an antidepressant drug for occasional use is the fact that it has low cardiovascular toxicity, and antiepileptic properties, and appears to exert its therapeutic effect quite rapidly.

Trazodone

Trazodone is a newly introduced antidepressant drug with, again, a quite novel type of structure (*Figure 9.11*). It is absorbed rapidly orally and is excreted as metabolites in urine and faeces. Trazodone is mildly sedative, has no anticonvulsant properties and is not anticholinergic. It differs from tricyclic antidepressants in

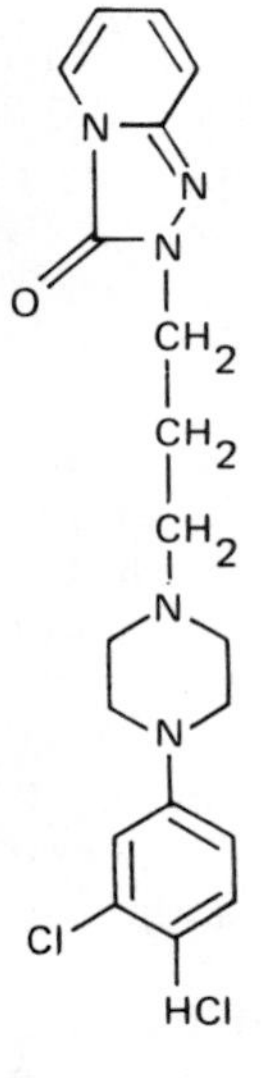

Figure 9.11 Trazodone

being free of re-uptake blockade activity at the presynaptic membrane of noradrenergic or serotoninergic neurons. It blocks 5-HT receptors in the CNS and may decrease the sensitivity of central beta-receptors. Initial data on the drug suggest few side-effects, absence of cardiotoxicity and effectiveness as an antidepressant.

Flupenthixol

Flupenthixol is a thioxanthene neuroleptic (*Figure 9.2*), and therefore its appearance as an antidepressant compound might be unexpected. Its value as an antidepressant has been reported in a variety of depressive states by a number of groups giving doses much lower than that used for the drug's neuroleptic properties. The general characteristics of the neuroleptic compounds have been described elsewhere in this chapter (pages 169–176). Flupenthixol has been used as an antidepressant in trials in both outpatient departments and general practice, and seems to have a wide spectrum of antidepressant activity. Further studies are needed to characterize both its spectrum of activity in the various types of depression and the optimum dose ranges. It is now claimed that flupenthixol decanoate given intramuscularly as a maintenance therapy is like lithium in preventing recurrences of affective illness. If these claims are substantiated by further studies, flupenthixol and flupenthixol decanoate, at the low level of administration suggested, will prove to be extremely safe and trouble-free additions to the antidepressive armamentarium.

Electroconvulsive therapy (ECT)

Though not quite fitting into the area of psychopharmacology, a discussion of ECT has been included here. ECT and chemical convulsive therapy were introduced by Cerletti and Bini and by Meduna in 1938, on the basis of the mistaken idea that epilepsy and schizophrenia were incompatible illnesses. Since then ECT has come into use mostly for the treatment of the depressive phases of affective illness—i.e. those illnesses characterized by depression; diurnal variation of mood; sleep disturbance; loss of appetite, weight and libido; retardation; delusions of guilt or catastrophe; paranoid, nihilistic and somatic delusions; etc.

Efficacy of ECT

The evidence for and against its efficacy is confused, many of the studies being uncontrolled and/or with groups of patients of various diagnosis. Where the studies have been controlled, ECT has emerged as being particularly useful for the depressive phase of affective illness, especially of recent onset. The MRC trial of 1965, for instance, showed ECT to be significantly superior to imipramine, phenelzine and placebo at 4 weeks (i.e. it has an advantage in the early stages of treatment). The superiority to imipramine was lost at a later date of assessment. Interestingly, in this trial males showed equal early response to ECT and imipramine, and it was the females who had the significantly better response to ECT.

An assessment of all the evidence, which cannot be discussed in detail here, led to the conclusion in recent reviews by the Royal College of Psychiatry, by Kendall and others, that ECT is clearly better than placebo and more rapidly acting, or at least as good as tricyclic drugs.

There still remain some 15–24 per cent of patients who do not respond to treatment with ECT. Some have past histories of prolonged illness and/or have been ill for a long time in the current episode, but further work is needed here.

Could ECT (when successful) be due to a placebo response to the drama of anaesthetic, etc? A recent trial in Edinburgh and another by West giving 'dummy' ECTs to some patients did not support the placebo view. The fit seems to be necessary and there is a lesser response if the duration of seizure is shortened.

Other means of inducing convulsions (e.g. Indoklon) are as effective as ECT, and photoconvulsive treatments also may be as good as ECT.

Effects of ECT

Given that a convulsion produces such a profound and acute alteration in cerebral activity, it is not surprising that there is a large literature on the systems in the brain at least temporarily altered by this treatment.

Recently interest has centred on the observation that ECT increased the sensitivity of dopaminergic and noradrenergic agonists in mice after pretreatment with reserpine. Subsequently these observations have been extended to 5-HT and other transmitter systems, and one view is that some complex changes induced in postsynaptic receptors by spaced ECTs increasing their sensitivity may be important in the therapeutic actions of ECT. This view has not gone unchallenged. Other workers were unable to replicate their findings but produced results pointing to a decrease in noradrenergic beta-receptor activity.

In man ECT is modified by atropine and a muscle relaxant. Under these conditions there is tachycardia and rise in blood pressure to up to 200 mmHg, and cerebral blood flow is doubled. Transient arrhythmias, especially in patients with previous cardiac pathology, occur frequently, but are usually brief. The EEG develops a diffuse slowing, an increase in voltage and a reduction in fast activity lasting for 8–12 weeks. Unlike antidepressant drugs, there is an increase in REM sleep but a decrease in total sleep.

SIDE- AND UNWANTED EFFECTS

Headache and mild confusion are common as an immediate aftermath of ECT. Some patients complain of aches in their muscles, usually in the jaw, neck or shoulders.

The most controversial problem is that of the effect of ECT on memory. Occasionally, patients say that they lose 'islands' of memory for remote events at least temporarily (several weeks) after bilateral ECT. Patients may lose memory for a period of confusion following the seizure, and for several weeks have difficulty in learning new verbal and non-verbal material. Again this is more marked for bilateral ECT than for unilateral ECT to the non-dominant hemisphere.

The most important possible deleterious effect of ECT is on long-term memory. Recent testing suggests that any defects from unilateral non-dominant ECT have gone by 3 months, and from bilateral ECT at 7 months in patients under 65. (Patients over 65 seem to have cumulative defects in this area with bilateral ECT and probably ECT should be limited to unilateral only in this group.)

It is not possible to say whether changes in cognitive function occur with ECT which are too subtle for our tests, or whether there is a subgroup in whom ECT produces some longer-term defects.

A complication is that cognitive impairment from depression and from chronic or subchronic illness may provide a background of marked to mild cognitive impairment against which it becomes difficult to assess any additional effects of ECT, and it should be remembered that psychotropic drugs themselves may contribute to cognitive problems.

Morbidity from ECT is mostly cardiorespiratory, but fortunately nowadays is rare. ECT may provoke angina, cardiac failure, arrhythmias or coronary thrombosis in those predisposed by pre-existing susceptibility. The occasional person may develop aspiration pneumonia, or have a pulmonary embolism or a period of prolonged apnoea. ECT is said to predispose to the dissemination of tuberculosis from an active but hitherto localized pulmonary lesion. Other rare complications include cerebrovascular accidents, status epilepticus, subconjunctival haemorrhage and bleeding from a peptic ulcer.

Patients usually excluded from ECT are those with acute respiratory infections, cardiac failure, aneurysms, myocardial infarction within 3 months and those with cardiac pacemakers. Other contraindications include osteoporosis, major fractures, brain tumours and active peptic ulcers.

Mortality

Mortality from ECT is probably in the range 3–9 per 100000 treatments and tends to occur during or immediately following ECT. This makes it a safe treatment, especially when the expected mortality from affective illness by suicide is 10 per cent in 5 years and 15 per cent in 10 years. In the three years following ECT mortality from suicide is lower than in those treated inadequately with antidepressant drugs or given neither drugs nor ECT.

Unilateral versus bilateral ECT

The duration of a fit may parallel efficacy but the amount of electrical energy passed may be related to memory loss. In an attempt to minimize the effects on memory, unilateral ECT to the non-dominant hemisphere has been helpful in this area, and unilateral ECT is the treatment of choice in the over-65s.

The evidence taken together, however, suggests, but by no means conclusively, that bilateral ECT is more effective than unilateral ECT. If ECT is reserved for the most pressing clinical condition, then some clinicians will favour bilateral treatment at least in patients under 65. This is a subject requiring further study.

Choice of patients with affective disorder for treatment with ECT

If the physical contraindications to ECT have been excluded, which patients should be selected for this treatment? With the advent of new antidepressant treatments and a growing skill in the use of both the established drugs and prophylactic compounds, the number of patients requiring ECT should be decreasing, until eventually it should become almost obsolete. This point has not been reached yet.

Most clinicians reserve ECT for the following:

(1) Patients who are a major risk for determined attempts at suicide.
(2) Patients with severe illness accompanied by psychotic symptoms such as delusions, where ECT is the treatment of choice.
(3) Where there is intolerance to a drug or drugs (unlikely with the breadth of choice), where the illness is drug-resistant, or when the patient comes to reject drug treatment.
(4) When there is a past history of failing to respond to drugs, but of an early improvement with ECT.

Uses of ECT in conditions other than the depressive phase of affective illness

Schizophrenia ECT has a limited use in patients with features of secondary endogenous-type depressive illness, but the evidence in favour of using it in acute or chronic illness is not well established.

Mania There have been few studies of ECT in this condition, although one extensive retrospective survey suggested some benefit for mania. The number of ECTs required was rather large. Ashcroft has suggested its brief use initially in the most severe form of mania when drug treatment has been rejected. Mania not controlled by neuroleptics is uncommon, but when it occurs the patient may die from exhaustion if not given ECT.

Puerperal psychoses Many patients with puerperal psychosis respond well to ECT.

Other conditions Treatment with ECT of other conditions has not been established.

Lithium

Studies of the pharmacological properties of lithium salts in man have been bedevilled by a number of problems. The essential features of its therapeutic use in man are that it is given as a long-term or relatively long-term treatment, and that this is in doses which give 12-hour plasma values generally in the region of $0.5–1.2$ mmol/ℓ. Acute effects are relatively unimportant in this context, but many of the studies have been on animals with an exposure to the drug of from hours to a few days. Fairly prolonged metabolic readjustments occur with continued treatment, and these short experiments in animals may be quite irrelevant to the use of lithium in man. Secondly, the dosage given in acute experiments in animals may be many times that of the day-to-day maintenance levels, and if given i.p. or i.m. will give rapid fluctuation of concentrations not seen in oral therapy in man. Finally, species differences—for instance, the difficulties of maintaining comparable plasma concentrations in rats and man, and interpreting the data therefrom—and the spuriousness of results from animals in lithium toxicity were not appreciated at first. However, these deficiencies are being or have been remedied, and the information on the effects of lithium both in man and in animals at relevant dosage schedules is increasing almost exponentially.

Lithium carbonate was discovered in 1817, and first introduced into medicine in the middle of the nineteenth century in the belief that the high solubility of lithium urates which might be formed would help in the alleviation of gout. Lithium bromide was used in the 1920s as a sedative and lithium salts were used in the 1940s as a substitute for people on low salt diets. This latter use of lithium was a disastrous error on the grounds that salt depletion is the condition most likely to give rise to lithium toxicity. Indeed there were fatalities from the use of lithium in these patients.

In 1949 Cade claimed that lithium salts could be used to suppress mania, an observation which was soon confirmed by other workers. The next step in its use in psychiatric treatment was by Schou and Baastrup, who described an effect of long-term treatment which attenuated or prevented attacks of mania or depression. A controversy followed as to whether this claim was valid, but subsequent trials have supported the original findings.

Lithium has been tried subsequently in other conditions—cyclothymia, hyperactivity syndromes, sociopathy, aggression, the premenstrual tension syndrome, alcoholism, addiction, etc., but the main discussion of the clinical use of this drug will be confined to affective illness, where most of the work has been done to date.

Pharmacology

Lithium is one of the group IA alkali metals which include sodium, potassium, rubidium and caesium. It has an atomic weight of 6.94 and forms highly soluble salts. In solution the radius of the hydrated lithium ion is the largest of the group IA metals, and in this form it compares in some of its properties with the group IIA divalent cations such as magnesium. This resemblance between lithium and group IIA divalent cations may be of some biological importance, because magnesium is the cofactor of many enzymic processes, and calcium, another group IIA cation, also has important biological roles. At therapeutic doses in man, the concentration of lithium in cells is comparable to that of magnesium.

The establishment of resting potentials and the processes underlying action potentials have been described in detail elsewhere in this book and will not be repeated here. During the resting potential lithium ions do not pass easily into the cell, but accumulate slowly, probably via entry through the sodium channels. The process is so slow that equilibration with the intracellular compartment may take 6 days or more to complete. Once inside the cell, lithium is extruded by the 'cation pump', a mechanism dependent on Na^+-K^+-ATPase which evicts sodium from the cell in exchange for potassium against the concentration gradients. Lithium reduces the efficiency of this process, but its transport outwards is so much slower and less efficient than that of sodium that the cells accumulate lithium slowly, while tending to lose potassium and sodium. The concentration of lithium within the cell thus becomes higher than that in the extracellular fluid in some tissues. It follows, therefore, that lithium might work therapeutically via changes in the properties of cell membranes as influenced by its effects on the distribution of electrolytes.

One of the ways by which cellular function is modulated is by the action of hormones. Fat-soluble hormones can cross cell membranes with ease, but this does not apply to the amino acid/amine and polypeptide hormones. These hormones often react with the enzyme adenylate cyclase in the cell membrane which converts ATP to cAMP ($3',5'$-adenosine monophosphate), which is part of a chain of events which lead to alterations in cell function (*see* page 70). In many tissues adenyl cyclase is inhibited by the presence of even quite low concentrations of lithium. This includes the brain, where the enzyme is in plentiful supply in the nuclea, in the mitochondrial fractions and in membranes. It may be that the inhibition of adenyl cyclase is due to competition with magnesium, the cofactor needed for conversion of ATP to cAMP, and that it is at this point that lithium is responsible for its effect on this process. Lithium is probably also inhibitory at a site further down the chain of events leading from hormone interaction with adenyl cyclase to the resultant alteration in cell metabolism.

Returning to the theme of magnesium and calcium, several authors have stressed the number of magnesium-dependent enzymes involved in a wide series of functions which may be inhibited by lithium. These include both Mg^{2+}-dependent ATPase, which may be needed for the phosphorylation of Na^+-K^+-ATPase (and therefore cationic transport at the cell membrane), and many of the magnesium-dependent enzymes involved in glycolysis.

Calcium and lithium probably interact in the region of the synapse (*see* below).

Synaptic vesicles are manufactured in the cell body and in noradrenergic neurons take up noradrenaline there, and in the terminal bulbs after their transportation down the axon. Stored catecholamine in the synaptic bulbs releases amine into a mobile presynaptic pool under the influence of Mg^+-ATPase. In this pool it can be degraded by MAO to inactive deaminated compounds.

After release of amines following an action potential, the amines are mostly reabsorbed across the presynaptic membrane or destroyed by catechol-*o*-methyl transferase (in the case here of catecholamines). In the short term, lithium causes increased deamination within noradrenergic systems, increase in re-uptake of the amine from the synaptic cleft and raised turnover. Lithium is known to be concentrated in synaptosomes as compared with some other areas of the neuron. In long-term experiments with lithium on rat brain, the management of noradrenaline has returned to nearer normal, perhaps with adjustment at a lower level of activity of noradrenergic function. One investigation suggested an inhibition of release of noradrenaline during chronic lithium treatment which could be antagonized by calcium. The general view at the moment is that the acute effects of lithium on noradrenaline in the brain are not continued into chronic treatment, but that some effects, perhaps a marginal 'quietening' of noradrenalergic function, may persist.

The changes in 5-HT are not entirely clear in long-term treatments. Turnover may be changed up or down, depending on the region sampled, but with decreased turnover being the most common findings. Other workers have suggested increased tryptophan uptake by synaptosomes, a decrease in tryptophan hydroxylase activity, but an increased production of 5-HT from tryptophan. Platelets from patients on lithium show an increase in 5-HT uptake as compared with those from normal controls, and there is evidence appearing suggesting reduced uptake by the platelets of patients with endogenous depression.

Lithium influences the endocrine system in several ways. One of these is that of partially blocking the effect of aldosterone, which results in an increased secretion of the hormone after several weeks, and possibly a slight increase long term. Lithium gives rise to an antidiuretic hormone (ADH)-resistant polyuria which initially was attributed to the blocking of ADH-sensitive adenyl cyclase in the kidney. The mechanism may be more complex than this, and may be associated also with specific histological changes in the collecting tubules.

Lithium acts on the thyroid gland to a significant extent in a few per cent of patients by blocking the action of thyroid-stimulating hormone (TSH), impairing coupling of iodotyrosines and interfering with release of the hormone. A number of patients develop low T4 or T3 levels, sometimes but not invariably associated with raised TSH levels, and move to the lower ends of the euthyroid range or become frankly hypothyroid. A smaller number show overt hypothyroidism to a greater extent than might be expected from the laboratory changes.

Weight gain is a complication for some patients. It may be partly central in origin, but otherwise its origins are not clear. Early in treatment there may be an increase in insulin release, but there are no consistent changes in, for instance, glucose tolerance curves during chronic therapy. Perhaps there are complicated and subtle changes in metabolism preceding the inhibition of many hormones using Mg^{2+} as cofactor which therefore alter energy mechanisms.

Absorption and distribution of lithium

Lithium is readily absorbed from the intestine and when given by other routes of administration. Its passage into cells is rapid in kidney and liver, but slow in brain, bone and muscle, which accounts for its slow equilibration in the body. Overall, lithium tends to accumulate in the cells, so that the lithium space is greater than that calculated from total body water. Distribution of lithium in the brain itself is non-uniform. The slow entry of lithium to the brain is also coupled with a slow exit time, a fact of some importance in patients who are in lithium toxicity.

Manic patients have a high tolerance for lithium and retain lithium, so that it is likely that it may enter their cells more rapidly than in control groups. It has been suggested that this rapid entry of lithium to cells in mania may also apply to depressed patients.

When lithium is taken by mouth as a single dose, most individuals have a peak level in plasma about 2 hours later, with a range of from 1 to 4 hours. The formulation of the drug used may affect bioavailability (e.g. slow release forms), but the two most commonly used drugs in the UK do not seem to differ much in this respect.

Of the lithium ingested, 90–95 per cent is excreted in the urine, the remainder being lost from the body in sweat, faeces, sputum, seminal fluid, and milk in the feeding mother. Some may be sequestered long-term in bone matrix.

The lithium ion passes freely through the glomerular capillaries, and 80 per cent is reabsorbed in the proximal tubules. Lithium and sodium may compete for the transport mechanism, because in sodium depletion more lithium is absorbed and in a sodium-enriched diet more lithium is excreted. The lithium remaining after absorption in the proximal tubule is concentrated in the loop of Henle, but is not reabsorbed like sodium in the distal tubules.

However, as the concentration of lithium in plasma rises, although it is not reabsorbed like sodium in the distal tubules, it begins to inhibit distal sodium absorption. This sets up a situation with positive feedback:

(1) A high lithium level decreases sodium reabsorption in the distal tubules.
(2) This results in failure to conserve sodium in the body.
(3) Sodium depletion leads to compensatory activity by the proximal tubules in which the uptake of Na^+ and of Li^+ is enhanced.
(4) This leads to a rise in blood levels of lithium and further wastage of sodium from the body.
(5) The net result is progressive lithium toxicity.

One of the effects of lithium is to give rise to a polydypsia/polyuria syndrome mentioned above, associated with histological changes in the collecting tubules and inhibition of the effect of ADH. There is argument about possibly central actions of lithium contributing in a less significant way to thirst and polyuria.

There is a relatively small gap between therapeutic and toxic ranges, with tolerance of lithium varying between individuals and falling with age.

Treatment with lithium

As mentioned earlier, lithium has been tried in a wide variety of conditions—acute depression, mania, aggression, emotional instability in children, thyrotoxicosis, premenstrual tension, alcoholism, cluster headaches, granulocytopenia, inappropriate secretion of ADH, etc. Its more or less established uses to date are confined to therapy of mania, the prevention of recurrence of affective illness, impulsive aggression, hyperthyroidism and granulocytopenia.

The question arises as to what is the appropriate dose of lithium. Lithium levels in plasma need to be monitored frequently at first and then at several-month intervals where long-term treatments are to be given. For a manic episode the plasma range of 0.8–1.2 mM/ℓ (or even slightly higher in young subjects) is acceptable provided that the dose is reduced *pari passu* with the break in mania, at which time tolerance for the drug declines. For long-term preventative or 'prophylactic' treatment the ideal dose range is a matter of some controversy. The range 0.8–1.2 mM/ℓ used to be the aim, and still is in some groups. Others are working in this range and reducing the input later when emotional stability has been maintained for a while, while yet others are trying a range of 0.4 or 0.9 to see if protection is afforded at these levels. Certainly, lower levels are often mandatory in the older age group where tolerance to lithium is limited.

The levels of lithium in plasma are those found 12 hours after the previous dose on a twice a day dosage schedule (the drug is given twice a day to avoid high plasma peaks).

Side-effects of lithium

People take time to acclimatize to lithium, so it is wise to introduce it in slowly progressive increments, starting at a low dose. In the initial phase of treatment there may be abdominal discomfort, nausea and loose stools, fine tremor, polyuria and polydipsia. Later patients may continue to have the tremor and polyuria or develop oedema, these later effects usually indicating too high a dosage. Many gain weight, and a few develop goitre.

Toxic levels may follow reduction in salt intake, where there is too high a dosage, in suicide attempts with lithium, and when some diuretics are taken. The signs of toxicity are coarse tremor of hands, vomiting and diarrhoea, polyuria and polydipsia, dizziness and dysarthria, sluggishness, progressing eventually to coma, with hypertonic muscles and hyperactive deep reflexes, generalized tremor or fasciculation. Sometimes there are epileptic attacks, and in the absence of knowledge of the cause, diagnosis of the cause may be made difficult by asymmetry of signs.

Monoamine oxidase (MAO) and monoamine oxidase inhibiting drugs (MAOIs)

Monoamine oxidase is an enzyme occurring widely in the body in brain, liver, heart, kidney, intestine, smooth muscle, blood vessels, etc. Monoamine oxidase is found in plasma, but elsewhere is situated on the outer surface of the membrane of mitochondria. In the brain it is present both in some neurons and in glial cells, and is in particularly high concentration in the regions where there are aminergic neurons.

Since monoamine oxidases catalyse the conversion of amines to inactive compounds and monoamine oxidase inhibitors block this enzyme, the presence of MAOIs is usually followed by increased levels of these amines.

When monoamine oxidase inhibitors block the monoamine enzyme system in the brain in this way, with those used therapeutically up to now, concentrations of 5-HT, noradrenaline and dopamine all rise, but the most powerful effect is on serotoninergic cells where the increments are proportionally higher in all the species studied to date. It is likely that in many of the described actions of MAOI, 5-HT plays a slightly more prominent role, but of course the other amines are involved as well.

In some systems when amine levels are modified, 5-HT and catecholamines act together, and in others they function antagonistically. Not all the effects of MAOIs can be ascribed to the three amines discussed above. There are many others in the brain some of which are normally present in only the most minute quantities under normal circumstances, but whose concentrations during exposure to MAOIs can rise to significant levels. For instance, MAOIs can result in the appearance of significant levels of octopamine and tryptamine.

Monoamine oxidase occurs in at least two forms—MAO-A and MAO-B. MAO-A is selectively inhibited by the drug chlorgyline; and noradrenaline, 5-HT and dopamine are mainly deaminated via the enzyme. MAO-B is selectively inhibited by deprenyl, and α-phenylethylamine and benzylamine are degraded mainly via this enzyme. Tryptamine, kynurenine (a metabolite of tryptophan) and tyramine are deaminated equally by the two enzymes.

The use of a selective blockade of MAO is already in use therapeutically (e.g. in the potentiation of dopamine in the treatment of Parkinson's disease using deprenyl, but this area is still in its infancy).

With inhibition of MAO, concentrations of amine rise in the nervous system to a steady state and remain at a limiting value. This is probably determined by negative feedback, one aspect of which is inhibition by the free amine of its corresponding hydroxylase. At the levels of amines achieved in the cell in response to MAOIs, they are released in larger aliquots during an action potential. This may produce negative feedback on production of amines via autoreceptors on the presynaptic neuronal membrane.

Noradrenaline and dopamine are sensitive to feedback, which starts at a concentration of 150 per cent of baseline values. 5-HT is less tightly controlled— there is little negative feedback at 200 per cent of baseline concentrations, but there are significant changes appearing from 300 per cent upwards leading to an associated decrease in turnover of 5-HT and a slowed firing rate from raphe cells.

According to some authors, monoamine oxidase inhibitors have little effect on amine levels until about 80–85 per cent of the enzyme has been destroyed. This fact has been ignored in the great majority of clinical trials, and even when dosage has been flexible, it has been impossible to evaluate the data because the proportion of patients in the group who are 'over the threshold' has not been known. This has made it particularly difficult to assess trials of these kinds apparently showing a good response to treatment in 'atypical patients', and a less satisfactory response in endogenous illness (*see* below).

Structure of MAOI

Most of the known MAOIs fit into the following pattern:

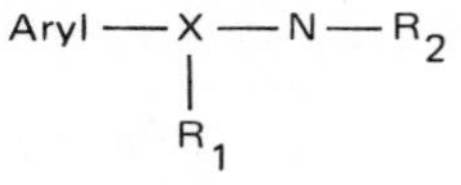

$$\text{Aryl} - \text{X} - \text{N} - \text{R}_2$$
$$\mid$$
$$\text{R}_1$$

The X moiety may be a cycloprophyl group, as in tranylcypromine, or an aliphatic group of 1 or 2 carbons and R_2 may be hydrogen or a more complex structure. *Figure 9.12* gives examples of some of the more widely used MAOIs. The structure of the MAOIs is not dissimilar to that of the normal substrates of MAO, and it is thought that there is an initial reversible binding of the drug to the enzyme followed by binding at greater affinity which becomes irreversible.

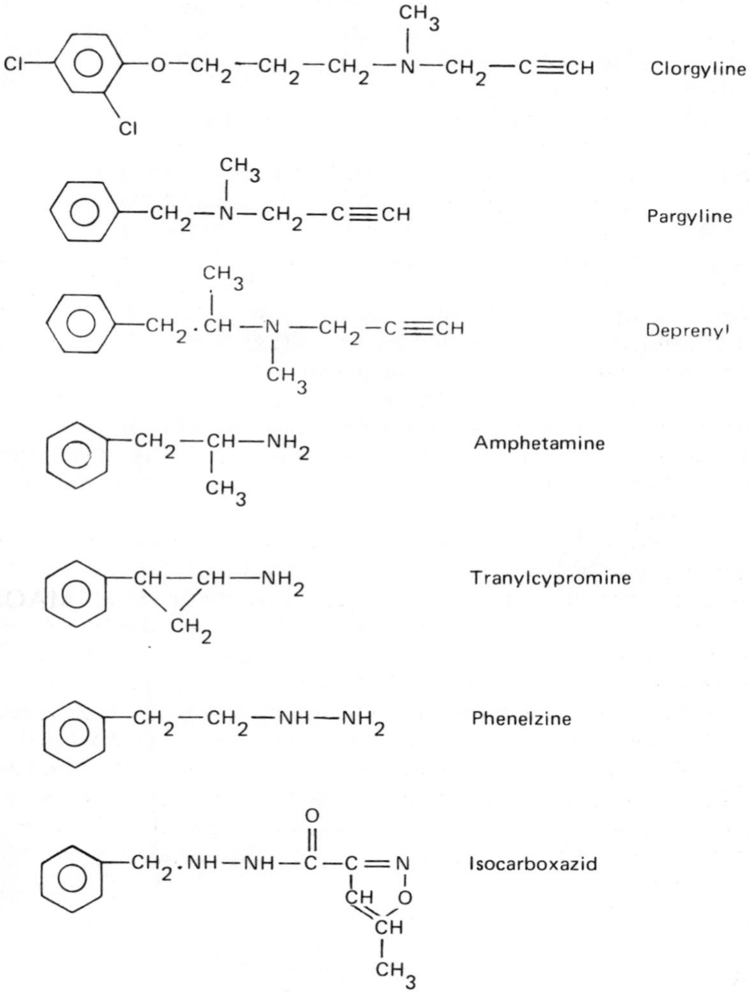

Figure 9.12 Monoamine oxidase inhibitors (and amphetamine)

Within the lesser known MAOIs are two, deprenyl and chlorgyline, which are rmarkable for their degrees of substrate specificity. Chlorgyline is active mostly with 5-HT (rather then phenylethylamine) and deprenyl is similarly most effective with phenylethylamines rather than 5-HT as stated above.

The process of monoamine oxidase inhibition is irreversible, so that there is no reactivation of function of the enzyme until new molecules have been synthesized and have been delivered to the terminals in synaptic vesicles.

MAOIs inhibit paradoxical sleep and the associated ponto-geniculo-occipital waves, in an action which is dependent on 5-HT, catecholamines (possibly adrenaline) and other neurotransmitters.

Growth and sexual development of the young of some species and sexual functioning in some adult animals are modified by MAOIs, in complex ways which depend variously on hormonal modifications involving luteinizing hormone, the gonadotrophic releasing hormones and other hormones (e.g. growth hormone, hydrocortisone). The changes in adults include interruption of pregnancy and oestrus, changes in weight of sex organs, alterations in sexual activity and inhibition of ovulation.

A series of interesting studies have been made of behavioural syndromes dependent on 5-HT. These require the presence of a critical level of 5-HT in the brain, and they mimic some of the behaviour patterns seen with indolamine hallucinogens (LSD, *N,N*-dimethyl tryptamine, etc.) to the extent that these two classes of substance have been assumed to work via the same receptor sites. These behavioural syndromes have been induced with non-selective MAOIs, with MAOI and 5-HT precursors (tryptophan or 5-HTP), MAOIs followed by reserpine, or MAOI drugs blocking and uptake of 5-HT across the presynaptic membrane. The pattern varies slightly with the mode of induction and the species, but it consists essentially of an excited hyperactive state; disruption of normal patterns of movement, exploration and social interaction; and also characteristic movements. For instance, rats treated with MAOIs and tryptophan have side movements of the head, head twitches, tremor and 'piano playing' with the forepaws. Once again the pattern is mainly 5-HT-dependent, probably with lesser participation of the catecholaminergic system.

An exaggerated extreme syndrome is seen under some circumstances when MAOIs are combined with amine re-uptake blockers such as the tricyclic antidepressants. The syndrome includes hypermobility, excitation, tremors and hyperpyrexia, and a very similar syndrome picture may follow the use of MAOIs alone.

With the tricyclic drugs this toxic reaction takes place following *previous* use of MAOIs, so that time has allowed larger pools of amines to accumulate in the nerve terminals and increased overflow and release into the synaptic clefts. If these larger quantities of freed amines cannot be reabsorbed across the presynaptic membrane and inactivated intracellularly by MAO, they presumably spend longer at higher concentrations in the synaptic cleft, overstimulate the neurons taking the aminergic input and lead to what is potentially a dangerous series of events.

Use of MAOIs in man

The use of monoamine oxidase inhibitors in psychiatry was initiated by two drugs used for the treatment of tuberculosis—isoniazid and iproniazid. Both, especially iproniazid, proved to have mood-elevating properties and, following initial trials by

Delay and colleagues, this class of drugs was introduced into psychiatric treatments by Kline and his associates in 1957. Currently the main MAOIs in clinical use in psychiatry are isocarboxazid, nialamide, phenelzine and tranylcypromine.

Some monoamine oxidase inhibitors were hydrazide derivatives of hydrazine (e.g. phenelzine), and attempts were made to produce compounds similar to amphetamine with a view to increasing central stimulating activity. The structure of amphetamine has been included in *Figure 9.12* for comparison.

As discussed above, monoamine oxidase inhibitors block the enzyme monoamine oxidase, but they also have less well-defined actions on other enzymes. As far as the catecholamines are concerned, the enzyme catechol-*o*-methyl transferase seems to be of more importance in dealing with circulating catecholamines.

Another function of monoamine oxidases as in animals is that of protection of the body from ingested indirectly acting sympathomimetic amines in food, as mentioned earlier. Intestinal and hepatic monoamine oxidases destroy these amines, preventing their gaining access to the systemic circulation and thus giving rise to hypertension induced by the release of endogenous catecholamines.

The means by which the clinically available MAOIs produce irreversible inactivation of monoamine oxidases is by forming stable complexes with the enzyme, but the process of synthesis of new supplies of amine is unaffected by these drugs. Thus, their effects given clinically are relatively prolonged.

At the usual dosage of MAOIs given therapeutically there is little effect on tissue levels of amines at first, but if sufficient is given to block MAO by the critical amount of 80+ per cent, with the passage of time (several weeks), there are measurable rises in their concentration in the brain, heart, intestine, etc. With the rise in brain levels the amounts of amine transmitters released rises. MAOIs also increase the effects of exogenous amines and their precursors, and of course, this effect is the basis of the hypertensive crises when indirectly acting sympathomimetic agents are ingested, or are administered by other routes.

Indications for the use of MAOIs are by no means straightforward, and are beyond the scope of this book.

Some of the difficulties in interpreting the clinical data as far as affective disorder is concerned is that there are still relatively few trials comparing patients with straightforward uncomplicated affective illness, where the dose has been matched individually to a group of randomly selected patients comparing MAOI with a tricyclic or similar drug, and where peripheral inhibition of MAO has been assayed.

It seems possible that many antidepressant agents may be less specific than we thought originally, and that drugs—for instance, tricyclic antidepressants such as amitriptyline or clomipramine—act on more than one narrow spectrum of psychiatric condition, e.g. via sedative and antidepressant properties. This may apply also to the MAOIs where there is most evidence for its value in neurotically anxious and depressed individuals, in 'atypical' depressions and phobic states.

The as yet imperfectly answered question is whether MAOIs are useful in 'classical' affective illness, as are tricyclics. It seems likely that at the dosages usually given this group are not as highly effective as, say, tricyclic drugs, but few trials have compared unselected patients of this type, matched drug input to produce peripheral measures of monoamine oxidase inhibition at the 80–85 per cent level and then compared responses. Certainly in the trials of MAOI and MAOI plus tryptophan in affective illness both drug and drug plus amino acid were useful treatments, the latter being more rapid than the drug alone.

To speculate, it would be most interesting if MAOIs shared with drugs such as clomipramine an ability to act on more than one psychiatric state, depending on dose given—possibly being anxiolytic at low dose and antidepressant at higher levels. This remains speculation, and the problem remains unresolved.

There are relatively few other uses of MAOIs as yet, although the use of selective MAOIs could introduce a new era for these drugs. For instance, deprenyl needs no dietary precautions because of the continuation of MAO-A in the gut. Selective MAOIs may allow much better tailoring of drug to psychiatric condition. Otherwise their uses have been confined to neurotic anxiety and depression, endogenous depression, premature ejaculation and the treatment of angina.

Side- and toxic effects

In common with some other antidepressant drugs, MAOIs are powerful suppressors of REM sleep, which 'rebounds' on discontinuing the drug.

Monoamine oxidase inhibitors are readily absorbed and are metabolized rapidly, but have effects which are relatively long-lasting.

Probably the hydrazine monoamine oxidase inhibitors are predominantly metabolized by acetylation, and in the UK about half of the population are genetically 'fast acetylators'. With such individuals it may be difficult to achieve therapeutic levels in the lower range of doses with drugs such as phenelzine, but not all the data support this view.

The mild side-effects of MAOIs often diminish as treatment continues. They consist of fatigue and drowsiness (and paradoxically nervousness, restlessness and a 'driven' feeling in others). They may also cause oedema, gastrointestinal upsets, muscle twitching, sweating, blurred vision, increased appetite and a gain in weight. The blood pressure near the upper limit of dosage may fall on standing (postural hypotension), but a dosage at this level may be necessary for a favourable clinical outcome. Headache is a problem with some patients. There may be changes in sexual function—delayed ejaculation or impotence in men, and anorgasmia in women.

Where a MAOI is acting in an amphetamine-like way and producing an increase in 'drive', patients have difficulty in sleeping. This is most common with tranylcypromine, which usually therefore is given in the morning and at mid-day, but the patient may habituate to the property of the drug with time.

At toxic levels of overdosage patients may have marked hypotension, and become either euphoric or agitated. This may be associated with hallucinosis and hyperreflexia. Others become hypertensive. The so-called hypertensive crisis, however, is generally the result of ingesting indirectly acting sympathomimetic agents, usually tyramine. For instance, there is tyramine in matured cheese (not cream or cottage cheese), hydrolysed proteins and yeast extracts, pickled herrings, some wines (notably Chianti), broad bean pods, banana skins and poorly stored protein foods (where bacterial breakdown of the proteins has been allowed). Of course, indirectly acting sympathomimetic drugs or substances which give rise to them can give the same reaction—with substances such as amphetamine, ephedrine, phenylephrine, phenylpropanolamine, fenfluramine (and other amphetamine-like antiobesity agents) and L-dopa. The hypertensive crises induce a severe rise in blood pressure, severe headache, muscle spasms and hyperpyrexia. This may progress to cerebral haemorrhage, shock or uncontrollable hyperpyrexia.

Other drugs which react with MAOIs include hypoglycaemic agents (which are potentiated), tricyclic and some other antidepressants (severe toxic reaction if given sequentially without a break between the two therapies) and pethidine.

With prolonged use, notably of tranylcypromine, the patient may become habituated to the drug and experience discomfort on its withdrawal. These side-effects are unpleasant but not too prolonged, except in those rare cases where the drug has been abused.

Recent views on affective illness, largely based on psychopharmacology

As new information has accrued on the properties of first- and second-generation antidepressants, and on the characteristics of aminergic and other neuronal systems, so hypotheses to explain affective illness largely based on drug responses have been proposed. The difficulty remains that most of the work is on normal *in vitro* or *in vivo* systems. These findings may not apply to the individual with affective disorder, and it is difficult to integrate the findings of basic studies with a clinical syndrome whose primary abnormality is unknown.

Some effects of drugs on aminergic synapses

(1) The tricyclic antidepressants block the presynaptic uptake of noradrenaline and/or 5-HT as discussed above.
(2) This will lead to increased availability of amines in the synaptic cleft and tend to decrease the sensitivity of the postsynaptic receptors (β-adrenergic in the case of noradrenergic neurons), and presynaptic α_2-receptors (in the same system).
(3) By blocking the presynaptic receptor release of amine will be increased.
(4) This will lead to larger aliquots of amines liberated onto postsynaptic β-receptors which in chronic treatment with tricyclic drugs become less sensitive.

The question is which of the various actions will predominate and what will be the overall effect on aminergic activity.

One hypothesis based on studies of the effect of amphetamines on appetite is that tricyclic drugs produce changes acutely, but that the status quo is restored ultimately. In this view this 'new balance' is held, making the cell less sensitive to its own controlling mechanism and therefore more stable. How this would affect response to incoming signals from other systems is speculative.

The view that chronic treatment with tricyclics leads to a return to pretreatment levels of activity in noradrenergic neurons does not apply to all studies, which have found different 'balances'—e.g. hippocampal cells with an inhibitory input of noradrenergic fibres increased rate of firing when treated chronically with desimipramine.

The view is that contrary effects of antidepressant drugs on noradrenergic systems may nullify each other but cause the system to be limited in its capacity to change, so that movement from 'the norm' becomes difficult. This is an interesting hypothesis discussed in greater detail in Chapter 15.

Similar views have been forwarded for serotoninergic neurons. Lithium in chronic therapy appears to have a stabilizing action by increasing 5-HT transmission but limiting excessive amine release. This latter effect may occur in part by the enhancement of intracellular levels of the precursor of 5-HT, 1-tryptophan, accompanied by decreases in tryptophan hydroxylase activity, so that the capacity for increasing 5-HT production is present but 'curbed'. In short-term experiments with lithium there is increased production and turnover of intraneuronal 5-HT, but possibly reduced storage of 5-HT and interference with stimulus-coupled release of 5-HT. With more prolonged treatment the behavioural responses (exploratory behaviour in rats exposed to changes in external stimuli) return to nearer normal, with some evidence of enhanced dopaminergic activity and 5-HT receptor super-sensitivity. This receptor supersensitivity is confined by greater ease of desensitization of the receptors on exposure to stimulation by the transmitter.

There is a further most interesting development in the interaction of 5-HT and noradrenergic systems, in that when the noradrenergic neurons are treated with drugs enhancing presynaptic uptake in this particular system, this may indirectly block the manifestations of abnormal activity in 5-HT systems.

This widening of views raises many possibilities. We already know and have discussed elsewhere patients with unipolar illness with abnormalities in excretion of 3-methoxy-4-hydroxyphenylglycol (MHPG), temporary mood response to amphet-amines, and recovery with imipramine, but not amitriptyline (apparent norad-renergic depressives?). Others have abnormal levels of MHPG, absence of response to amphetamines (short-term) and imipramine (long-term) but recover on amitriptyline. This points to depressives of noradrenergic and serotoninergic type and suggests exploration for the greater success of antidepressants with differing properties.

Clearly, the old view of simplistic aminergic interactions and drug effects has to be abandoned in favour of more complex models.

Chapter 10

Addiction

Definition

The use of drugs to modify experience and behaviour is a human custom of extreme antiquity. Most cultures tolerate the use of one or more drugs, while the use of others is socially unacceptable or illegal. A number of words are used to describe the problem of drug addiction or misuse, and three different concepts covered by this term should be differentiated.

Physical tolerance. The body's ability to destroy the drug increases (metabolic tolerance) or target cells in the brain become less sensitive (cellular tolerance), and the two processes may occur at the same time. This leads to the need for increasing doses of the drugs and to physical withdrawal symptoms if and when the drug is withdrawn suddenly. This makes it difficult or almost impossible for the addict to stop taking the drugs himself without medical assistance.
Psychological dependence. The second concept is psychological dependence. This is the drive by the addict to seek out and take the drug continuously or episodically to experience its psychic effect and/or to avoid psychic distress. While all addictive drugs produce psychological dependence, only some produce physical dependence.
Physical, social or economic damage. Finally, it should be remembered that even when the taking of drugs has led to neither physical or psychological dependence, the habit is expensive and destructive in a number of ways and may lead to physical, social or economic damage.

To some degree these three concepts can be regarded as stages, physical dependence being unlikely to occur without psychological dependence and the psychological dependence without socioeconomic damage.

Aetiology

The problem of drug addiction has attracted considerable research interest and there is a wide range of theories to account for aetiology. While all the drugs involved are active on the brain and produce changes in sensation and emotion, only some show the phenomenon of physical tolerance. Addiction of any kind does not appear to occur naturally in animals other than man, but it can be induced either by forcibly administering the drug until tolerance has been established or (particularly in the case of alcohol) by subjecting the animal to physical or psychological stress. In addition, epidemiological studies have shown that, at least as far as alcohol is concerned, there are inherited racial and cultural differences in addiction rates, and interest has focused recently on the possibility of the existence of metabolic differences which would account for this. Finally, there is the question of whether or not addiction occurs only in personalities who are vulnerable in some way. With regard to the drugs to which addiction occurs, fashion is probably as important as pharmacology, and political and socioeconomic decisions can have an influence. In the case of alcohol addiction, it has been argued that as alcohol becomes cheaper more is drunk and addiction and other problems increase.

The rest of this chapter will be concerned with discussing the pharmacological properties of individual addictive drugs. The drugs have been arranged in groups which share common properties, starting with those which are most commonly used or abused.

Nicotine

Nicotine is almost certainly the most frequently used drug in Western society. This may well be because, unlike all the others, the state of chronic intoxication is neither obvious nor socially unacceptable. The dangers of smoking over a long period of time have been realized only relatively recently, although it is not clear whether these are related to nicotine itself or to the other substances in tobacco smoke.

Initially tobacco smoking produces pallor, dizziness, sweating and nausea, which pass off rapidly if the subject persists. This indicates the development of tolerance to the constituents of tobacco smoke, probably nicotine. It is not clear whether or not there is a withdrawal state, but it is noticeable that many addicts show the classical symptoms of having to take their drug first thing in the morning upon waking before they feel able to undertake their tasks. Some nicotine users report symptoms, which are presumably withdrawal, of shaking, depression, restlessness, constipation and sleep disturbance, which indicate physical dependence. Certainly tobacco smoking and probably the nicotine content of tobacco produce marked psychological dependence, and most smokers have the greatest difficulty in discontinuing the habit once it has become established. The behavioural components of the smoking process have been shown to be gratifying and rewarding in their own right, but it is unlikely that they account for all the dependence produced.

Nicotine has many well-known actions but principally it affects the brain, the cardiovascular system, the adrenals and the gastrointestinal tract. It raises the level of cerebral arousal and prepares the cardiovascular system for activity while relaxing the skeletal muscles. It increases the rate of habituation to non-significant stimuli, and it is presumably this combination of relaxation with arousal which the smoker finds psychologically rewarding. In small doses nicotine stimulates the sympathetic ganglia and many other sites of synaptic transmission, although in larger doses it paralyses them. It provokes the secretion of adrenaline. It has an antidiuretic effect by stimulating the pituitary to produce antidiuretic hormone. It increases the motility of the gastrointestinal tract, but tolerance to this effect is rapidly acquired. Large doses produce rapid death from respiratory paralysis;

interestingly, if the nicotine content of a cigar were injected intravenously, it would almost certainly be a fatal dose.

Nicotine in the blood stream is rapidly cleared by the liver, where it is converted to inert cotinine. It is possible that there is a difference between cigar smoking, where the nicotine is absorbed through the mucosa from alkaline smoke, and cigarette smoking, where acid smoke has to be taken into the lungs for the nicotine to be absorbed through the alveoli. The former produces a steady relatively low blood nicotine level, whereas, because of rapid absorption from the alveoli and rapid clearance, the latter produces short-lived peaks of nicotine in the blood reaching the brain. These peaks may be more stimulating than lower but more constantly raised blood nicotine level. The blood nicotine levels are rarely assayed and, at present, the best objective indicator of a subject's level of smoking is the blood carboxyhaemoglobin level due to the concomitant inhalation of carbon monoxide.

Alcohol

The use of alcohol is inextricably interwoven with the entire fabric of Western society, and it is not surprising, therefore, that its use is widespread. There is broad awareness that alcohol can produce liver damage. It can also lead to peripheral neuritis, and recently it has been shown that prolonged and heavy consumption produces a reduction in brain volume, which, surprisingly, is often reversible with abstinence. There is an increased liability to digestive disorders and to cancer of both the upper gastrointestinal tract and the liver. Finally, there is a relationship between alcoholism and certain kinds of cardiomyopathy, but not coronary artery disease. As alcohol can be used as a source of energy and therefore reduces the need for the intake of other foods, vitamin deficiency may be responsible for some of these disorders. In the case of peripheral neuropathy, this has been known for some time, but there is now evidence that liver damage may be due to the way in which alcohol dehydrogenase monopolizes the supply of oxidized nicotinamide adenine dinucleotide (NAD^+), which it needs as coenzyme. The latter is then unavailable for other processes, including the metabolism of fat.

Tolerance to regular alcohol consumption occurs rapidly, and it is both metabolic and cellular. In the short term, cellular tolerance is the more important, as is shown by the fact that intoxication is more obvious at the same alcohol level when it is rising during a drinking bout than when it is falling afterwards. In the long term, induction of enzymatic breakdown occurs in the liver, mainly involving the microsomal enzyme system.

Alcohol is broken down in the liver by alcohol dehydrogenase, by catalase and by the microsomal ethanol oxidizing system.

Alcohol dehydrogenase, using NAD^+ as a coenzyme, breaks down alcohol to acetaldehyde. The acetaldehyde is then broken down by aldehyde dehydrogenase to acetic acid, which can be used to provide energy by the normal oxidative processes. There are probably several forms of alcohol dehydrogenase, and an especially active form, rare in Europeans, is found in 85 per cent of the Japanese population. It has been shown that the Japanese population is more liable to develop facial flushing and has lower rates of alcoholism than have Europeans. This is comparable with the use of Disulfiram and citrated calcium carbimide as treatments for alcoholism which interfere with the action of aldehyde dehydrogenase and cause acetaldehyde to accumulate in the body, producing unpleasant flushing, among other symptoms. The fact that alcohol dehydrogenase is present in the liver in most species of mammal is interesting; presumably as the natural taste for alcohol in mammals is very rare, it may have evolved to enable them to eat fermenting vegetable manner with impunity.

The other two metabolic pathways play a smaller part in alcohol breakdown. Catalase oxidation of alcohol involves hydrogen peroxide and is limited by the very low rate of generation of this agent in the liver. Under normal conditions, it probably accounts for less than 2 per cent of the breakdown, but there is speculation that it may account for more under conditions of chronic intoxication. The microsomal ethanol oxidizing system uses oxygen and reduced nicotinamide adenine dinucleotide phosphate. This system is particularly liable to induction both by alcohol and by other drugs, including barbiturates, and may well be the system responsible for cross-tolerance with these other groups of drugs.

Despite decades of research, the essential effects of alcohol on the nervous system are by no means fully understood. On the behavioural level, however, increases in concentrations of alcohol in the blood impair mental functions, starting with the most complex and progressing to the most basic. This used to be described as descending from the cortex to the medulla, but it is doubtful whether this is any longer an accurate description, although it is a good way to remember the effects. It should be borne in mind that an overdose of alcohol, approximately a bottle of spirits, if taken in one dose, will produce death from respiratory depression. At the cellular level, it is known that alcohol affects the turnover of some neurotransmitters, including noradrenaline and dopamine, but the effects reported seem to vary and it is not clear in what particular way this is linked with the behavioural changes observed. The second theory, which does not necessarily exclude the first, is that alcohol has a direct effect upon neuronal membranes by interfering with their lipid structure and thus in some way modifying their ability to transmit impulses. Potency correlates with fat solubility for a considerable number of anaesthetic agents, and this action of alcohol may be similar.

Physical dependence upon alcohol is believed to be accounted for by the development of cellular tolerance which, upon alcohol withdrawal, enables the affected pathways to overact, which results at the most extreme in delirium and convulsions. Either theory of cellular action could satisfactorily account for this phenomenon. Physical dependence can be induced in animals by forcibly administering alcohol to them, and once tolerance has developed they will continue to seek alcohol to prevent the development of withdrawal symptoms.

There can be little doubt that psychological dependence upon alcohol also develops and can occur in the absence of physical dependence. Psychological dependence may be due to the use of alcohol to escape from unpleasant mental stimuli, but, particularly in Western societies, cultural factors are also important. It can be extremely difficult for an individual to find a leisure activity at which the consumption of alcohol is not an integral part. In animals, stress, physical or physiological, can be used to induce a preference for alcohol solutions when normally they would be rejected.

Interest is now focusing upon the effects of acetaldehyde, the first breakdown product of alcohol. In the liver, as has been mentioned, alcohol may take up almost the entire supply of oxidized cofactors and must competitively interfere with almost every other hepatic function. It is possible that by appropriating the available aldehyde dehydrogenase other biogenic amines which have been oxidized to their respective aldehydes might react to produce abnormal metabolic products. Two of these of particular interest are tetrahydropapaveroline, a morphine-like compound, and a number of tetrahydroisoquinolines, especially one called 'salsolinol'. The induction of a morphine-like compound might link alcoholism to the opiate addictions.

It has been found that following injection of very small quantities of salsolinol into certain sites in a rat's brain the rat's preference for alcohol is greatly increased. It would obviously be interesting if chronic alcohol consumption could produce a substance in the brain which led to the psychological tendency to consume more alcohol.

The aetiology of alcoholism is not fully understood, as stated above, but there is now some evidence that genetic factors are important. The morbidity risk for alcoholism for a person with one alcoholic parent is approximately 25 per cent (but this might be due to imitation rather than inheritance). In one study 71 per cent of monozygotic twins were found to be concordant in their drinking habits, compared with only 32 per cent of dizygotic twins. Recently a study of sons of Danish alcoholics who were adopted in early life showed that they were four times more likely to become alcoholic than were comparable adoptees without alcoholic biological parents. Unfortunately, except for the racial variants in alcohol dehydrogenase activity, no other metabolic factors have been found which might account for the aetiology of alcoholism.

Barbiturates

These sedative drugs have very similar effects to alcohol on the intact animal. The sedative action requires the presence of two alkyl side-chains of fewer than six carbon atoms. If the side-chains are longer, they tend to be convulsants (*see Figure 10.1*). If one or more of the side-chains is reactive, then the drug tends to be anticonvulsant.

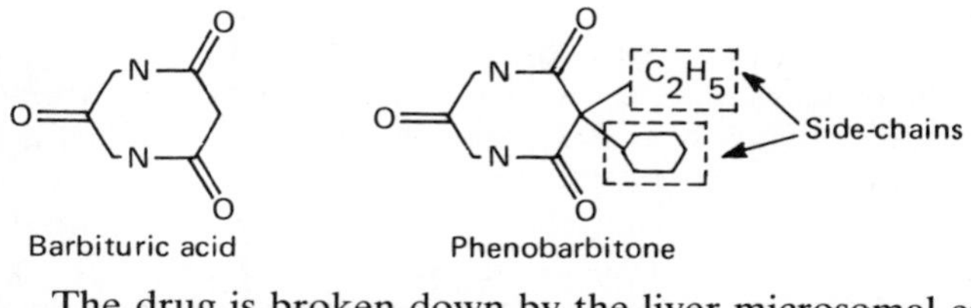

Barbituric acid   Phenobarbitone   *Figure 10.1*

The drug is broken down by the liver microsomal enzyme system by oxidation. This microsomal system is the secondary system in the breakdown of alcohol but the main pathway for the breakdown of barbiturates and many other drugs, which accounts for cross-tolerance, as this microsomal system is easily induced. Usually, the larger side-chain is oxidized first. It can be seen from the above that if drugs of this group are taken in combination with alcohol or other sedative drugs, as they often are, the rate of breakdown may be either increased because the enzymes have been induced by the previous doses or reduced because there is partial competition between them. This is not in itself sufficient to account for their tendency to additive interaction and, in addition to this metabolic tolerance, it is known that for barbiturates cellular tolerance also develops sufficiently rapidly to account for a significant part of a recovery from a large dose of a long-acting barbiturate.

There are a large number of barbiturates available with varying durations of sedative action. These variations are due mostly to the varying rates at which they are broken down in the liver, except for the ultra-short-acting barbiturates used as anaesthetics, which are fat-soluble and are removed from the blood stream into the fat stores and later released in subanaesthetic doses to be broken down by the liver. Only Phenobarbitone is markedly anticonvulsant.

The exact site of action of the barbiturates is unknown. It can be demonstrated that the ascending reticular activating system is particularly sensitive to their effects. Low doses block some synapses and higher doses may increase the sodium conductance of the axons, thus producing a block to nerve impulse conduction. Presynaptically barbiturates may well block the uptake of calcium on which transmitter release depends. They may also mimic the action of gamma amino-butyric acid (GABA) on presynaptic terminals, as in some sites such as in the dorsal route ganglia this effect is blocked by GABA antagonists. Barbiturates also block the postsynaptic response to transmitter release, particularly in selected parts of the cortex, where they affect postsynaptic excitatory noradrenergic synapses but not inhibitory ones or cholinergic or serotoninergic synapses.

In the brain-stem they appear to block the postsynaptic response to acetylcholine. They have been shown to reduce the turnover of some monoamines, but this might well be a secondary rather than a primary effect. The GABA-agonist effect might well account for the anticonvulsant properties.

Behaviourally, increasing doses of barbiturates, like alcohol, produce increasing mental confusion, inco-ordination and eventually death from respiratory failure. Tolerance occurs rapidly both to these effects and to the use of barbiturates as hypnotics.

Other sedative drugs

All other sedative drugs can be addictive both physically and psychologically. All hypnotics tend to produce dependence, both for the induction of sleep and in susceptible persons, by daytime abuse as well. A number have proved such severe problems that they have had to be withdrawn from the market—for instance, methaqualone. It is convenient to include here also solvents taken by inhalation (glue sniffing). Many of the solvents involved are either general anaesthetics in their own right or closely related to them chemically. They probably have an effect similar to that of alcohol on neuronal transmission, interfering with the lipid membrane. Most of them seem to produce the same progressive clouding of consciousness as do alcohol and barbiturates. Unfortunately, some of them are extremely toxic, particularly to the liver. It is possible that some of them also have hallucinogenic properties.

Recently, even the benzodiazepines have come to be regarded as addictive. This is an example of the potential of so many drugs which alter mental processes to also have a potential for addiction. There is very little tolerance to benzodiazepines; certainly liver enzymes are not induced, and there is some evidence that as the dose is increased, there is no further increase in the effect. These drugs may act by blocking the action of a protein or another substance, which interferes with the action of GABA on its receptor site. If this is so, then at maximum interference raising the dose of benzodiazepine further is not going to have any additional effect, as it will not produce any further quantities of GABA to bind with its receptors. Locating the binding sites of benzodiazepines with a radioactively labelled form has now shown them to be widespread throughout the entire brain, including the cerebellum, thus refuting the original idea that they were confined to the ascending reticular activating system.

Owing to its anticonvulsant action it is probable that the abrupt withdrawal of large doses of benzodiazepine may precipitate convulsions. Whether the anxiety and tension felt when the drug is stopped are withdrawal symptoms or are a return of the original anxiety state for which the drug was prescribed, is not clear. Certainly, when benzodiazepines are used as a hypnotic, on withdrawal there is a rebound of increased REM sleep which persists for some weeks. It is possible, therefore, that physical tolerance does occur and thus physical dependence is possible. Certainly, there can be considerable psychological dependence. Whether or not abuse is liable to lead to socially unacceptable behaviour is more doubtful, although the benzodiazepines can reduce self-control, particularly when combined with alcohol. Therapeutic doses impair driving skills and, again, this effect is magnified by alcohol. In this respect, it is particularly important to remember that many benzodiazepines have a long half-life in the body, often because they are broken down to pharmacologically active metabolites which may remain in the body for longer than the parent compound.

Opiates (*Figure 10.2*)

This group of drugs has been used for medicinal and other purposes since antiquity. Crude but active extracts are taken direct from the opium poppy. While modern medicinal opiates are pure substances, those used by addicts, especially if obtained from illegal sources, vary greatly in their purity, both because of inefficiency in the method of preparation and because of subsequent deliberate dilution by sellers to increase their profits. For this reason 'street morphine' or 'street heroin' is often one-tenth or less the strength of the pure drug obtained from a medical source. The drugs can be taken orally, but addicts prefer to inject them, especially intravenously, as the rapid onset of action produces a particularly pleasant sensation. Tolerance and physical dependence occur rapidly with all these drugs. Physical withdrawal symptoms take the form of shaking, piloerection, restlessness, nausea, diarrhoea and sneezing. While these sensations can be very unpleasant, they are never fatal.

All the opiate drugs have a characteristic T-shaped molecule with a definite structure–activity relationship. It is the L-isomer which is active. Specific opiate antagonists can be produced by substituting a chain onto the nitrogen atom in this molecule.

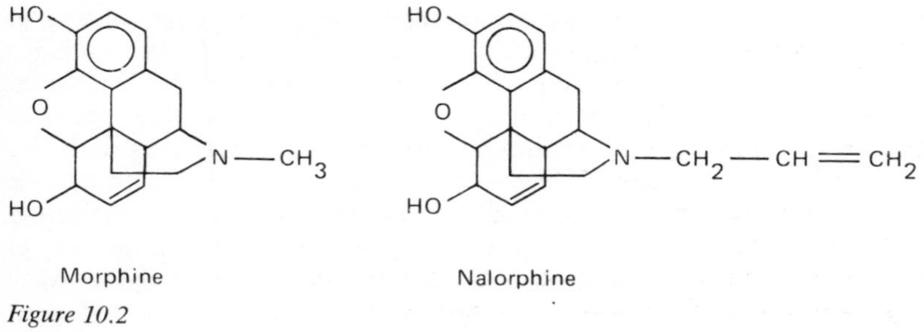

Morphine   Nalorphine

Figure 10.2

These specific agonists and antagonists show such a strong relationship between structure and activity that it was felt that there must be specific receptors within the CNS. These have now been located in a number of structures in the brain and the spinal cord associated with pain transmission. These areas include the dorsal horn of the spinal cord, the grey matter surrounding the ventricles and the aqueduct in the brain-stem and the midbrain. There are also receptor-rich areas in the striatum and the amygdala. The former are believed to be involved in pain reception and the latter with emotional reaction to it. Small quantities of morphine have great effects if injected directly into these areas and also can produce tolerance and withdrawal. Small quantities of sodium increase the binding of antagonists while decreasing that of agonists, and have led to the suggestion that the receptors exist in two forms. (For further details of the receptors *see* Chapter 4.)

More recently still, the naturally occurring transmitters have been discovered which bear a distinct structural affinity to the opiate drugs. These include two pentapeptides turned 'enkephalins' (leucine- and methionine-enkephalin) and larger molecules such as β-lipotrophin which are produced by the pituitary and are probably forerunners of β-melanocyte-stimulating hormone. The methionine enkephalin structure occurs within the sequence of its molecular formula. Other endorphins are still being described. These probably play a part in the natural modulation of pain perception. Interestingly, it has been shown that their concentration increases after the administration of placebos.

Clinically, opiates lead to sedation and euphoria, although the latter may only occur in certain individuals. Some people following opiate ingestion report their sensations as pleasant, whereas others describe only an unpleasant sedation. There is considerable variation between species of animals, and in some, hyperexcitability is produced. Autonomic effects are always produced, and these include nausea, respiratory depression, constipation and pupillary constriction. The reverse effects occur during the withdrawal syndrome.

Analgesia is produced by reducing both the transmission of and emotional reactions to pain impulses. This is probably the mechanism in which the endorphins (endogenous morphine-like substances) are involved. The natural system interacts with other brain neuroregulators and can be blocked by disruption of serotoninergic activity. It can also be activated by electrical stimulation both locally and peripherally.

There is no evidence of metabolic tolerance. Cellular tolerance occurs rapidly but always disappears completely. It has now been shown that it is not produced by an increase in the number of opiate receptors. Possible mechanisms include hypersensitivity in the postsynaptic receptors which are the targets of the opiate-inactivated neurons. Alternatively, there might be a disturbance in balance between susceptibility to the agonists and antagonists. Thirdly, it has been shown that opiates increase the levels of enkephalin circulating and this has been postulated as the mechanism of tolerance.

Stimulants

These include cocaine and the amphetamines. These drugs probably block catecholamine re-uptake and breakdown, leading to an excess of the transmitter at its receptor site. They produce stereotyped behaviours in animals and also in man, with increased energy and restlessness. There is often euphoria and reduction of fatigue but they do not act as effective antidepressants. They tend to depress the appetite, and therefore were at one time used for the treatment of obesity. They were, however, found to be addictive (*see* below), so they are no longer used medically, except for the use of cocaine as a local anaesthetic and some amphetamine-like drugs in the treatment of asthma and respiratory congestion. Interestingly, prolonged overdose of both drugs tends to produce a paranoid psychosis which can be very difficult to distinguish from schizophrenia.

Tolerance does not develop to these drugs and therefore there is never physical dependence. However, because their euphoriant action is highly rewarding, psychological dependence can and usually does develop rapidly.

Cocaine

This complex molecule is still only obtainable from plant sources and is very expensive. In the blood stream it is metabolized rapidly into a number of components by serum esterases and therefore has a short half-life of about 20 minutes. Intravenous injection, therefore, has a brief effect only, but absorption from the nasal mucosa, in sniffing, is slow and thus the effect of cocaine taken this way is more prolonged. Cocaine inhibits the presynaptic uptake of the catecholamine neurotransmitters but it does not potentiate their release. It acts strongly in the striatum, where the tricyclic antidepressants, another group of catecholamine re-uptake inhibitors, have little or no effect, and this may account for their difference in action. The drug also prevents the feedback inhibition of dopamine synthesis and it also inhibits the production of 5-hydroxytryptamine (5-HT). Cocaine inhibits monoamine oxidase. These actions suggest that its action is to increase the quantity of monoamine neurotransmitters, particularly dopamine, in the synaptic cleft and delay their removal.

Amphetamines

These are a group of drugs more closely related to the catecholamine neurotransmitters, with rather longer side-chains. They presumably selectively block their re-uptake and breakdown in the synaptic cleft but not their activity at the receptor site. They were developed as improved remedies for asthma, in which a similar drug, ephedrine, is still used because it has far less central activity. The risk of amphetamine-like central activity in asthma remedies, nasal decongestants for the relief of colds and appetite suppressants must always be borne in mind.

Amphetamine itself occurs in two main forms, of which the dextrorotatory isomer is the active one. Some amphetamines are excreted in the urine unchanged and some as a deaminated product, benzoic acid. Hydroxylation can also occur to the active products, norephedrine and hydroxyamphetamine. Addicts excrete more of these products except benzoic acid than controls. Similarly, acidification of the urine greatly enhances excretion, particularly of unmetabolized amphetamine.

The behavioural effects are those of the group. It is possible that tolerance develops for all the effects but it is particularly marked for appetite suppression. However, the depression and lassitude claimed as withdrawal symptoms may equally well be due to the overactivity induced by the chronic misuse.

Biochemically, amphetamine stimulates the release of catecholamines from nerve endings, it inhibits monoamine oxidase and blocks neuronal re-uptake from the synaptic cleft, causing persistence of all the 'released' monoamine neurotransmitters. It leads to a reduction of the synthesis of dopamine, noradrenaline and 5-HT in the striatum.

Hallucinogens

D-Lysergic acid diethylamide (LSD), etc.

LSD and other drugs such as psilocibin and mescalin, which occur naturally, all produce intense visual hallucinations, with mood changes and alterations in the other sensory modalities. They may act on the 5-HT inhibitory system, which appears to be of particular importance in the visual cortex and in other areas controlling mood and perception. They may activate inhibitory receptors on the body and dendrites of the first cells of this system in the same way as 5-HT. These first cells use 5-HT as a transmitter to inhibit second cells in the system. LSD and others drugs which are actively hallucinogenic do not have nearly as marked an inhibitory effect on the second cells as does 5-HT or non-hallucinatory substituted compounds of LSD. Therefore, the second cells are released from the control of the first and overstimulation occurs.

There is an interaction between LSD and the dopaminergic system. It can be shown experimentally to affect dopamine-sensitive adenylate cyclase, which suggests a direct postsynaptic action. Terminals in the caudate and limbic system appear to be sensitive to it.

While psychological dependence on these drugs can probably occur, there is no evidence of tolerance or any form of physical dependence. Dependence with these drugs may be far more of a habit than the satisfaction of a drive.

Cannabis

The active constituent of cannabis is mainly tetrahydrocannabinol. It is obtained from the plant *Cannabis sativa*, which can be easily grown in warm countries and in greenhouses in the UK. It is usually consumed in a relatively impure form, often in a similar way to tobacco and mixed with it. It seems probable that the drug, in some way, interferes with the cholinergic and serotoninergic systems in a rather similar fashion to both the LSD and the anticholinergic hallucinogens. There is no evidence of tolerance or physical dependence, and even psychological dependence may be relatively uncommon. It is undoubtedly abused widely in areas where it is easy to obtain because of the warm climate, and in these areas the production of permanent brain damage has been claimed. This matter is by no means settled, but it is usually stated in the UK that it does not do so and that any association with such illnesses as schizophreniform psychosis is due to patients in early illness being drawn into a cannabis-smoking society. It should be noted that in Middle Eastern countries it was believed to induce maniacal violence in soldiers, and our word 'assassin' comes from 'hassasheen'; in the UK a section of society ascribe to it a peaceful, dreamy state of 'universal love'. It would seem that its psychological effects are very greatly influenced by the expectancy of the individual taking the drug.

Anticholinergic drugs

It has long been known that overuse of these drugs can produce confusion, amnesia and hallucinations. They differ from LSD in that the hallucinations are less vivid and the confusion is considerably more marked. There are also peripheral symptoms of cholinergic blockade, including tachycardia, dryness of the mouth, dilated pupils, narrowing of vision and a dry, hot skin. While it is well known that these actions are due to a blockage of cholinergic receptors, the distribution of these receptors in the brain is not well known at all. Memory is presumably involved, as these are the only drugs in this group to produce amnesia. There is little evidence of tolerance, but because of the unpleasant peripheral side-effects, these drugs are not often abused on a long-term basis.

Chapter 11

Electroencephalography

Principles of recording

The electroencephalogram (EEG) is a graph of the voltage between two points on the intact scalp against time. This has been taken to reflect the neuronal activity of the underlying cerebral cortex. The recording apparatus is usually calibrated so that 1 cm of vertical deflection represents 100 μV and in one-third of a second the paper moves 1 cm horizontally. The amplification involved in this recording is of the order of a million times, and therefore the recording is very sensitive to interference both from external sources and from the electrical activity of the patient's skeletal and cardiac muscles. To interpret the recordings, it is important to be able to recognize these artefacts, especially those due to the heart and movements of the eye. The exact origin of the electrical activity being recorded on the scalp is not known, but the predictable changes in cerebral activity during sleep, following drugs and as a result of brain pathology encourage the view that these alterations are a reflection on the functioning of the underlying brain.

The normal EEG

The normal EEG is symmetrical and shows the electrical activity as waves of varying rates. These waves have been classified into: delta waves (less than 4 Hz*); theta waves (4–7 Hz); alpha waves (8–13 Hz); and beta waves (more than 13 Hz). The normal EEG contains a mixture of alpha and beta waves (*see Figure 11.1*). The alpha waves are usually more prominent at the occipital poles and when the eyes are shut, and can be abolished, at least temporarily, by opening the eyes or performing any mental task. There is a wide variation among normal individuals between those in whom alpha activity is present most of the time even when the eyes are open, and the individual is thinking, and those in whom the alpha activity is almost totally absent. Rarely alpha activity may not occur at all. The EEG record of one individual is relatively stable, but when measured at different times, allowance must be made for changes produced by maturation in the young and by sleep and other alterations of consciousness.

In the new-born infant delta waves predominate but the record tends to be irregular. As the child matures, the mean frequency of the record becomes faster

*1 hertz (Hz) = 1 cycle per second.

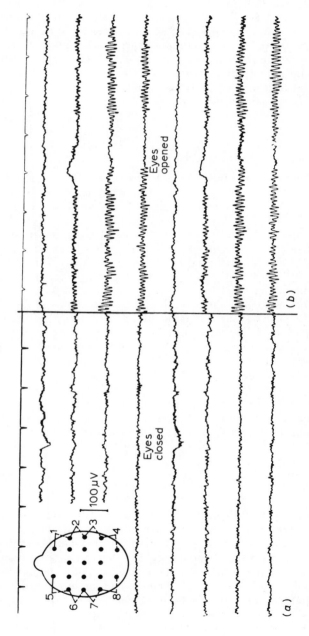

Figure 11.1 (a) M-type alpha subject. Man aged 27 years. EEG: complete absence of alpha rhythm. Low voltage beta components not affected by eye closure. (*b*) P-type alpha subject. Man aged 18 years. EEG: well sustained 11Hz alpha rhythm diminished for only about 1 second following eye opening

and more regular. Theta waves usually appear at about 18 months, and by 5 or 6 years the amounts of theta and alpha activity are approximately equal. Noticeable delta activity is usually abnormal in a normal adult subject, but some theta activity may persist into adulthood in some perfectly normal individuals. A slow and irregular EEG, with marked theta activity, is sometimes referred to as 'immature'. It is claimed to be more frequent in individuals with psychopathic personality disorders. It is not known whether this pattern reflects a generalized cerebral immaturity. This problem is complex because both the assessment of a psychopathic in contradistinction to a normal personality and of a mature as compared with an immature EEG are largely subjective.

Sleep

In the initial period of sleep or drowsiness the alpha rhythm at first becomes more persistent, then gradually declines during progress to deeper stages of sleep, when slower rhythms appear. In the deepest stage of sleep high-voltage delta activity is the main feature of the EEG. During normal sleep there are other patterns, which include spindle-shaped bursts of fast activity, and in light sleep bursts of high-voltage slow waves as a response to auditory stimulation. These latter are called 'K'-complexes. The first period of a normal night's sleep is characterized by this type of EEG pattern, but later in the night this is interrupted by periods of 'paradoxical' rapid eye movement (REM) sleep. As the name implies, there are marked movements of the eyes which give rise to electrical artefacts in the frontal channel, otherwise the EEG is of the type associated with light rather than deep sleep, even though the patient is unusually difficult to wake. This period of sleep has been shown to be associated with dreaming, although it is now known that dreaming is not confined to REM sleep. Drugs alter the amount of time spent in REM sleep (usually four or five periods of about 20 minutes each per night), and most hypnotics suppress it. When hypnotics are stopped, there is nearly always a period of REM rebound with more prolonged and active REM sleep and the patient complains of excessive dreaming. This may take several weeks to subside. Other drugs, including antidepressants, also may have this effect.

Epilepsy

The EEG is of great value in the investigation of epilepsy. While it may be possible to confirm the clinical diagnosis of epilepsy by demonstrating epileptic activity in the EEG, normal recordings, even if repeated many times, cannot exclude it. Abnormalities associated with epilepsy which may be found include both signs of brain damage, which will be dealt with later, and the slowing and irregularity found following epileptic fits. However, a clinical diagnosis of epilepsy can only be confirmed when epileptic activity itself can be demonstrated in the EEG, either going on to produce a fit during the recording or mounting up towards a fit but not reaching it. The EEG is seen to become slower and more synchronous and to increase in voltage. These changes produce waves narrow at their base relative to their height which therefore have a sharp or spiked appearance (*see Figure 11.2*). There can be either continuous spikes or alternating spikes and waves, the latter

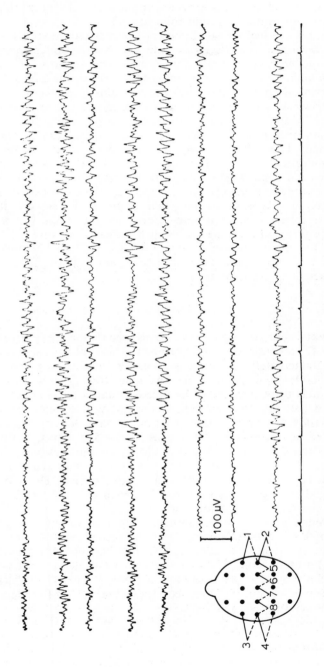

Figure 11.2 Psychomotor epilepsy—commencement of seizure pattern. Man aged 28 years, became vacant and unresponsive during above part of recording; subsequent chewing movements. EEG: initial 9–10 Hz alpha rhythm replaced by bilateral rhythmical 5–6 Hz theta activity, best seen in the temporal regions and a little more on the right side

100µV

occurring classically at 3 Hz being pathognomic of petit mal epilepsy. This is a form of idiopathic subcortical epilepsy characterized clinically by 'absences' (loss of awareness) of a few seconds' duration rather than fits.

Even more important is the fact that if epileptic activity is recorded, it is often possible to determine its origin. The EEG may show whether the epileptic activity spreads from a point on the cortex or alternatively appears synchronously in all channels. The latter would point to a focus in one of the subcortical centres in the thalamus. Clinically, cortical epilepsy may show the Jacksonian spread or an aura, whereas subcortical epilepsy is characterized by the sudden auraless onset of a convulsion or absence. Rarely, a cortical focus activates a subcortical focus, producing secondary subcortical epilepsy and this pattern of spread can be followed on the EEG recording. The differentiation between cortical and subcortical epilepsy is of great importance in their treatment, as optimum therapies are by different drug regimens and cortical epilepsy may be the first sign of a brain lesion requiring direct treatment. Unfortunately, some of the episodes of cortical epilepsy which are clinically the most atypical may have their origin in the temporal lobes. As the cortex of these lobes is rather isolated from the rest of the brain, it is probable that seizures starting in them are less likely to spread to involve the entire cortex and therefore be manifested as convulsions. In addition, because the temporal lobes are tucked away under the rest of the brain, it is very difficult to record the electrical activity of this cortex.

Brain lesions

While there is uncertainty as to the origin of the waves seen on the EEG recording, it certainly appears as if dead brain cells produce no electrical activity, and as if the damaged brain cells immediately surrounding them produce slower and more irregular waves of a higher voltage than healthy ones (*see Figure 11.3*). The irregular slow activity may be widespread or localized. Often, if the slow activity is localized, it indicates the site of the lesion, but an expanding lesion may press the opposite pole of the brain against the skull, to produce slow activity there, and this may be considered erroneously to be a focus of damage. Thus, both false localization and false lateralization are possible. Slowly growing lesions produce much less disturbance than do rapidly growing ones and may reach a very considerable size without producing any visible changes in the EEG. Head injuries and vascular lesions tend to produce a generalized disturbance at first, but later the EEG may give some assistance in their localization.

Intoxication and delirium tends to produce slowing and irregularity of the electroencephalogram. Eventually in severe cases the record will be filled with diffuse irregular delta activity. In some conditions such as hepatic coma the degree to which this change is present is one of the most accurate indicators of the degree of biochemical disturbance and has been used to monitor it (*Figure 11.4*). Changes are non-specific for the various causes of these conditions and appear to reflect only the underlying disturbance of brain activity.

Provocative techniques

A number of techniques are available which increase the likelihood of enhancing abnormalities to make them visible in the EEG, and to this end most routine

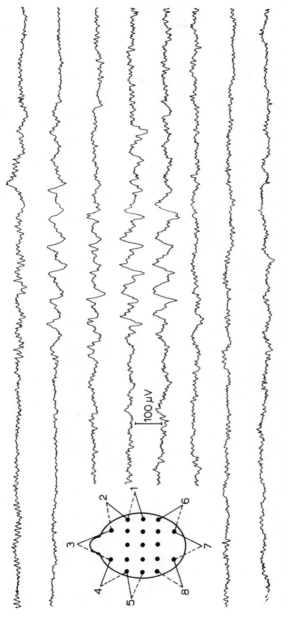

Figure 11.3 Glioblastoma, left frontal region. Man aged 24 years with headaches for 3 months. EEG: bilateral rhythmical delta discharge in frontal regions, more evident on left side. More 10 Hz rhythm in right temporal region than in left

230

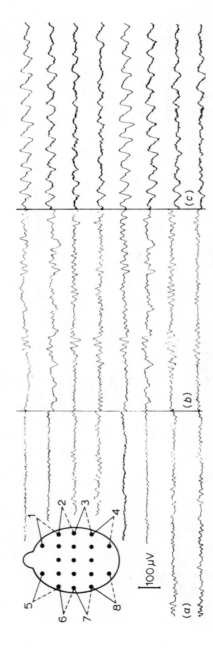

Figure 11.4 Hepatic encephalopathy (portal systemic encephalopathy). Man aged 33 years. (*a*) Mental state normal. Blood ammonia 200 µg/100 ml. EEG: occasional slowing of alpha rhythm below 8 Hz with random theta components posteriorly. (*b*) Some clouding of consciousness. Blood ammonia 280 µg/100 ml. EEG: widespread theta activity at 5–6 Hz (eye movement artefacts in channels 2 and 6). (*c*) Patient frankly delerious. Blood ammonia 500 µg/ml. EEG: high voltage rhythmical delta activity at 2 Hz, frontally predominant

recordings utilize both hyperventilation and flashing lights of various speeds. Hyperventilation reduces the p_{CO_2}, which leads to constriction of the cerebral arterioles and reduces the oxygenation of the brain.

Special electrode placements may help, and these include the insertion of needle electrodes under the interior surface of the skull to record the activity of the temporal lobes. At operation electrodes may be placed directly on the brain or even inside it. Most recently, miniaturization of components has made it possible to produce an electroencephalographic recording device so small that it can be worn by the patient while he goes about his normal everyday activities. The recording is usually made on a tape cassette (rather than on paper), and this is later projected on to a television screen. It is possible in this way to examine the electrical activity over considerable periods of time such as a complete 24 hour cycle and to detect disturbances associated with naturally occurring events which would not otherwise have been suspected.

Evoked potentials

The electroencephalographic response to any single stimulus is normally invisible among the overall electrical activity being recorded. However, if a pattern of electrical activity following a stimulus is repeated and this repeated stimulus is superimposed and added, the 'noise' (activity not related to the stimulus) tends to cancel itself out and that which is due to the stimulus summates and becomes visible. These 'evoked potentials' have been studied in a number of settings in relation to psychiatry, neurology and other medical subjects. Their greatest use so far, however, has been in fields such as demonstrating the effectiveness of a hearing-aid in a very small child who cannot speak, and making an early diagnosis of multiple sclerosis by demonstrating delayed conduction in the optic pathways.

Of more interest to psychiatry is the so-called contingent negative variation or expectancy wave. When after a signal the individual is required to respond on receipt of a second stimulus to perform an action such as pressing a button, a negative potential change occurs over quite large areas of the brain which lasts several seconds and which is often most in evidence on the vertex. Consistent differences in the development of this wave with the presence of various psychiatric disorders, including psychopathy and schizophrenia, have been claimed but the method is not yet sufficiently refined or accepted to have entered clinical practice.

Acknowledgements

The figures are produced by kind permission of Kiloh *et al.* (1981).

Chapter 12

Neuropathology of dementia (chronic brain syndrome)

Introduction

The well-recognized clinical picture of organic brain disease due to gross pathology can be divided into the acute brain syndrome or delirium and chronic brain syndrome or dementia, both of which are due to widespread brain dysfunction and damage; and a small number of recognized syndromes in which damage to a particular part of the brain produces a recognizable clinical picture. In the investigation of these states it must be remembered both that they can be caused by almost every disease to which the brain and the body is prone and that in the acute stage and sometimes in the chronic, localized lesions causing swelling and distortion of the brain, or obstruction to the drainage of the cerebrospinal fluid, will, because the brain is contained in a rigid box, produce generalized symptoms.

The investigation of these conditions demands that, as the first priority, the degree to which disease in the rest of the body might be contributing be established. Whatever is present should be treated, and this is particularly important in the acute states. Following this the search for a treatable cause of dementia is governed by the balance between the chances of finding such a cause and the distress the investigations will cause to the patient. They will also to some degree be governed by the expense and availability of certain tests. For example, the American Consensus Committee on the investigation of dementia recommended that the 'work-up' could not be considered as complete without computerized axial tomography. This chapter will consider the pathology of a number of conditions causing dementia which are important, either because they are common or because new knowledge is becoming available, or because they are treatable. Because they cause dementia, they are all likely to present to the psychiatrist.

Senile dementia and Altzheimer's disease

Senile dementia now represents the biggest challenge to the psychiatric services. The percentage of the population over 65, and even more the percentage over 75, is at present increasing rapidly and it is in these age groups, particularly the over-75s, that dementia becomes increasingly frequent.

The relationship between Altzheimer's disease and senile dementia is arguable, but there is no doubt that they show a common brain pathology, with argentophile plaques and neurofibrillary tangles. To some degree these changes develop in all brains with age, but it is only in cases of dementia that these changes become widespread and prominent. Occurring before the age of 65, prominent changes of this type are called Altzheimer's disease, although they also occur in Down's syndrome. After the age of 65 they are called manifestations of senile dementia. It is also difficult to dissociate this pathology and factors which might be relevant to its causation from arteriosclerotic dementia, which nearly always co-exists to a greater or lesser degree in the population of Western countries, where a significant percentage survive to the age at which the pathology becomes common. Ninety-eight per cent of patients over the age of 80 have significant arteriosclerosis due to atheroma.

At post mortem examination or computerized axial tomography (CAT) the brain is seen to be shrunken, with narrow gyri, wide sulci and dilated ventricles. This is usually widespread. Histologically there is diffuse neuronal loss, with an increase in glial tissue and pigmentation. Small infarcts are usually co-existent, but the basic Altzheimer's pathology is the presence of characteristic neurofibrillary tangles and argentophilic senile plaques. There is a positive correlation between the number of plaques and the degree of dementia, but this is only observed when a large number of cases are considered, though in individual cases there can be surprising disparity.

Recently Altzheimer's pathology has been the subject of very considerable research interest, and it has been fairly clearly demonstrated that there is a lack of cholinergic activity in brains showing this pathology, which suggests a defect in the acetylcholine transmission system. All surveys tend to agree about this deficiency. Other transmitter deficiencies have been reported, but there is far less agreement. Probably the most frequently reported of these is low noradrenaline concentrations, especially in the locus coeruleus.

Interest also centres around the neurofibrillary tangles, which have only ever been observed in the human species. Tangles can be produced in animal brains, particularly by increased concentrations of aluminium, but they are produced from a single strand, not a paired one, and there does not appear to be any increase in aluminium associated with Altzheimer's pathology in human brains. The Altzheimer tangles, which are paired helical filaments, are formed from a protein which appears to be normally present in the brain, even in the young. It is most probable that this protein takes up a different configuration and it is suggested that the change may be comparable with that of amyloid formation, where normal protein takes up a beta pleated form which is very resistant to subsequent enzymatic breakdown.

There may be some relationship between the argentophile plaques and those of amyloid and other degenerative illness known to be caused by viruses. The possibility that senile dementia might in fact be caused by a slow virus infection has been raised, but there is as yet no evidence to support this view. However, recently a case of another degenerative condition, Jacob Creutzfeldt's disease, which was arrested by the antiviral agent amantadine has been reported. It has been suggested that the plaques may be the cause of the reduced cholinergic function, but this reduced activity has been demonstrated to be in the axons rather than the cell bodies where the plaques occur.

Arteriosclerotic dementia

Atheromatous degeneration is very common in the cerebral arteries, both on the larger branches of the circle of Willis and on smaller branches within the brain. The brain is affected by a large number of small infarcts giving this condition its other name, 'multi-infarct dementia'. The brain at post mortem or on CAT scan may appear relatively normal, but it is usually somewhat shrunken and it may appear irregular in shape, classically having a 'chewed appearance' due to the numerous small infarcts.

Infarcts may be caused directly by blockage of an artery by atheroma; or if an artery is only partially occluded and there is a lowering of blood pressure beyond the obstruction, there may be a reduced supply of blood which is insufficient to sustain the peripheral brain tissue. Once there is necrosis of brain tissue, there is a risk that there will be further haemorrhage into the infarcted area, and there is controversy as to whether haemorrhage takes place only under these conditions. Perhaps with a lower sensitivity to anoxia, the glial tissues tend to survive under adverse conditions in which neuronal cells cannot. These glial cells eventually remove the neuronal debris and replace the infarcts by a dense mass of fibrous tissue.

Dementias not associated with old age

Pick's disease

The atrophy here is more patchy, particularly affecting the frontal and temporal lobes, so that there is a different pattern in the CAT scan. In the affected areas there is neuronal loss and glial fibrosis, but some neurons may be seen to be swollen, with eosinophilic, agyrophilic or metachromatic inclusions.

Huntington's chorea

It now seems probable that in chorea there is overactivity in the dopaminergic nigrostriatal tract compared with the underactivity in Parkinson's disease. Drugs which improve chorea tend to decrease this activity (i.e. phenothiazines and alphamethylparatyrosine) and it is made worse by such drugs as L-dopa and bromocryptine. Pathological changes are most marked in the caudate nucleus and the globus pallidus, the head of the caudate nucleus being particularly shrunken; often this shrinkage is visible on CAT. There is generalized loss of brain tissue and thinning of the cortex, but this is not so marked by comparison with the degeneration in the deep structures and the dementia produced has been described as subcortical, as opposed to the cortical type of Altzheimer's disease. Clinically, subcortical dementia is said to be marked by emotional and personality changes and impairment of recent memory. Features such as aphasia, apraxia and agnosia, which may occur in cortical dementia, are never seen in this type.

It has been suggested that the disease might be caused by depletion of the GABA system. However, it seems probable that the biochemistry is far more complicated than this. In chorea, basal ganglia dopamine and noradrenaline are increased, whereas choline acetylase, GABA, substance P, enkephalins and angiotensin-converting enzymes are all decreased. The exact nature of the defect is not yet known and a number of theories are being tested; possibly the most interesting of these is that an inborn error of metabolism leads to an abnormal glutamate receptor which, after a period of failure requiring overstimulation, leads to a breakdown of the system. It is also interesting to note that some of the biochemical changes observed in the basal ganglia in Huntington's chorea have also been claimed to be found in parts of the limbic system in early schizophrenia.

Trauma

Whether or not the skull is fractured by a blow, the brain is accelerated within the skull and moves relative to it. The brain may be damaged immediately under the blow, or at the opposite pole where it hits against the skull, or by movements of different parts of the brain relative to each other, which may all cause rupture of blood vessels. Rotational force is therefore particularly damaging in the relatively large human cortex. It is possible that even without movement, pressure waves being transmitted through the brain, which is of a gel-like constituency, may cause damage. This type of damage is particularly likely to occur in the elderly, where the brain is shrunken and therefore has more room to move inside the skull. Concussion, with a loss of consciousness and even, in addition, retrograde and anterograde amnesia, may occur in the absence of any visible brain damage. However, repeated concussion—e.g. punch drunkenness in boxers—may show multiple small haemorrhages, broken nerve fibres and brain atrophy. The relationship between concussion and minimal disruption of the brain not obvious at post mortem remains unclear, and there are widely varied views on the pathology of post-concussional syndrome, or compensation neurosis, as it may be called by others.

Subdural haemorrhage

This is usually produced by the rupture of a superficial cortical vein crossing the subarachnoid space to enter a dural sinus. It is, therefore, again commonest in the elderly, where this space is largest and there is most room for the brain to move. Possibly because in the elderly there is more fluid surrounding the brain, there is often no history of loss of consciousness or injury. The haemorrhages are usually frontal or parietal and do not cross the midline. Rarely they are bilateral. Bleeding is venous and develops slowly, the brain accommodating and showing signs of atrophy under the haemorrhage. The haemorrhage gradually develops a thick fibrous membrane and at times may eventually be replaced by a fibrous sac containing a clear brownish fluid.

Infections

Investigations of the CSF will often suggest or rule out infection. This is probably not a common cause of dementia, but while treponemal infection is now rare, it cannot be forgotten.

Dementia is produced in the quaternary stage of treponemal infection after many years and is often called general paralysis of the insane. The brain is atrophic, especially in the frontal region; the meninges are thickened; and granular ependymitis may be seen in the fourth ventricle. The cortical changes may be visible on CAT scan, but the diagnosis would usually be made from positive serological changes being found in the CSF. This condition, again, can at least be arrested and may be partially cured by treatment with penicillin.

Almost all other brain infections are capable of causing dementia but few of these are common. However, the causes range from trypanosomes to tapeworms.

Normal-pressure hydrocephalus, sometimes called low-pressure hydrocephalus

This condition, which usually has its onset in later life when the skull can no longer expand, is believed to be most frequently caused by old infection around the base of the skull. It is not certain that this is true for every case and its aetiology is largely unknown. The clinical picture usually presents in middle life, with gradually increasing dementia and frequently a disturbance of gait; on neurological examination this reveals signs of long tract damage in the upper motor neurons serving the legs. On radiological examination the ventricles are shown to be dilated. However, to distinguish a case of this type from atrophy it is necessary to inject a radioactive substance either into the lumbar cerebrospinal space or directly into the ventricles and to observe the rate at which it either enters or exits from the ventricles, showing that communication between the lumbar and ventricular spaces is impeded. It is accepted that the condition is caused by partial blockage of the drainage of the ventricular CSF, and this probably accounts for the frequent association with basal infections which have long since been recovered from. Treatment by means of the drainage operation produces almost total remission of symptoms, and its importance, although it is a rare condition, lies in the fact that it is one of the recoverable causes of dementia.

Intoxication

Probably the most important type of intoxication in clinical practice is alcoholism. Recently CAT scan has made it plain that many more heavy drinkers than was realized show signs of brain atrophy. More encouraging is the fact that when abstinence is achieved, after some months the brain often appears to recover its normal volume. This atrophy appears to be generalized.

Other poisons may show more localized damage. An interesting argument concerns the development of Korsakoff's syndrome, which has a typical clinical picture of short-term memory failure with confabulation. The lesions here appear to be associated with deficiency of thiamine and to be centred in the corpora mamillaria, the posterior colliculi and the peri-aqueductal grey matter. These sites have been noted to have a high transketolase activity.

In addition to alcoholism, the disease is seen in dietary deficiency, gastric carcinoma and hyperemesis gravidarum. Whether alcohol intoxication in the absence of vitamin deficiency can produce these lesions is debated.

Conclusion

As can be seen from the above, a large number of very varied conditions can produce brain damage which presents to a psychiatrist usually as dementia but occasionally as delirium. Only a few of these conditions are treatable, and the psychiatrist always has to balance, particularly in the elderly, the disadvantages of numerous and unpleasant investigations against the possibility of overlooking a treatable lesion. Recent advances in the understanding of the clinical pathology of some of these lesions inevitably leads to hope that it may be possible to help in some of these cases. The understanding of the chemical pathology of Parkinson's disease, where degeneration is most marked in the substantia nigra and the red nuclei, led to the understanding of the defect in dopamine transmission and to the development of L-dopa as a treatment of the condition. Possibly, eventually a similar understanding of the biochemistry of senile dementia with Altzheimer's pathology might lead to a treatment for this most widespread of psychiatric conditions. So far experiments with choline administration and other measures designed to remedy the apparent disturbance of acetylcholine transmission have proved totally ineffective.

Finally, it should be noted that it is now being suggested that in some schizophrenics (Crowe's type II syndrome) there is a dementing process, which can be demonstrated by visible shrinkage of the brain on CAT.

Chapter 13

Aggression

Introduction

The first problem with the term 'aggression' is that it is used in so many ways that it has to be defined and limited in its breadth of meaning. By aggression is usually meant behaviour which, accompanied by (a) enhanced arousal, has (b) the potential for producing physical or psychological harm, (c) the intent to do so and (d) motivation on the part of the victim to avoid this harm if possible. It is very difficult to compare aggressive behaviour in the different species, and attempts to understand human aggression from observations on animals has limitations. Nevertheless, it is worth looking at animal studies as an initial step, and starting with a possibly wider view of aggression than that given above, which is perhaps most appropriate to humans.

Some of the conditions under which 'aggression' may occur in animals

(1) Predatory. Here the animal is behaving in the sequence of events (e.g. stalking, attacking) leading to killing of the victim for food.
(2) Spontaneous aggression between males in a number of circumstances—establishing the male hierarchy in a troop of animals, maintenance of that hierarchy, establishing or changing pair bonds (e.g. baboons, chimpanzees) during oestrus, obtaining a harem (seals).
(3) Aggression induced by irritability, fear, anxiety or pain.
(4) Aggression used to maintain individual or group rights to a feeding or nesting territory.
(5) Protection of prey.
(6) Protection of an infant.

To this could be added data on chimpanzees, etc.:

(1) Redirection of aggression where a dominant male attacks a subdominant male, who, in turn, may attack an individual further down the hierarchy.
(2) Failure to comply with a request—e.g. to groom the subsequent aggressor.
(3) When a member of the troop has a strange appearance (because of disease).
(4) When a head of the hierarchy is establishing himself.
(5) When a favoured food is in short supply.

Baboons undertake threats and attacks:

(1) While protecting the troop from predators, usually leopards, cheetahs or lions.
(2) In the resolution of disputes between males.
(3) In the formation and maintenance of consort pairs.
(4) In the allowing of favoured sleeping sites in trees, especially if a predator is in the vicinity.
(5) In acquiring highly prized foods.
(6) While exploring strange or dangerous locations.
(7) In contact with other troops, especially at the limits of their current territory.

In lower animals aggression can similarly be seen as predatory, spontaneous, provoked by fear or pain, territorial, protection of food, prey or young, and also, it must be added, in experimental situations.

In the great majority of species in their natural habitat, intraspecies threats and aggressive acts are brief and are accompanied by 'inhibitory' or 'linking' processes which prevent the attack going on to severe damage to either animal. The process may be largely ritualized and followed by withdrawal (flight) of the 'loser'.

The process in chimpanzees and baboons involves threats, attacks of varying severity, submission and the 'reassurance' of the victim by the aggressor. There are large repertoires of threatening behaviour, varying severity of attack, a large variety of acts of submission, followed by some movement or act by the aggressor to 'reassure' the victim.

Advantages to the species of aggression

The evolution of aggression is paradoxically most obvious in animals whose survival depends on co-operation between and living together of a number of individuals.

(1) High aggressivity among the dominant members ensures maximum safety. It is the powerful dominant male baboons which will protect the troop from natural predators (the large cats), who will explore dangerous territory or the boundaries between the troop's present territory and that of another troop.
(2) The formation of a troop defended in this way ensures access to food and water, and the optimum use of available territory. It also ensures powerful leadership, a stable predictable social environment for the young, protection to the young and differential reproduction (selection of the genes of the most physically powerful and dominant animals).

Factors causing abnormal levels of aggression

Many of our ideas of aggression in animals derive from either captive individuals or colonies or from domesticated or laboratory species. Under some circumstances these animals become 'abnormally' aggressive, but the conditions producing this unusual violence can exist in the natural habitat.

(1) Overcrowding causes increased aggression in a number of species. This probably has a number of causes—lack of 'personal' space, disturbed male-to-female ratio, lack of 'escape distance' (i.e. the individual who is subjected to threat cannot 'absent' himself from the aggressor).

(2) Unfamiliar appearance: an animal with an unusual appearance through, e.g., disease or injury.
(3) Introduction of unfamiliar adults to a colony.
(4) Parental or peer deprivation. An infant monkey separated from its mother and not allowed to interact with its peers becomes socially maladroit and aggressive. Such an individual introduced into a colony provokes much fighting. Sexual functioning is abnormal. but female 'deprived monkeys', if artificially inseminated, will neglect or kill their offspring.

Time of appearance of aggression

The first appearance of aggressive behaviour can be quite early in an animal's development and can be observed in, for instance, the young of cats and dogs. Young chimpanzees will threaten larger animals if their mother is nearby and is higher in the dominance hierarchy.

The anatomy and physiology of aggression

Immediately the area of behavioural observation is left (and this field has large unexplored areas), the other facets of aggressive behaviour become less and less clear, and there is no clearly established anatomical or physiological basis. However, it is known that at a primitive level the crude mechanisms for escape and attack are represented in the mesencephalon. Higher structures are important, and there is an inhibitory pathway arising either from the forebrain or the limbic system, which passes to the septum and the medial hypothalamus. Lesions of the medial hypothalamus give an immediate but transient reduction in the threshold for inducing rage; long-lasting reductions are obtained with lesions of the ventromedial nucleus. Stimulation of the medial hypothalamus in cats gives clawing defensive movements, but stimulation of the lateral hypothalamus gives the movements of predatory activity (stalking, etc.). Cats with lesions of the hippocampus and the cingulate gyrus seem to be particularly friendly, but those with damaged amygdaloid nuclei gradually develop a decreasing threshold for rage. Usually animals with bilaterally removed amygdaloid nuclei are passive and non-aggressive. The pathway probably concerned starts from the amygdaloid and passes to the hypothalamus by the ventral amygdalofugal pathway. While stimulation of the amygdaloid can provoke rage in some species, it suppresses predatory activity. In monkeys stimulation of the posteromedial nucleus of the thalamus decreases the 'authority' of dominant monkeys, and stimulation of the caudate nucleus will inhibit their aggression.

Neurotransmitters in aggression

Little is known about the neurotransmitters and other pathways involved in aggression. Among the many which could take part there are definitely three, but these are only likely to be a small part of the total. They are 5-hydroxytryptamine (5-HT), noradrenaline and gamma aminobutyric acid (GABA). Decreasing GABAergic function blocks predatory behaviour (mousekilling in rats), which is reversed by potentiating GABA activity. From what little is known of monoaminergic function in aggression, it seems that stimulation of the noradrenergic system facilitates 'affective aggression'—that type of aggression discussed briefly below, which is associated with a major increase in emotional responses/ autonomic activity, etc. Conversely, it decreases predatory aggression. Recently it has been suggested that aggression can be enhanced by the induction of beta adrenergic receptor supersensitivity. Blockade of the production of 5-HT plays a role similar to but not quite identical with that of stimulating noradrenergic function.

Arousal during aggression

In animals which seek other species as a source of food, the hunting pattern of aggression is distinguished from intraspecies aggression. In the former interspecies or 'predatory aggression' is not accompanied by widespread activation of autonomic/hormonal responses, although the animal may be highly motivated and have concentrated attention on 'the kill'. In the other situations where aggression is shown, the animal may have the type of autonomic overactivity and hormonal responses characteristic of preparation of the individual for 'flight or fight' described for anxiety/high arousal states. Thus, there is sympathetic activity, secretion of adrenaline and noradrenaline, and production of ACTH and corticosteroids. This prepares the whole organism for the increased neuromuscular/ endocrinal/cardiovascular and other responses necessary for the coming encounter. This is an important part of aggression with a high endocrinal component.

Role of hormones in aggression

This is a very complex subject, in which differences between the species are sufficiently variable to make comparisons between them impossible. In general, however, exposure of the fetus or neonate to testosterone possibly sensitizes its brain to future exposure to testosterone, and perhaps to 'paying attention' to learning experiences (in higher animals) which facilitate more aggressive behaviour. Absence of this exposure to testosterone may lead to the more female type of behaviour development. However, the effects of testosterone on the brain may be dependent on its conversion there to oestrogens (e.g. in rodents—similar evidence is lacking in primates and in man).

Whether aggressive activity is proportional to testosterone levels in adult life or whether there is a threshold level beyond which aggression does not increase is a matter for debate. Certainly, dominant monkeys tend to have higher testosterone levels than those lower down in the hierarchy. Since 'demotion' can be accompanied by decrease in the hormone, and a fall in the hierarchy can follow artificially reduced levels, 'cause and effect' become confusing. Some authors have said that highly aggressive monkeys have generally higher levels of production of 17-hydroxycorticosteroids and aggressive mice have larger adrenals than less aggressive animals. Others have pointed out, however, that corticoid levels are usually higher and production levels increased in the less dominant animal. Adrenalectomized mice lose aggressiveness; moderate replacement of steroids enhances aggression, but high doses decrease aggression.

Sex hormones play a part in aggression in rodents by their effect on the production of pheromones. One pheromone is characteristic of males and is aggression-promoting, and another (or the absence of the male pheromone) inhibits antagonistic behaviour. The male pheromone is dependent on testosterone and is present constantly, and the female pheromone (or the absence of the male factor) is independent of the oestrus cycle.

There is an additional pheromone in male mice—an 'aversive' pheromone, which presumably leads to 'distance' or avoidance between the males.

Experimentally, in the short term ACTH increases aggression in mice but over a longer period leads to a reduced antagonism. Various investigations suggest that aggression and submission are not the opposite ends of a continuum controlled by the same mechanism but depend on different processes in the body.

During encounters between mice defeat leads to enhancement of adrenocortical activity, while the victor shows no such changes. During fighting luteinizing hormone (LH) and follicular stimulating hormone (FSH) fall to a greater extent in the defeated animal, and the fall in FSH lasts longer.

Modulation of aggression

Without understanding its basis, man has known for centuries that strains of animals can be bred for increased or decreased aggressiveness, and then can be trained further—in other words, there is both a genetic and a learned component. Examples of this are the selection of aggressive breeds of dogs and bulls for fighting or, in the former, for defence of property, etc.; and the selective breeding of cavalry horses, fighting cocks, etc. Conversely, the antagonist temperament of earlier versions of the bulldog have disappeared in the present strain.

Hamburg, in his observation of the chimpanzee, acknowledged the role of the innate mechanisms and their modification by sex hormones in aggression, but also stressed the importance of learned responses based on observation by the young, imitation and their practice (this, of course, applied to a number of areas of behaviour).

Human aggression

Human beings have a remarkable propensity to various forms of violence, and there is no shortage of theories to account for this, from the evolutionary ones to those postulating unfavourable factors imposed by the growth of 'civilization'.

Some have started from the assumption that man started as a gatherer–scavenger, as an individually vulnerable creature. This led to group formation, and skills in group defence could be turned to intraspecies aggression. Others have suggested that, in contrast to primates, humans were omnivorous. Male–female differential development favoured the evolution of a male suited for a hunting group which developed increasingly effective aggressive methods involving tools. Survival demanded the potentials for the extremes of co-operativeness (for hunting, for forming a self-protective group) and aggression (for hunting and maintaining territory).

Other theories concentrating on the possible role of civilization have stressed the facts that man can apply aggression more and more effectively; that there are psychological mechanisms in man as a complex being in a complex society not present in animals; that the group co-operation/submission developed in our nature persists (witness the Charge of the Light Brigade); that tools have developed to the present horrific possibilities; and that the inhibitory mechanisms preventing actual bodily harm present in animals seem to be ineffective on many occasions. This is despite the fact that man has a rich repertoire of submission gestures. The ability to kill or injure at a distance will render these ineffective, but aggression by man at short range is also often not inhibited by submissive behaviour.

Where the role of 'civilization' is stressed, what appears is partly the implications of living in large complex urban groups. Factors postulated as potentiating the tendency to aggression are crowding, mobility (which reduces the development of social relationships involving mutual altruism), the complexity of societies in which each person has to relate to so many different individuals (a wider group of strangers than encountered by any hunter–gatherer tribe), the tendency of the young to disperse so that tasks are not shared with their relatives, and the trend for there to be delay in reproduction.

The psychological mechanisms associated with aggression in man include frustration, irritability, anger, anxiety, hatred, 'displacement' (i.e. venting of aggression from one person or situation to another), projection, repression, anger 'turned inward' against self, paranoid ideas and delusions, prejudice and animalization— the tendency in humans to designate others as lesser beings: as 'vermin', 'beasts' (prison slang for sexual offenders), 'pigs' (members of the police force), 'criminals', 'nutters', etc.

The latter processes of 'animalization' have been a marked feature of aggression against 'out groups' throughout human society and were typified perfectly during the Nazi era in Germany; it is easy to think of current parallels.

The learning process is of the greatest importance in higher animals such as primates and in humans, and can only be touched on briefly here. The reader is referred to the work of the Harlows, Hinde, Bowlby and others. Bowlby was a pioneer in demonstrating the importance of separation of children from parents on future emotional development. In the 'learning' process of aggression in childhood can be included divorce and other separations from parents, poor quality of parenting and lack of affection, illegitimacy, institutional life and aggression as a form of punishment.

The latter factor tends to produce aggressive children. As in primates, the learning process extends to observation, imitation and practice, and there is increased aggression in families and societies where a high level of 'antagonism' is the norm. Watching violence (e.g. on television) can be followed by imitative aggression, and children may acquire a repertoire of learned violent patterns which may only manifest themselves when the situation is such as to evoke it.

Training in childhood, adolescence or adult life and habituation to violence can modify behaviour completely, and many examples of this can be quoted—military training, training people for 'special groups' requiring the use of directed aggression, etc.

The role of hormones, particularly sex hormones, in human aggression is not clear. In young, but not older, men hostility has been found to be correlated with testosterone levels. On the other hand, comparison of testosterone levels in hostile or aggressive prisoners and in non-aggressive prisoners has not produced consistent findings by different workers. Men, however, are more aggressive than women, and women exposed to androgens in infancy tend to be 'tomboys', to favour rough games and play, but are not outside the normal range of girls' behaviour. Again, it may be that it is early exposure to androgens which sensitizes the brain to 'attention' to aggressive learning patterns. The adult aggressive tendencies may be the sum of a biological predisposition to acquiring violent patterns of behaviour plus the experience of exposure to specific social learning situations.

An earlier example is the famous one of two adjacent tribes—the peaceful Arapesh, who discouraged anger and aggression, and the more aggressive Mungudumor tribe, whose whole mode of life from the age of suckling onwards was directed to fostering the maximum of anger, antagonism and later warlike attitudes (smaller, more extreme forms of Athens and Sparta?). It should be noted that the behaviour applied, in both cases, to both men and women in the tribes. This argues against the theory that testosterone produces the alleged typical aggression of man.

Special factors fostering aggression in humans

Overcrowding has already been mentioned; to this can be added social frustration. During the depression of the late 1920s and the 1930s robbery, suicide and lynching all increased in the USA, and this occurred also in their crowded big cities in the 1960s and the 1970s. Oddly, perhaps, homicide in general and, understandably, alcoholism increased during prosperity.

As stated above, in past and present societies where robbery, violence and murder are or were commonplace, this is the accepted norm. This can be seen, for instance, in prison subcultures and in underprivileged males in lower social groups.

The situation is complicated by the selection of 'victims', which is not wholly random. It has been found that some policemen are assaulted more frequently than others, and victims of violence and murder are not necessarily 'chance' but may have some characteristics making them more vulnerable.

Illness and aggression

Any condition leading to loss of brain 'tissue'—accident, tumours, dementia, encephalitis—especially if involving the basal ganglia, the hypothalamus and the limbic system may predispose to uncontrolled violence. Part of the pattern may be the beginnings of disinhibition.

Epilepsy is generally believed to be associated with violence, but the correlation between the two is much less than belief implies. This is true also of schizophrenia, where, despite the presence of paranoid ideas, the acting out of the hostile thoughts or auditory hallucinations is rare. Depressive illness is often accompanied by paranoid ideas and/or feelings of inferiority and unworthiness. Again this may lead to acts of violence but perhaps it is more usual for, say, a mother or a spouse in psychotic depression to murder the relative before suicide or attempted suicide, as an act of love in the presence of delusions of catastrophe ('the world is terrible, so we will leave it together'). Morbid jealousy, 'the Othello syndrome', can lead to physical or psychological violence or murder. Sometimes it is based on alcoholism, dementia, brain diseases, schizophrenia, depression or a personality disorder.

Psychopathic individuals form a section of those committing violent crimes. Puerperal psychosis is a major, but not the only, cause of infanticide and the association of aggression with premenstrual tension is well known.

However, the greatest danger to an individual is in the home. At its worst it carries the rubrics 'baby battering' or 'granny bashing'. Many of those practising this behaviour were themselves similarly treated—brutalized in childhood—and fit into the sociopathic group.

Drugs and other modifiers of aggression

Some drugs can induce or decrease aggression. The former include amphetamines, apomorphine, cannabis combined with deprivation of food, L-dopa with a peripheral decarboxylase inhibitor. With amphetamines violence may occur also during amphetamine psychosis. Alcohol, barbiturates and chlordiazepoxide given chronically can produce or release aggression in some circumstances. As regards alcohol, violence can be a feature of disinhibition of the intoxication stage, but post-alcoholic violence in the irritable 'hangover' period may be equally important. Lithium has been used as an anti-aggressive drug.

Psychosurgery—the bilateral removal of the amygdaloid nuclei—has been tried on pathologically aggressive individuals. The effect on personality would require further research, quite apart from the doubtful ethics of the procedure.

Hunger can be a trigger of aggression, but chronic starvation reduces people to an apathetic immobile depressed state. This has been used as a means of enabling a small number of guards to cope with large populations confined in concentration camps.

Biochemical changes and aggression

This is a meagrely researched area to date. However, in patients with personality disorders, aggression scores were signi'icantly negatively correlated with levels of 5-hydroxyindole acetic acid (5-HIAA) and positively correlated with 3-methoxy-4-hydroxyphenolglycol (MHPG), with no correlation with homovanillic acid. As much as 85 per cent of the variance was contributed by 5-HIAA + MHPG, but the major contributor was 5-HIAA (80 per cent of the variance of aggressive scores).

Recently, increased levels of plasma-free and conjugated phenylacetic acid have been found in detainees serving long terms in prison for violent crimes, as compared with pair-matched non-violent control prisoners. Phenylacetic acid is the major metabolite of phenylethylamine, an amphetamine-like substance.

The role of GABAergic neurons in animals has been discussed above.

Drugs and aggression

Date on drugs are mostly from animal experiments. Some of these investigations have been directed to the aminergic systems, and it has been found that imipramine, desimipramine, amitriptyline, clomipramine and mianserin (all antidepressant drugs) decrease predatory killing by rats. Surprisingly, maprotiline was inactive, so this was probably not an effect on the noradrenergic systems. Presumably, it could be a serotoninergic or cholinergic mechanism. With one of the active compounds, imipramine, the effect was observed by injecting it directly into the amygdaloid nuclei. Chlorpromazine had no effect in this experiment. Clearly, this is an area requiring further exploration—could these drugs be making the animals more irritable, for instance?

Three drugs—maprotiline, amitriptyline and mianserin—decreased the isolation-invoked aggression of mice, but with at least two of these there is a sedation effect, which is an uncontrollable variable.

Chlorpromazine, benzodiazepines and peripheral beta-receptor blockers can reduce aggression; benzodiazepines, however, sometimes have an opposite effect. Sulpiride selectively decreases 'isolation' aggression in mice, but is inactive in 'muricidal' behaviour in rats.

On the whole, these and similar observations on drugs and aggression are subject to too many possible explanations to be of much specific use at present in this area.

Premenstrual tension

Of the women in the childbearing period of life, as many as 40 per cent are suffering from premenstrual tension. This syndrome is variable in its length and severity, but, among other things, is characterized by depression, irritability, anger, anxiety and often loss of energy. Of the crimes of violence committed by women, many occurred during this time, as compared with few in the preovulatory phase.

It is interesting that women who suffer from both premenstrual tension and affective illness can often distinguish between 'normal depression' and that of premenstrual tension, and between the depression of the premenstrual phase and that of endogenous illness.

Alcohol and aggression

There is no doubt that alcohol plays a part in aggression in man, but beyond this statement is considerable doubt about exactly how these two phenomena interact.

Alcohol is associated with a wide spectrum of behaviours in which violence of some form is a part. It is associated with traffic accidents, with injury to pedestrians, with people arrested for felonies and with homicide. Conversely, alcohol is associated with the victims of aggressive crimes, with suicide and with people killed in various kinds of violent accidents. Many rapists and many of those molesting children sexually have often taken alcohol beforehand. Some apparent victims of accidental violent deaths have taken alcohol, and some of these may be 'hidden' suicides. Wife battering and assaults on children occur about twice as often in families where there is a member with alcoholism, and it is surprising how often a pattern set up in one generation continues into the next.

Whether acute alcohol intake acts by disinhibition, releasing previously controlled aggression, or evokes and promotes aggression is not yet clear. In chronic alcoholism the presence of impotence in the male and alcohol-induced paranoid ideas may be contributing factors. There is, however, another facet to alcoholism: where it seems to act directly as a provoker of aggression is in post-alcoholic violence, a phenomenon only recently recognized as relatively common. Here the aggression is probably a manifestation of irritability of withdrawal and/or of the 'hangover', as mentioned above.

Chapter 14

Anxiety

Introduction

Anxiety is not an easy subject to discuss with any degree of coherence, because, like so many other areas of normal and abnormal emotion and the associated biological mechanisms, there are so many incomplete areas of information. The uncertainty begins with the very nature of anxiety. Anxiety is a normal emotional state concerned with optimal functioning and with threatening situations. It is an emotion which is likely to be an evolutionary development concerned with survival in the widest sense of the word.

Some authors distinguish pathological anxiety from 'normal' anxiety and 'fear', considering them to be different in some way (e.g. anxiety may be 'free-floating'— that is, not attached to any object or situation). Others say that pathological anxiety differs from 'normal' anxiety only in its frequency, severity and duration, that its triggering factors are minimal and are not available to superficial appraisal, and that it impairs well-being and efficiency. Otherwise these authors suggest that abnormal anxiety is indistinguishable from normal anxiety and fear, which lie on a continuum of the following kind.

Cognitive elements involving:

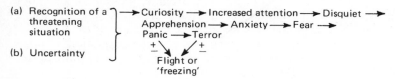

This progression, as with other emotions, carries with it increasing levels of arousal, a result which has some unfortunate implications for the experimentalist, in that measures of the emotion and of the degree of arousal may be inseparable.

Neuroanatomy and neurophysiology of anxiety

It is not possible to set down a definitive neuroanatomy and physiology of anxiety—only some of the facts, facets and hypotheses.

Anatomy

It is likely that two regions of the brain play a major role in anxiety, of which one is the cortex. It recognizes and analyses the event provoking the anxiety. It is the recipient of whatever are the afferent signals to the cortex which evoke the emotion of anxiety, heightened arousal and the awareness of both. The areas of the brain which probably are the recipients of the cortical signals of awareness of threat, and the evokers of the efferent emotional/arousal mechanisms, include parts of the limbic system. Its efferent connections probably relay to the neocortex partly via the hypothalamus.

The region of the limbic system which gives main evidence of involvement with anxiety is the amygdaloid nucleus, stimulation of parts of which . evoke fear responses in animals and overwhelming anxiety in some humans. Moving away from the limbic system, stimulation of the medial dorsal nucleus of the thalamus elicits crouching and 'escape' in cats, and an area of the posterior hypothalamus near the mamillary bodies is associated with 'flight mechanisms'. In general, dorsal and posterior areas of the hypothalamus are concerned with flight mechanisms and are the link with the peripheral components of anxiety (motor and autonomic), and some of the physiological components to muscular exercise.

The reticular formation and ascending noradrenergic and serotoninergic fibres are the main pathways mediating the level of cortical arousal during anxiety. The term 'level of arousal' here is taken as the state determining the 'intensity of behaviour and motivation' and the level of alertness present. It is a factor in the liveliness and degree of exertion of effort which is experienced and displayed by an individual. Anxiety has an additional component. Centrally there is the cognitive uncertainty and discomfort about a novel, problematical or potentially threatening situation. This produces an autonomic/peripheral/hormonal response via (a) the autonomic nervous system, (b) the systems concerned with muscle tone and activity, and (c) release of corticotrophin-releasing factor by the hypothalamus and the resultant liberation of adrenocorticotrophic hormone (ACTH), which itself has central as well as peripheral effects.

The autonomic nervous system (activated by its 'head hypothalamic nuclei') is responsible directly or via the liberation of catecholamines from the adrenal medulla for the peripheral effects. These are cardiovascular and visceral changes, sweating of the hands, increased heart rate, increased blood flow through the muscles, decreased blood flow through the skin, tremor, dilation of the pupil, reduction in salivary secretion and a raised blood pressure. The release of catecholamines by the adrenal medulla is not specific to anxiety; it can occur in a whole variety of 'arousing' emotions, including anger, sexual activation, hypoglycaemia, etc. With the release of catecholamines, free fatty acids and glucose from the liver are liberated from adipose tissue into the blood.

In some ways the adrenocortical response is considered to be a longer-term response to stressful circumstances, but in prolonged, severe stress probably both hormonal systems take part (see Chapter 8). Such severe stress may be accompanied by raised erythrocyte sedimentation rate and increased protein-bound iodine, and other changes.

As mentioned above, ACTH may have an effect in anxiety quite separate from that of adrenocortical stimulation. The injection of ACTH in animals evokes 'anxiety-like' behaviour and the substance is found distributed mainly to the hypothalamus, the amygdaloid nucleus and the hippocampus. Some ACTH fragments have a similar effect. Corticoids released by ACTH do not mimic this action, and, in any event, the results of ACTH injection are too rapid for mediation via steroids and adrenalectomized animals have an 'anxiety reaction' identical with that of control animals. Thus, ACTH has a direct action on the central nervous system.

A drug which blocks synthesis of 5-hydroxytryptamine (5-HT) produces the anxiety profile. ACTH increases turnover of 5-HT, but has no effect on behaviour of rats with lesions of the main ascending 5-HT pathway. In addition, a benzodiaze-pine given chronically increased 5-HT and decreased 5-hydroxyindole acetic acid levels and blocked the behavioural effects of ACTH. The suggestion, as yet unproven, is that ACTH may act on anxiety processes via modulation of the activity of serotoninergic neurons.

The appearance in anxiety/fear

Anxious individuals look tense and apprehensive, the muscles are tense and they will be unable to relax. They sit on the edge of the chair, jump at unexpected noises, and may have some tremor of the hands. The eyes are wide open and the pupils are dilated. They may lick their lips (because of dry mouth) and be restless and fidgety. Movements are sometimes impulsive and poorly coordinated.

During fear, the person will be motionless at first, with eyes and mouth open, sometimes breathless, sometimes in a crouching position, and will have a pale sweaty skin and a raised pulse rate. The superficial muscles shiver, breathing is hurried, the mouth is dry, and if the fear is not overwhelming, the individual may yawn. As fear increases, there may be trembling of the muscles, starting with the lips, the hair 'stands on end' and the voice becomes husky or indistinct or fails altogether. The individual may be restless, pace up and down and be unable to act in any directed meaningful action.

As fear merges into terror, the pulse rate rises, sometimes to the point at which there may be temporary cardiovascular failure and faintness; there is a deathlike pallor, laboured breathing, dilatation of the nostrils, gasping, convulsive move-ments of the lips, a hollow trembling cheek, gulping, protruding eyes with dilated pupils, and sometimes rolling of the eyes. The muscles are rigid, the hands clench and unclench, and the arms may be held over the head as if to avoid some danger. The person may have uncontrollable flight and/or defaecate or urinate.

Animal studies

Some of what we know about anxiety and fear comes from human work—such as the knowledge that some people experience severe fear on stimulation of the amygdaloid nucleus or parts of the hypothalamus. Much of the information on the subject, however, has come from animal studies where 'fear behaviour'—flight or freezing—is equated with similar emotions in man. Some of the 'fear behaviour'—e.g. cessation of the current activity, flight or freezing—is general to complex and even less complex organisms; other behaviours are specific to the species.

The animals used most in these studies are rodents, especially rats, where an aversive stimulus, the threat of which should evoke 'anxiety', is coupled with a neutral stimulus to condition 'fear responses'. Conditioned responses of various complexity have been coupled with anatomical, physiological, pharmacological and other experiments to try to establish the various bases of anxiety. Such experiments are difficult to interpret. Applying intracranial stimuli, or giving drugs with multiple effects on arteries, motor activity and sensory processes, or ablating parts of the brain may produce what appears to be a clear-cut answer, but which has a quite different meaning from the one given, or may not be extrapolated easily to man. This is in no way to be taken as a denigration of the considerable amount of useful and detailed work in this area which has contributed to our knowledge of anxiety.

Evocation of anxiety

While the preceding sections may have given the general impression of anxiety being evoked by threatening situations, the position is more complex than that.

Some fear responses are innate—that of darkness in diurnal animals and of light in nocturnal creatures. Babies fear strangers. Many species seem to have an innate fear of heights or of rapidly expanding objects.

Fears can be attenuated by adaptation, and habituation, or, conversely, can be reinforced. New fears can be learned and subsequently attenuated or reinforced.

Sight of the natural predator is a familiar phenomenon in 'at risk' species, and there are interesting reports of lack of fear of man in animals who have hitherto not been exposed to his 'aggressive habits'.

Anxiety as a psychological drive

Unlike other emotions, anxiety has the important function of being involved in a drive mechanism, which is needed in part for the accomplishing of certain tasks. The behaviour evoked by anxiety is in part directed to increasing that drive (completing the task in hand, etc.), so that anxiety secondarily reinforces the behaviour. Here the Yerkes–Dodson law applies. With increasing anxiety the efficiency of the individual rises to a maximum, reaches a plateau but falls progressively as the anxiety level increases further. There is thus an optimum level of anxiety below and above which efficiency is reduced.

Pathological anxiety in man

The difficulty of defining pathological anxiety was discussed earlier—it is that anxiety considered to be excessive in severity of frequency which impairs functioning and/or which has no superficially identifiable cause. It may have no immediate 'object'. Perhaps 3–5 per cent of the population have pathological anxiety, with women outnumbering men by 2 to 1.

It may invoke a whole range of somatic symptoms—'tightness' in the head, 'butterflies', tenseness of the muscles, etc.—which in part are a reflection of the somatic changes accompanying the condition. In others anxiety may have few if any secondary somatic effects.

It is often secondary to other psychiatric conditions—depersonalization, depression, hypochondriasis, hysteria, psychosomatic conditions, schizophrenia, acute brain syndrome, alcoholism, obsessional states, etc. It is an intrinsic part of the various phobic conditions.

Physical causes of pathological anxiety must not be forgotten—such as hyperthyroidism, hypoglycaemia, phaeochromocytoma, the premenstrual tension syndrome, disorders of calcium metabolism, and others. Drug abuse (amphetamine, hallucinogens) and withdrawal states from 'hard' drugs evoke anxiety reactions.

While considering anxiety, it is important to distinguish between what has been described as 'trait' anxiety and 'state' anxiety. 'Trait' anxiety occurs in the individual with a life-long predisposition—a natural tendency to react with anxiety. 'State' anxiety is the anxiety occurring at a point in time in an individual, and therefore it may be either a relatively new experience for that person, or an episode in a life-long tendency to have the 'trait' of anxiety.

Habituation in anxiety

Observation of 'habituation' in the experimental situation may be one of the most useful studies of anxiety. Given one of a series of experimental stimuli, patients with anxiety show two features which differ from those of control subjects. First, the physiological changes take longer than controls to return to baseline values. Second, if the same stimuli are repeated, normal subjects tend to habituate—that is their responses tend to become less and less with repetition. This occurs to a much smaller degree, and more slowly, in anxious subjects, who thus show impairment in their ability to adapt to recurrent stimuli of this kind.

The antecedents of the anxiety

The antecedents of the anxiety-prone person are passing beyond the scope of this book. There are scattered references in animal studies to effects of subjecting a maternal rat to various manipulations on the behaviour of its offspring, and the possible effects of experiences in the neonatal animal during a critical period of development on its subsequent emotionality. For human and primate studies, the reader is referred to writers such as Bowley, Anderson, Hinde, Murray Parkes, and to authors who have dealt with overwhelming stress and other factors in the genesis of 'anxiety'. Most standard textbooks of psychology discuss the studies of anxiety in people under stress (parents of children with mortal illness, soldiers in battle or under stressful training, the differences in anxiety between the leader of a group and the others, etc.).

Psychophysiological measures in anxiety

The somatic concomitants of anxiety have been used to assess anxiety in controls and in patients with various anxiety conditions. The main problem mentioned above is that most of the changes monitored are non-specific—more features of various degrees of arousal than of anxiety itself. Nevertheless, the area of study has been fruitful.

Two strategies have been employed. By taking normal controls and subjecting them to 'stress', features of 'state' anxiety can be observed; whereas by investigating patients with anxiety, the phenomenon of 'trait' anxiety can be assessed.

(1) *Cardiovascular system* This has provided a rich field for methodology in the investigation of anxiety arousal: pulse rate, radiotelemetry of the ECG, blood pressure, finger pulse volume and forearm blood flow.

(2) *Skin conductance* Changes in the conductance of skin are largely determined by activity or inactivity of the sweat glands, and, in particular, palmar skin conductivity has been used in the assessment of varying levels of anxiety/arousal. A consistent finding has been low levels of conductance at rest in palmar skin in patients with anxiety as compared with controls.

(3) *Muscles* Activity in muscle is increased in anxiety but not consistently in all groups. The most 'reliable' muscle groups differ between studies but probably include the frontalis muscle, the masseter and the forearm extensors. The assay procedure is the measurement of isometric tone by surface electromyography. At rest, muscle activity in anxious individuals tends to be higher than in normal controls.

(4) *Other measures* Respiration tends to become rapid in anxious patients and the efficiency of respiration is reduced. Attempts have been made also to assess anxiety by salivary flow, in view of the well-known 'dry mouth' experienced during fear.

Drugs and anxiety

A number of drugs have been used to control anxiety, foremost of which are the benzodiazepines. Besides being anxiolytic, these compounds are also anticonvulsant and muscle relaxants. Their function seems to be tied to that of the gamma aminobutyric acid (GABA) system (*see* Chapter 4). By displacing the natural inhibitor of GABA activity, this system is released to greater activity.

One recent theory is outlined below.

Alcohol, meprobamate and barbiturates are anxiolytic but do not bind to the benzodiazepine receptor. Another group of drugs with anxiolytic properties has been largely ignored. Tertiary amine tricyclics reduce anxiety well in advance of their antidepressant effect, and the same may apply to monoamine oxidase inhibitors, mianserin and trazodone.

The question to be asked is: Where is the final common pathway for the anxiolytic response onto which these diverse agents converge? The behaviour analogue of anxiety in man in animals was warning of impending punishment, of stimuli warning of frustrative non-reward and of novel stimuli. Similarly, in man anxiety was elicited by threat of pain, by loss or failure and by unfamiliar circumstances. The accompaniments were increased arousal, increased attention to environmental clues, especially novel ones, and inhibition of current behaviour (especially rewarded behaviour).

It was argued that the area of brain mediating this 'conglomerate' of actions was the septohippocampal part of the limbic system and its ascending noradrenergic and serotoninergic afferents. There was some controversy as to whether the ascending noradrenergic pathways were part of the neural substrate for reward and reinforcement or, on the contrary, mediated responses to stimuli warning of frustrating non-reward.

It was claimed that natural rewards (in contradistinction to electrical stimuli) suggested the non-reward hypothesis, and that animals deprived of the noradrenergic pathway could still learn and perform reward responses. The animals, however, had retarded extinction of the responses and lost the partial reinforce-ment effects produced when randomly non-rewarded stimuli were mixed with rewarded stimuli.

The hypothesis was that the septohippocampal system had a cognitive role in anxiety, being a match–mismatch comparator which monitored current activity and desired goals. Discrepancies (punishment, non-reward, failure) were recorded, as were threats of discrepancies. Current activity was stopped while there was a search for alternative actions.

It cannot be overemphasized, however, that much of the activity of the CNS is occupied by the process of match–mismatch comparisons, looking at the differ-ences between the actual and the expected, or memorized, event from the simplest psychological control mechanisms to the problems of abstract thought. However, in this view, the septohippocampal system was an organ of hesitation and doubt which, if it become overactive, could lead to anxiety.

The effect of benzodiazepines in anxiety was postulated to be at the GABAergic afferents to the nucleus coeruleus or the GABA terminals in the lateral septal area of hippocampus. The hypothesis said little about the possible sites of action of barbiturates or meprobamate, although barbiturates can potentiate GABAergic function. The anxiolytic effects of some antidepressants were congruent with this hypothesis, but the role of the amygdaloid nucleus in anxiety was not covered in this discussion.

A possibly different kind of anxiolytic agent has been used in the form of beta-blocking drugs such as propranolol. It is not clear as to whether such compounds are acting centrally as well as peripherally. The ascending reticular activating system contains many noradrenergic neurons whose actions may be reduced by propranolol, which blocks the postsynaptic receptors.

Of course, there are also other beta receptor sites in the brain. For the moment let it be assumed that the main actions of propranolol in anxiety are in controlling the level of functioning of the peripheral sympathetic nervous system.

Propranolol and other similar drugs will prevent such somatic manifestations as palpitations, tremor, diarrhoea, etc. It is assumed that in anxious individuals with prominent somatic symptoms, interrupting them with beta-blockers breaks a feedback loop which otherwise would perpetuate the anxiety. In other words, by taking away the anticipated somatic accompaniments of anxiety, the experience of anxiety is lessened, and perhaps with learning may be less on a future occasion. In general, beta-blocking drugs are inactive in those with free-floating anxiety not associated with bodily symptoms. This might suggest a peripheral only action for the drugs but this presupposes a level of understanding of anxiety which we do not possess yet.

The uses of beta-blockers have been extended to the control of 'normal' mental stress—public speaking, artistic and sporting performances, etc.—in which exces-sive metabolic and cardiovascular activity is prevented. This is of value in its own right. It may be of particular benefit to those in whom acute 'normal' stress may be harmful—for example, post-coronary thrombosis. The main contradictions are low cardiac reserve and asthma.

Chapter 15

Affective disorders

Introduction

One definition of affective disorders is that they are a group of phasic illnesses in which the main abnormality is in changes in mood, and the other symptoms are more or less secondary to this, and in which there is a return to full normality in the periods of remission.

An alternative definition is an extension and modification of the one proposed by Hamilton. In this definition these illnesses are defined as phasic changes in vitality, showing themselves psychologically in the cognitive and affective spheres, somatically in loss of drives for food, sex and work, and in both areas in changes in rhythms.

The problem of the classification of depression is one which continues to be a subject of much debate in an area where there have been outstanding work by Roth and colleagues, Paykel, Kendall, Winokur and others. For the purpose of this chapter, which is concerned with the biological and pharmacological aspects of mood, the unipolar/bipolar classification will be accepted tentatively, although this is almost certainly incomplete, and the material will be confined to a discussion of those features of unipolar affective discorder (recurrent or endogenous depression) where the patient has depressive illnesses only, and of bipolar affective disorder (manic depressive psychosis) where there are attacks of both mania and depression. The difficult and unresolved question of the extent to which these illnesses are separate from other forms of mood change or are one end of a continuum will not be discussed here. An important feature of both types of illnesses is intervals of normality between episodes.

Symptoms

It is also not the purpose of this chapter to discuss the finer points of phenomenology of affective illness—a discussion which might occupy a chapter itself. A brief description of the clinical characteristics is necessary, however, because the spectrum of symptoms has influenced studies into the treatment and aetiology of these conditions, and therefore has some bearing on attempts to understand the underlying processes.

Mania

Mania is a mental state associated usually with euphoria, a feeling of heightened energy and well-being, and an excess of enthusiasm and energy. Patients with mania are expansive and talkative; their speech is rapid, discursive and often with a content in which open-ended associations are made which lead to a rapid flitting from one subject to another, sometimes in an amusing way (flight of ideas). The trends of thought have a logical basis which can be traced. They may make frequent puns, and have 'clang associations' (words or phrases chosen by their sounding similar to previously used words rather than by an association of meaning). Such is the pressure of thought and distractability that the degree of heightened activity in mania may not be harnessed to any consistent task. In hypomania, however, the forceful and energetic organization of the environment may be only too evident and exhausting to people in the vicinity of the patient. With increasing mania, grandiose ideas and plans take over, and unrealistic schemes may be set in motion which may wreak havoc on the financial and other affairs of the patient and his or her family. Some patients become sexually overactive and promiscuous. The need for sleep decreases and the individual may be too busy to eat, and engage in increasing activity and plans. Not surprisingly, the old and frail may become dangerously exhausted, and death from exhaustion, though rare, is not unknown even now. Religiose delusions or delusions of grandeur may intrude at this stage. Later the delusions become more bizarre and may be associated with hallucinations and ideas of reference.

Perhaps the most uncomfortable form of mania for the patient is where it is combined with some depressive thought content and symptoms, the so-called 'mixed affective states'. Superficially, the patient seems to have typical manic behaviour but on closer questioning is disturbed and unhappy, with an underlying depressive mood state. This mixture of driven overactivity and depression seems to have a nightmarish quality for the patient.

Depression

The depressive phase of bipolar illness and the depression of unipolar illness are clinically indistinguishable (at least at the present time). The individual's mood is anything from mildly sad to a state of the most profound melancholia. This may be accompanied by feelings of mild to severe anxiety and apprehension. The patients' 'drives' are reduced, so that they lose interest in food, sex and work. With regard to the loss of interest in food, appetite disappears, many patients complain that food becomes tasteless and, unless they force themselves to eat, they tend to lose weight. Others, however, 'binge' as a form of compensation. They are indifferent to their usual pursuits and interests, and are very conscious of their inertia, lack of initiative and absence of mental or physical energy. In some patients all their processes, including thought, speech and movement, become slowed, while others, driven by a rising tide of anxiety, become restless and agitated. Thought processes become inefficient, so that simple tasks, planning or decisions become difficult or impossible, and concentration is almost invariably very poor. If anxiety reduces their ability to organize their thought processes still further, patients become unable to follow through their normal tasks consistantly. Many are aware of and are very distressed by an inability to feel for others.

What may loosely be described as disturbance of rhythm takes place. This manifests itself as the diurnal shift in mood (and other symptoms) seen in many patients, at least in the earlier stages of illness. Characteristically, they feel at their worst on waking but gradually improve as the day goes on, sometimes feeling almost normal by the evening, only to return to their nadir the following morning. Sleep also is often disturbed, and the patient may, in addition, wake earlier than is the usual habit. These sleep changes could be partly dependent on alterations in diet secondary to loss of appetite. Temperature and some hormonal rhythms are disturbed, and some excretory rhythms (e.g. 3-methoxy-4-hydroxyphenylglycol: MHPG) are abnormal.

These disturbances are accompanied by psychological symptoms which may be mild right through to gross psychotic states. They include feelings of worthlessness and hopelessness, self-blame and delusions of guilt and punishment, nihilistic delusions, delusions of catastrophe, hypochondriasis and poverty; paranoid ideas and ideas of reference. A feeling of hopelessness and the uselessness of life is almost invariably followed by suicide thoughts, which can move on to intention and action. Attempts at suicide are most common on passing into or coming out of illness.

The concurrence of a number of the symptoms, especially those present in the depressive phase, has played a part in the thinking on affective illness. The presence of depression of mood, with or without anxiety, anorexia, loss of interest in sex, cognitive inefficiency, disturbances in sleep pattern, lack of physical and mental energy, and the characteristic diurnal pattern of symptoms, together with the phasic nature of the illnesses, sometimes with seasonal and/or regular recurrences, have suggested a predominantly biological illness, probably based on limbic, hypothalamic and brain-stem structures.

Environmental and constitutional factors

Most psychiatrists work from the assumption that environment and constitution combine to interact in the aetiology of mood disorders. It is assumed that noxious environmental factors participate in the causation of depression to a greater or lesser extent, so that there is really no such thing as an 'endogenous' illness, which therefore is a misnomer. Certainly, there is an excess of traumatic life events, as compared with matched controls, preceding the first episode of affective disorders in a large proportion of cases, and subsequently life events, of which the illness itself is a major one, are difficult to evaluate as aetiological factors. The events are often loss, separation or threatening events, and may occur in clusters. It has been suggested recently that the effects of individual adverse life events may summate if they occur over about 6 months. Other precipitating events include virus infections, an operation, serious medical illnesses, a hormonal upset, etc. The effect of events must not be overestimated, however, because, as pointed out by Paykel, they are by no means overwhelming.

Later the overall pattern of recurrences will be discussed; it can be stated here that there is little understanding of what determines the regular recurrences seen in so many patients, sometimes on a seasonal basis. We also do not know whether in the whole group of affective illnesses there are subgroups in which 'events' play a part and others in which they do not.

Genetics of affective disorder

Despite the availability of quite a lot of information on the genetics of affective disorder, we are still ignorant about the mode of inheritance. According to Price, the view that transmission is dominant must be accepted on the available evidence, but, on the other hand, the dominant gene or genes cannot be fully penetrant. He also claims (but perhaps this is a more controversial point) that sex-linked inheritance can also be ruled out (*see* below). In fact, as yet there is no agreement as to whether affective illness is monogenic or polygenic.

There is no doubt, however, that hereditary factors do contribute to the illnesses. There is an increased familial prevalence of depressive illness and suicide, especially in first-degree relatives. People in the families of bipolar patients have a higher morbidity than those related to patients with the unipolar disorder. It may be, however, that if melancholic character structures and depressive reactions are added to the numbers with overt unipolar illness, the risk of this type of disorder or related characteristics is still high in unipolar families. The unipolar trait may manifest itself in depressive changes and personality traits more than in the form of depressive psychosis, whereas the abnormality in the bipolar condition is more often than not a psychosis. Perhaps only 50 per cent of depressive disorders in the families of patients with unipolar illness assume the proportions of frank psychosis.

With bipolar illness there is equal morbidity in male and females, but in unipolar depressions females outnumber males by 2 to 1, and this ratio is higher if the depressive traits and reactions mentioned above are included.

Among relatives of patients with affective disorder the morbidity risk is in the region of 10–15 per cent. For early onset probands (<40 years) the risk in first-degree relatives is greater, about 19 per cent as compared with late-onset probands (>40 years), where the risk is about 10 per cent. Risks are higher in the relatives of bipolar than in the relatives of unipolar individuals.

Winokur and his colleagues have suggested three subdivisions of the unipolar group: (1) depressive spectrum depressions with genetic links to alcoholism and antisocial personality; (2) pure depressive disease, in which there is a family history of depression, more depression in sisters, more suicide in parents, no association with alcoholism and suppression of cortisol in the dexamethasone suppression test; (3) non-familial sporadic depressions. These proposed groups require further investigation.

Twin studies have revealed 67–69 per cent concordance rates in monozygotic twins (MZ), and in the region of 13 per cent in dizygotic twins (DZ), which suggests a large genetic component. Splitting the group into unipolar (UP) and bipolar (BP) gave concordances of 72–74 per cent BP and 40–43 per cent UP—a significant difference. There were no differences between DZ pairs: BP 14–17 per cent; UP 11–19 per cent. These data underline again the predominant effect of genetic factors, especially in the bipolar families, but the simple dominant inheritance scheme could only operate on a basis of incomplete penetrance (variable manifestation).

The excess of females in unipolar families might suggest X linkage, but, paradoxically, the evidence for this has come from bipolar families. Linkage with deuteran or protan colour blindness or an Xg blood group on the X chromosome have been proposed, but this would imply absence of father–son transmission. This has been observed, so the question is unresolved—perhaps a proportion of bipolar families are transmitted by a gene on the X chromosome, but the identified markers are at opposite ends of the chromosome, which makes the situation rather difficult to understand. Father–son pairs are said to be commoner in bipolar I (severe mania) than in bipolar II (hypomania only) patients, so if there is X-chromosome transmission in some, it might be more likely in the latter.

Genetic evidence has accrued from several adoption studies where the biological parents' children are separated from them shortly after birth. This separates rearing practices and other environmental variables. There were high concordance rates (3 of 8) among a series of 12 sets of twins reared apart. In another study in children of parents with affective illness reared apart from their parents, there was a significantly increased incidence of affective illness in the children as compared with controls. Similarly, of 8 children of mothers with affective disorder who had been separated at birth and adopted, 3 had developed illness.

Where the criteria for the diagnosis of unipolar illness (which can never be 'absolute', because of the occasional late appearance of mania in a hitherto apparent unipolar illness) are strict, bipolar and unipolar families 'breed true' or very nearly so. For instance, in Perris's series the risk of the relatives of bipolar probands was 16.3 per cent for bipolar illness and 0.8 per cent for unipolar disorder. For the relatives of unipolar patients the risk was 10.6 per cent for unipolar illness and 0.5 per cent for bipolar.

In unipolar illness father–son transmission has been recorded, despite the excess of females in this condition.

Finally, it should be mentioned that a common genetically determined variant of brain protein, 'Pc 1 Duarte', is particularly common in depressive illness—a finding of unknown significance to date.

The HLA system is another area under examination as having possible genetic association with affective illness, without conclusive results so far. Attempts to compare evidence of affective illness with ABO groups also were inconclusive.

Some of the studies and conclusions on the genetics of affective illness have been criticized. It has been pointed out that most twins are concordant for unipolar or bipolar illness but one-fifth to one-seventh are 'mixed'. One of the problems is the diagnosis of unipolar illness, which is never an absolute one, only one of slowly increasing probability with the passage of depressive episodes without the occurrence of mania. It was also pointed out that in one adoption study 29 bipolar adoptees had a risk of 2.5 times that of the adoption parents in whom there was a high risk of unipolar illness (an odd finding). It was conjectured whether unipolar and bipolar illness could be seen as a single genetic unit, with mania latent.

Another possibility was that the unipolar and the bipolar groups may share parts of their genetic basis; one group of workers favoured a two-threshold model, the first giving rise to unipolar and the second, if passed, to bipolar disorder.

If the original unipolar–bipolar dichotomy is accepted, perhaps unipolar illness in a bipolar family is pseudounipolar, i.e. bipolar. It has been suggested that there were genetic differences in bipolar illness marked by whether or not they responded to lithium. It had been found that in monozygotic twins lithium was most successful in concordant bipolar pairs and least helpful in the affected one of discordant pairs. Taking the ratio of lithium concentrations across the red cell membrane, it was higher in concordant than in discordant pairs, and higher in the therapeutic successes with lithium than in the failures.

Clearly, there are many problems still to be unravelled in this area.

The course of affective illness

The study of the course of affective illness presents many difficulties—the problems of extracting accurate retrospective data, and the fact that a prospective study could last for a large part of the researcher's professional life. Much detailed work over a long period of time has been done by Angst and his colleagues and by Perris, who are the main sources of information on this subject. They have emphasized the methodological problems—the possibility that the material is not homogeneous, that data are from hospitalized patients and that the course of illness may be modified by drugs.

The median age of onset in bipolar illness is 34.7 years (a figure higher than that of earlier studies, because it includes those whose mania does not appear in early episodes). Those whose mania appears in the first few episodes have a lower age at first episode than those with a more delayed appearance of mania. The median age of onset in unipolar illness is 45.3 years. The range of age of onset of both illnesses extends from adolescence to old age, with unipolar illness having a flatter distribution curve than bipolar.

The length of the cycles—i.e. the interval between the onset of one illness and the beginning of the next—tends to shorten with number of episodes and with age, and to be shorter in bipolar illness. Episodes of illness tend to be longer in unipolar than in bipolar illness (medians of 5.1 months versus 4.4 months), with an average cycle length of 19.4 months and 33.2 months, respectively. Although, as stated, the natural overall tendency is for the length of the cycle to decrease with age and with increasing numbers of episodes, some patients can show periods of natural remission.

Over a period of assessment of 5 years, absence of relapse was seen in 44 per cent of the unipolar and 16 per cent of the bipolar patients. The remainder had died or had had further relapses. The chances of spontaneous remission in bipolar patients is low, even at an average age of 60 years.

Although bipolar illness is the 'more malignant' illness, depressive episodes tend to be longer in unipolar illness, with, as stated above, medians of 5.1 months versus 4.4 months and with 50 per cent of the episodes lying between 3.2 months and 11.5 months in unipolar and between 2.5 months and 7.6 months in bipolar illness.

Affective disorders as illnesses of 'biological origin'

It it is likely that affective illnesses are due to a biological abnormality. By this is meant that the core symptoms of an episode are due to biochemical/physiological changes or a sequence of changes in the brain which, if reversed, would lead to rapid loss of most of the symptoms. Again, it must be emphasized that this in no way devalues or negates the importance of psychological factors, including life events discussed above—a point which is of great importance in the understanding and treatment of patients both during illness and between episodes. The hypothesis, therefore, is that the evidence is in favour of the prime mover and primary effects being biological in nature, and that the main acute psychological symptoms are an integral part of the process initially, even if some manifestations and subsequent psychological and social changes may be secondary. If this is so, the influence of the life events, physical illness, etc., would be as a trigger to an underlying biochemical vulnerability.

The idea that affective illnesses are 'biological' rested initially on the following evidence (to which other data are accruing with time):

(1) Although the mode of inheritance is undecided, there is good evidence for a significant genetic component.

(2) In the most stringent studies unipolar and bipolar illnesses breed true. (This does not exclude the possibility of there being several different illnesses within the unipolar and bipolar rubrics.)

(3) Depressive illness can be precipitated not only by traumatic psychological events, but also by physical factors—the drug reserpine, virus infections, some endocrine upsets, etc.

(4) The treatments of choice for the core symptoms of an episode are antidepressant drugs or ECT, and for prevention of episodes lithium and tricyclics (unipolar only), irrespective of whether secondary psychological problems require other methods for their amelioration or whether psychosocial manipulations reduce the threshold to illness.

The amine hypothesis for affective disorders

The current stage of the development of our knowledge of affective illness starts with the so-called amine hypothesis. Reserpine was introduced into Western medicine in the middle 1950s and led to two observations.

In the first it was found that something like 6–15 per cent of individuals treated for some months for hypertension with high doses of reserpine became psychotically depressed. There do not appear to be any reports of the precipitation of manic episodes by reserpine. It is possible that those becoming depressed on therapy with reserpine have an inherited predisposition, but that does not detract from the original observations. At about the same time it was found that reserpine prevented storage of amine by the nervous system. The two observations on reserpine—its inhibition of amine storage and its depression-provoking propensities—were put together by Pare and Sandler in the amine hypothesis, in which it was suggested that depression was the product of lack of amines in the brain and of decreased aminergic activity.

Schildkraut and Kety noted the way in which amphetamines improved the mood of normal individuals and also potentiated catecholaminergic neurons. This suggested the model: reduced noradrenaline levels $\longrightarrow$ reduced noradrenergic activity $\longrightarrow$ depression of mood (and vice versa—enhanced noradrenergic activity evoked mania).

An alternative model came from the observation that prevention of destruction of amines with a monoamine oxidase inhibitor (MAOI) which increased amine levels in the brain combined with an excess of the precursor of 5-hydroxytryptamine (5-HT), the amino acid tryptophan, raised the mood of a group of chronic schizophrenics. When tryptophan was added to MAOI in the treatment of depression, recovery was accelerated both during the administration of the amino acid and subsequently. This suggested the model of reduced 5-HT levels and lowered serotoninergic function in depression, especially when followed by similar observations with tryptophan and tertiary amine tricyclics, and the finding that the 5-HT pathway was essential to recovery.

The two versions of the amine hypothesis gathered support from an increasing body of knowledge of the characteristics of aminergic neurons, and the behaviour of the first generation of antidepressants, all of which seemed to share the property of making more noradrenaline and/or 5-HT available in aminergic neurons.

However, although most of the initial data seemed to support the original hypotheses, with the passage of time various observations became difficult to reconcile with a 'simple amine' hypothesis:

(1) It became obvious from animal experiments that tricyclic antidepressants block uptake of amines at the presynaptic membrane (*see also Figure 4.16*). In theory, by blocking their re-uptake, released amines are allowed to remain longer in the synaptic cleft and thus have more chance of attaching to the postsynaptic receptor. This was proposed as their therapeutic action. Amine re-uptake blockade is both powerful and early in onset. Despite the rapidity of its pharmacological action, the antidepressant response is slow and is not complete for 4–8 weeks. There was dissociation between the proposed pharmacological action and the therapeutic effect.

In an attempt to explain this discrepancy away, it was suggested that perhaps time was needed to reach 'steady state'. This argument does not hold, because central side-effects appear within hours of taking tricyclic drugs and, in any event, recovery is far from complete when steady state has been reached. The

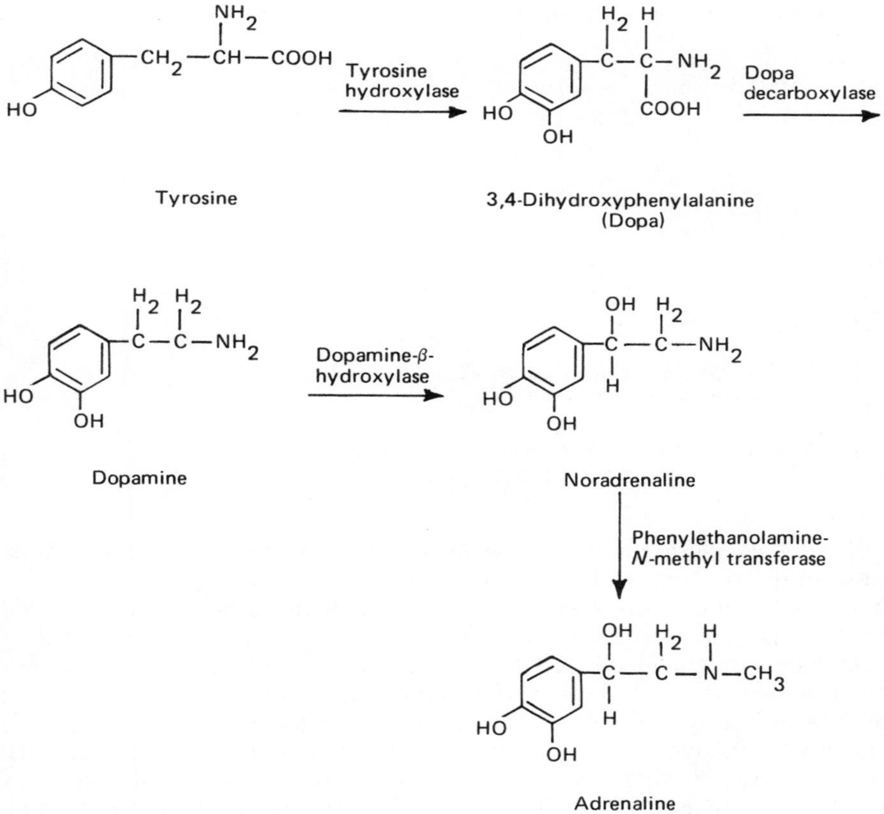

Figure 15.1 Pathways of biosynthesis of the catecholamines—dopamine, noradrenaline and adrenaline

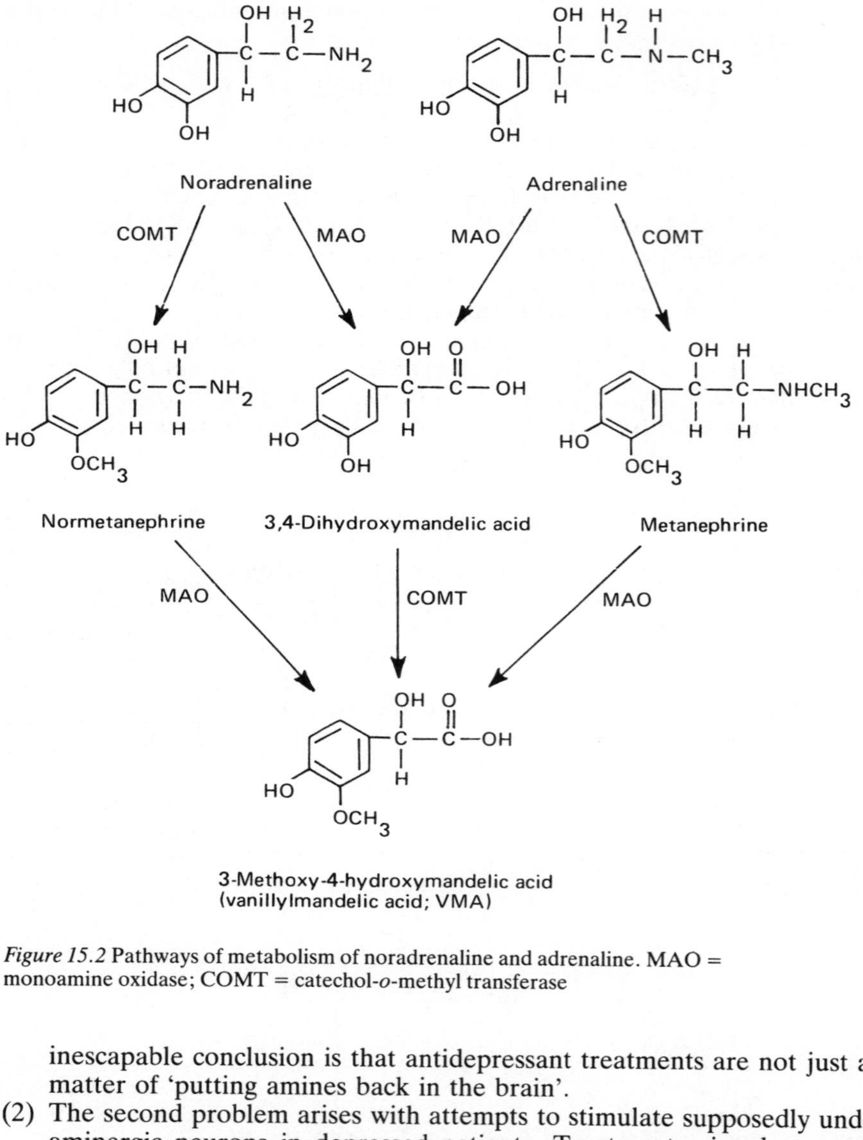

Figure 15.2 Pathways of metabolism of noradrenaline and adrenaline. MAO = monoamine oxidase; COMT = catechol-*o*-methyl transferase

inescapable conclusion is that antidepressant treatments are not just a simple matter of 'putting amines back in the brain'.

(2) The second problem arises with attempts to stimulate supposedly underactive aminergic neurons in depressed patients. Treatments aimed at potentiating catecholaminergic neurons include cocaine and also L-dopa (with or without inhibitors of peripheral decarboxylase inhibitors). Neither type of treatment was conspicuously successful in reversing the symptoms of a depressive syndrome (although L-dopa is a poor activator of noradrenergic neurons). Similarly, attempts to potentiate 5-HT function in patients with MAOI by giving L-tryptophan (*see* page 267), whatever effect they may have in the long term, did not abolish depressive symptoms in the short term. However, cadaver studies show that it takes 3 weeks to block MAO in the brain in humans, so perhaps an early response to tryptophan should not be expected.

(3) The final piece of evidence against the versions of the amine hypothesis in the form of 'reduced amines–reduced aminergic function' were the observations that neither selective depletion of 5-HT or noradrenaline nor unselective amine depletion (with reserpine) mimicked classical endogenous illness in normal subjects, again within the time when amine depletion should have been at its most complete.

It is necessary, therefore, to re-examine the amine hypothesis, and the first question to ask is whether amines have any part at all to play in affective illness. Do amines take part in the treatment and/or aetiology of these conditions?

As far as treatment is concerned, there is a mass of mostly circumstantial evidence implicating amines in the therapeutic process of all forms of antidepressant treatment which, on balance of probability, is unlikely to be refuted. Two pieces of rather more specific information make it very unlikely that some forms of antidepressant treatment are acting via the aminergic systems. The first is the finding already quoted for the actions of MAOI and some tertiary amine tricyclics. When synthesis of 5-HT was favoured by an excess of its precursor, the actions of both drugs were potentiated. This is a powerful argument in favour of involvement of serotoninergic function at some point in the therapeutic process. The second is the finding of a team in the USA which gave imipramine to depressed patients. In some they used an additional drug which blocked synthesis of noradrenaline and in others a compound which prevented production of 5-HT. The first group continued to get well, while the second began to deteriorate, which suggests that the integrity of 5-HT pathway was essential to the therapeutic response to imipramine. On the other hand, other data, such as the action of drugs which act almost exclusively on catecholaminergic systems, emphasize the value of these neurons as a point of application for relieving the depression of affective illness.

If we accept for the moment, therefore, that amines are involved in the therapeutic response to all or at least most of the antidepressant drugs, is it valid to go on to say whether they are acting on normal aminergic neurons, or is the pathological process distal to the aminergic neurons themselves, or even in some parallel system?

The paradigm for this argument is Parkinson's disease, which is due to disease of the dopaminergic neurons and to imbalance between them and the opposing cholinergic system. Initial methods of treatment of Parkinson's disease were directed to the normal neurons (anticholinergic drugs to bring their level of activity down to that of the pathological system). It was only later that the dysfunction of dopamine systems was recognized and manipulated directly in this illness.

Which of these two models applies in affective illness? Obviously, we must keep in mind the possibility that drugs may be acting on totally normal presynaptic or postsynaptic aminergic systems, but it does seem rather unlikely. If it were so, it would be anticipated that cocaine, L-dopa, L-tryptophan or, for that matter, tricyclic drugs would act far more predictably than they do—in a way comparable with that of anticholinergic drugs in Parkinson's disease. Obviously, we cannot at this stage disprove this possibility because the 'correct' balance may not be achieved by these substances but, again, on balance of probability, it is not the most likely explanation for affective illness. However, one group has made a quite convincing case, which has some experimental support, for the view that depression is a disease of perhaps localized cholinergic dominance (*see* below).

When the first versions of the amine hypothesis were advanced, little was known about the behaviour of aminergic systems and certainly the area of homeostatic mechanisms at work was virtually unexplored, so perhaps with this in mind new formulations may emerge. One way to arrive at such formulations is to look at the available data. We know, for instance, that secondary amine tricyclic drugs such as nortriptyline, protriptyline, desipramine, etc., act predominantly on the uptake mechanisms of noradrenergic neurons. It has never been proved that this is its beneficial pharmacological action but, as a working hypothesis, let us assume that long-term potentiation of noradrenergic function by re-uptake blockade is therapeutic. Many of our positive data on depressive illness are not in patients separated by the unipolar–bipolar dichotomy, but it must be assumed that the bulk were unipolar.

Two pieces of the jig-saw were mentioned above. One was the action of a blocker of 5-HT synthesis in preventing the antidepressant response of imipramine. This, as discussed above, suggested that the integrity of the 5-HT pathway was essential to recovery, at least during treatment with imipramine. There are no data to say whether this was true of other drugs. The second was the potentiation of MAOI by L-tryptophan. This suggested that whereas enhancing the availability of all monoamines might be therapeutic, producing overflow conditions at 5-HT synapses gave optimal conditions for recovery. This has to be reconciled first with the observations that two antidepressants (mianserin and amitriptyline) may also block 5-HT receptors, and that the drug maprotiline worked well in the presence of a blocker of 5-HT receptors.

In an attempt to account for all these data, it is our view that one type of unipolar affective illness could be due to overactivity of 5-HT receptors. Others have produced equally convincing hypotheses on changes of sensitivity of noradrenergic synapses.

Experimental and other bases of the catecholamine hypothesis

The general basis of the catecholamine hypothesis is that noradrenaline deficiency and decreased noradrenergic function underlie depressive illness, and that a converse situation holds in mania. Briefly, as stated previously, the argument started with observations on the effects and actions of reserpine and amphetamine, and depended heavily on the observed property of tricyclic drugs in increasing the availability of noradrenaline at noradrenergic synapses. This latter effect was absent in dopaminergic neurons, where the tricyclic group of drugs had no effect on uptake of dopamine across the synaptic membrane (a notable exception now is the drug nomifensine). Some of the attempts to evaluate the catecholamine hypothesis (e.g. by the attempted use of cocaine as an antidepressant agent, the use of L-dopa, etc.) also have been mentioned above. Other attempts to test the hypothesis have depended on a variety of studies of catecholamines in urine, in cerebrospinal fluid (CSF), etc.

Urinary studies

With urinary studies the problem is that metabolic processes are being assessed at third hand and there is considerable difficulty in evaluating the relationship between what is happening at aminergic synapses and what appears as a urinary metabolite. There seems to be considerable doubt whether the main metabolite of dopamine, homovanillic acid (HVA), when assayed in urine gives information of sufficient accuracy on central processes, and the same holds for a metabolite of noradrenaline, 3-methoxy-4-hydroxymandelic acid (VMA), which is mostly of peripheral origin. Some hope of measuring noradrenergic turnover in the brain was afforded by the discovery that 3-methoxy-4-hydroxyphenylglycol (MHPG) was the major metabolite of noradrenaline in the CSF, but unfortunately there is a significant concentration of this metabolite from somatic sources as well as that coming from the brain. Something between 25 per cent and 60 per cent may be of central origin.

With this in mind, the data on urinary studies are open to more than one interpretation, but the studies have been encouraging from a purely empirical point of view. Low levels of urinary MHPG have been seen in some individuals with unipolar affective disorder, and in bipolar depressed patients, who develop higher levels in the manic phase and on recovery. In unipolar depressives it has been suggested that the patients with low MHPG (Type A) had a deficit in central noradrenergic mechanisms, responded temporarily to amphetamine and had a favourable response to the noradrenergic potentiating drugs imipramine and desipramine. Type B had a normal or high excretion of MHPG, no postulated deficit in noradrenergic mechanisms, responded well to amitriptyline (a drug acting mainly on 5-HT neurons), had no elevation of mood with amphetamine and failed to respond to imipramine.

Cerebrospinal fluid

It would be anticipated that analysis of CSF should give more reliable data on noradrenaline from MHPG and dopamine from HVA levels. However, the MHPG from the spinal cord comes from neurons whose cell bodies are mostly in the brain-stem, notably the nucleus coeruleus. Animal studies have shown that CSF data can give information on amine metabolism in the brain, but there is the problem in humans that the usual source of cerebrospinal fluid is from a lumbar tap, and the question arises as to how representative this is of central processes and to what extent it reflects mainly spinal events. It seems likely that HVA concentrations on the lumbar CSF is largely of central origin, but that a proportion of the MHPG has risen from cells in the spinal cord.

A refinement to the techniques used in CSF studies has been the simultaneous administration of probenecid. This substance blocks the transport of HVA (and also of 5-hydroxyindolacetic acid) out of the CSF. This gives a more dynamic picture of amine turnover, in that the difference between baseline and probenecid-treated levels should give some idea of the rate of accumulation (and therefore of turnover of amines) in that time.

Unfortunately, studies of the CSF have not given a consistent picture of what is happening to catecholamine metabolism in the brain in affective illness. Most of the investigators have reported significantly reduced baseline levels of HVA in depressive affective illness but not all the studies have confirmed this. Similarly, some investigators of CSF HVA in mania reported increases, with reductions in recovery, and again these observations have not been supported by all studies. In studies of HVA in the presence of probenecid, bipolar and unipolar depressed patients tend to have lower levels of accumulation of HVA than do controls, and probably more reliance should be put on these data rather than the baseline data.

One suggestion is that HVA levels are related more to retardation than to the underlying change in mood, but decreased levels have been recorded in most studies of mania, and also decreased accumulation of HVA after probenecid. With regard to MHPG levels in CSF, the studies are divided between those who found levels in depression which were within the range seen in control subjects and those who reported reduced levels of CSF MHPG. One report suggested raised CSF MHPG in mania, returning to normal levels after treatment with lithium. Post-mortem studies have not cast much light on catecholamines. One suggested normal noradrenaline levels; another, decreased levels localized to the red nucleus.

Research into indolamines in affective disorder

As with the catecholamine hypothesis, there have been formidable barriers to effective attempts to delineate abnormalities in indolamine and/or its precursor, tryptophan, in affective illness. These include the sheer 'biological distance' between occurrences at serotoninergic synapses of neurons, which, after all, are only a tiny fraction of the total number of nerve cells, and metabolites or precursors in biological fluids; the complications imposed by the binding of tryptophan to albumin; and the small proportion of tryptophan passing down the indolamine pathway. There is a further problem imposed by the fact that as yet there seem to be few, if any, established observable peripheral events which are controlled by serotoninergic neurons and which can be used as a means of monitoring central serotoninergic activity in man.

Despite these difficulties, a considerable amount of work has been done on tryptophan/indolamines in affective disorder, and while there is only a minimal amount of clear-cut data, there are some indications that patterns of information may be emerging.

Urinary studies

Early attempts to study indolamine metabolism from urinary metabolite of 5-hydroxytryptamine (5-hydroxyindolacetic acid: 5HIAA) or tryptamine have not produced consistent results. Other urinary studies have concentrated on the metabolites of tryptophan. The major route of degradation of tryptophan is via the so-called kynurenine pathway (*Figure 15.3*), indolamine metabolism being only a very minor part of the turnover of this amino acid.

The first step in the pathway is catalysed by tryptophan pyrrolase, an enzyme whose activity is maintained at an increased level by the presence of significant increases in the level of its substrate, tryptophan, and whose activity is increased also by cortisol. Another powerful influence on tryptophan metabolism is its binding to albumin in the extracellular space. This maintains the bulk of tryptophan in plasma and interstitial fluid in protein-bound forms, leaving only a small fraction as non-bound, which has an important effect in putting tryptophan 'at a disadvantage' at the blood–brain barrier (*see* below).

The combination of the effect of substrate in maintaining tryptophan pyrrolase and the protein bound/non-bound fraction all combine to tend to keep concentration of tryptophan in non-bound forms at relatively low concentrations and within a smallish range of levels.

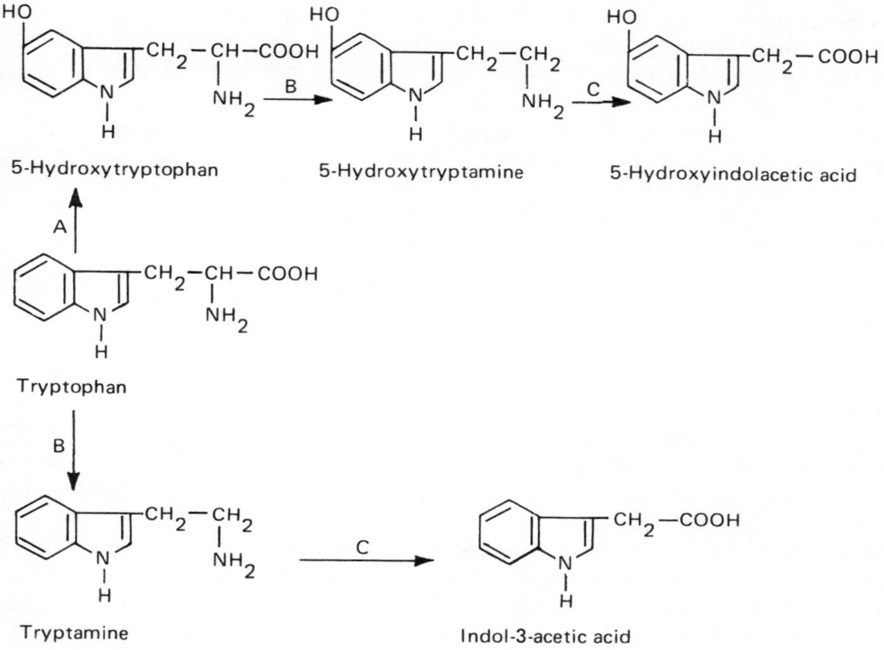

Figure 15.3 Biosynthesis and metabolism of indoleamines. A = hydroxylation; B = decarboxylation; C = oxidized by MAO

There have been several attempts to assess tryptophan metabolism via its products down the kynurenine pathway, and the results have suggested some increase in the baseline levels of xanthurenic acid and after tryptophan loading in depressive illness. Similarly, in two bipolar patients during the depressive phase more radioactive kynurenine was excreted following the injection of radioactive tryptophan than during manic or normal phases. These data suggest the possibility of increased catabolism of tryptophan via the kynurenine pathway, and since tryptophan pyrrolase is induced by cortisol, this mechanism has been proposed as being responsible.

It is rather difficult to accept the interpretation of these data as indicating a continued increase in tryptophan pyrrolase. For one thing, xanthurenic acid is only one of several metabolites, and presumably it would be necessary to measure them all to be certain that tryptophan pyrrolase activity had increased. A second point is that if metabolism by tryptophan pyrrolase is the only pathway of degradation of tryptophan (ignoring the negligibly small indolamine route), then, unless the patient were in a marked catabolic imbalance, input should equal output. The data could be interpreted as a temporarily increased degradation of tryptophan at the time of the experiment.

The blood–brain barrier has an important role in the control of 5-HT synthesis in the brain, because passage of tryptophan and of similarly sized neutral amino acids is competitive, so that they can be mutually exclusive. For instance, the ingestion of a protein meal may be followed by increases in the concentration of all the amino acids, including tryptophan, but because of the competition for re-uptake the levels of tryptophan in the brain may fall. Similarly, insulin, by decreasing the concentration of other neutral amino acids in plasma, may allow a rise in brain tryptophan. Several papers suggest that the ratio of tryptophan to competing amino acids may be reduced in affective illness.

These mechanisms owe their importance to the fact that the rate-limiting step for the synthesis of 5-HT in the brain is tryptophan hydroxylase, an enzyme not normally saturated with its substrate. Thus, a rise in brain tryptophan can increase 5-HT synthesis, and vice versa, although homeostatic mechanisms may limit the size of the changes.

Blood studies

PLATELETS

5-HT uptake

5-HT uptake by platelets is an active process depending on [Na] and a cAMP –adenylate cyclase system. It has been studied on the basis that a defective enzyme might be widespread in the body and that the platelet has some similarity in its properties to aminergic terminals.

The 5-HT content of platelets has a diurnal rhythm which varies with the season of the year, and one interesting study reported similar levels of platelet 5-HT in unipolar patients, but in the first half of the year the pattern of controls of higher 5-HT levels at 8 A.M. than at 4 P.M. was reversed in these patients. Patterns in the second half of the year were not different.

In this investigation 5-HT re-uptake and MAO activity were normal in unipolar patients and 5-HT levels and uptake tended to correlate. In bipolar II patients 5-HT level and uptake did not correlate, 5-HT levels were negatively correlated with MAO activity and 5-HT concentrations were raised whether the patient was manic, in normal mood or depressed.

Other investigations have not corroborated these findings.

Plasma membrane ATPase and adenylate cyclase activities are reported as normal, but in two studies V_{max} (the maximum rate of transport under given conditions) and $\bar{y}$ (overall uptake) for 5-HT were significantly lowered in both unipolar and bipolar depressed groups. K_m values (the Michaelis constant), a measure of the affinity of a substrate (in this case 5-HT) for its binding site, were similar to those of controls. Short periods on lithium in a small group did not affect the variables. A further study confirmed the decrease in V_{max} for unipolar patients, and showed that this abnormality remained after recovery, but that long-term treatment with lithium increased the rate of transport of lithium by platelets to above that of control values in both unipolar and bipolar individuals, and decreased the affinity of the membrane carrier for 5-HT.

Monoamine oxidase in platelets

Platelets contain monoamine oxidase in their mitochondria. This enzyme is probably of smaller molecular weight than that described for brain MAO and, although this is not finally established, is probably present in one molecular form belonging to the MAO-B group. There are large inter-individual differences in its activity which are genetically determined. Females have higher MAO activities in their platelets than do males, but the presence or absence of changes with age is undecided. Peak MAO activity occurs just before ovulation and there is a 'trough' in the postovulatory period. Iron deficiency anaemia lowers platelet MAO activity. The enzyme is blocked by the MAOIs and by high concentrations of tricyclic drugs. It is not affected by phenothiazines.

One early study in affective illness indicates low platelet MAO in bipolar illness compared with controls and unipolar patients, and a second indicates an increase in MAO activity in atypical depressives. It is difficult to compare the various studies of MAO activity in platelets, because of differences in methodology, but low MAO activities in the platelets of bipolar patients is a reasonably consistent finding in ill and recovered conditions. This is now complicated by the recent finding that platelet MAO activity was similar to that of controls in bipolar patients responsive to treatment with lithium, and that in patients refractory to lithium enzyme activity was reduced below that of controls and of those responding to treatment with lithium.

Reduced MAO activity in platelets may extend to the first-degree relatives of patients with bipolar illness.

The work done on unipolar patients is difficult to interpret, but a recent study found changes also in unipolar illness in the form of raised MAO activity, which was probably correlated with severity of illness. This was not seen in reactive illness. The data also confirmed the low activity of MAO in bipolar patients seen by others, and in both types of illness the changes continued on into recovery.

Lithium-treated patients had significantly higher MAO activity than did untreated patients in the bipolar but not in the unipolar group.

These data can be associated with the observation that an oral dose of tyramine when given to (presumably) unipolar depressed patients was followed by a reduced level of urinary excretion of the conjugated substance, whereas isoprenaline appeared in normal amounts in the conjugated form in urine. The explanation of this was that activity of monoamine oxidase was enhanced or the substrate was gaining greater access to the enzyme, thus converting it to other substances so that a smaller amount of tyramine was available for the smaller conjugated pool.

AMINO ACIDS

Tryptophan

Interest has focused on the amino acid tryptophan because it is the precursor of 5-hydroxytryptamine (5-HT) and of tryptamine. These two indolamines are responsible for only a small fraction of tryptophan metabolism. Most of it is involved in protein synthesis; and before or after this, is degraded via tryptophan pyrrolase in the liver via the pathway shown (*Figure 15.4*). This enzyme is inducible by cortisol and by an increase in the concentration of its substrate tryptophan in plasma. Both tranylcypromine and imipramine inhibit tryptophan pyrrolase in rat liver.

Tryptophan in plasma is present in two forms—as the free amino acid and bound to albumin. Dissociation of the tryptophan from binding can be very rapid.

To enter central metabolism for the synthesis of protein or the production of 5-HT, the amino acid has to cross the blood–brain barrier. The process requires competition with other amino acids (particularly the larger neutral ones) for carrier sites. Tryptophan is in some ways at a disadvantage here as being the only amino acid bound to protein, so its concentration in unbound form is low as compared with that of the other amino acids. As a result, tryptophan levels in the brain may fall after a protein meal because of the increased competition for entry from other amino acids.

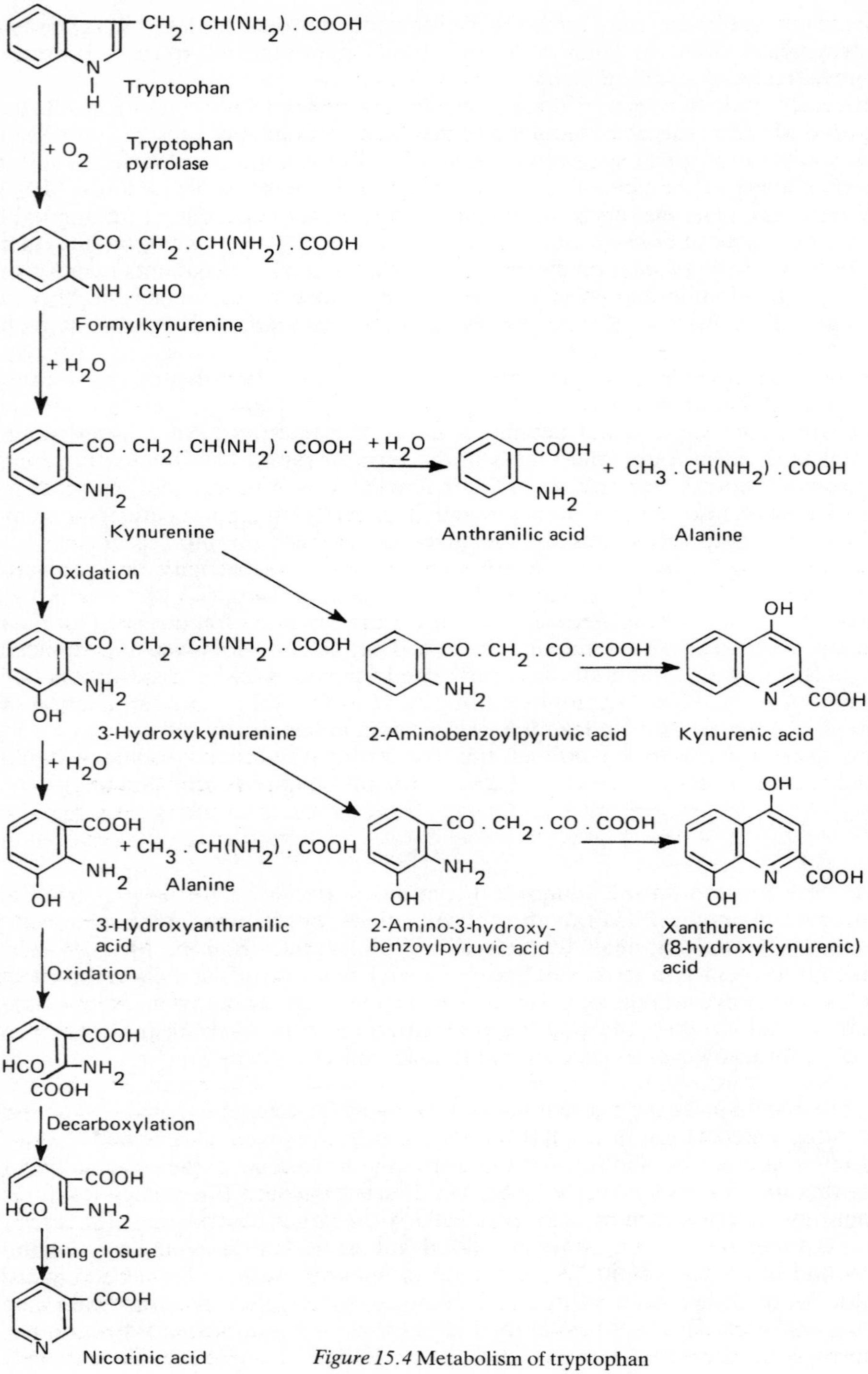

Figure 15.4 Metabolism of tryptophan

The first stage in the formation of 5-HT is 5-hydroxylation, the enzyme for which is unsaturated under normal conditions, so that the local concentration of tryptophan is one of the rate-controlling factors in the synthesis of the amine.

Therefore, interest in tryptophan and its metabolites (*see* above) has been continued. Initial reports of reduced fasting concentrations of a free tryptophan have not ben upheld by subsequent work, although the diurnal pattern of concentrations may be altered in unipolar patients. A possible exception is in the early puerperium, where there is evidence of a parallel between mood state and free plasma tryptophan concentrations.

Concentrations of total tryptophan in plasma have usually been similar to control levels. An interesting exception was in a study of the kinetics of tryptophan in unipolar and in bipolar depressives. Here the permission of both patients and controls was sought for what was a complicated and lengthy procedure. Inadvertently both groups may have been stressed to some extent, but what emerged was a lower total tryptophan level at the onset of the investigation in unipolar patients than in the controls. The bipolar patients did not show any differences in tryptophan concentration. When the test was done on recovered unipolar patients, the plasma levels of tryptophan lay between those of controls and those of ill patients. The difference between depressed unipolar patients and controls was significant but small. In further investigations larger falls in tryptophan concentrations in plasma were seen between stressed and unstressed controls, and stressed and unstressed depressives. This raised the question as to whether the change was common to both but whether unipolar individuals have an idiosyncratic tendency to be unable to maintain tryptophan levels during stress which is developed in full during illness. More likely perhaps is that the response to stress in both controls and depressives of a fall in tryptophan concentration is acting on a biochemically vulnerable system in the latter, or is occurring more frequently.

For ethical reasons this is a difficult hypothesis to pursue, but if confirmed, would explain much of the variability of the studies in tryptophan/indolamines—the results would depend very much on the 'ambience' of the environment in which the tests were done. To date, markedly reduced levels of tryptophan have been seen in female depressives awaiting their first of a series of ECTs.

One hypothesis for affective disorder, therefore, could be that there is a fall in tryptophan provoked by stress and which leads to a temporary but presumably repeated decrease in plasma tryptophan levels, and that this group of individuals cannot 'cope' with this biochemically. However, because of its competition with other amino acids at the blood–brain barrier, the effects of other amino acids should not be ignored. Indeed, there are preliminary data looking at the relationship of tryptophan to other amino acids in affective illness.

In 8 bipolar and 11 unipolar patients, 4 were in 'relative tryptophan deficit'—i.e. the ratio of tryptophan to the sum of the concentrations of three competing amino acids, valine, isoleucine and leucine, was significantly reduced. Recovery (4 female bipolar, 1 female unipolar) was associated with 4 out of 5 patients in either depression or mania with various regimens of L- or DL-tryptophan at high doses. In a single case study of a treatment-resistant bipolar patient there were high fasting concentrations of isoleucine, leucine and tyrosine, and the ratio of total tryptophan to the sum of valine, isoleucine and leucine was low in both depressed and manic phases. Large doses of L-tryptophan (100 mg/kg) give higher plasma curves than did normal controls despite enhanced catabolism of tryptophan to kynurenine, which suggests decreased transport into tissues. Valine, isoleucine and leucine rose abnormally at the same time postprandially. It is of interest with regard to this latter finding that tolerance curves to tryptophan, phenylalanine and tyrosine and peripheral utilization of glucose are decreased in depression.

An interesting observation requiring replication is that a group of depressives had a gaussian distribution of concentrations of plasma tryptophan before treatment, but when given ECT and largish doses of L-tryptophan, their plasma levels becomes bimodal—those that were initially low stayed low and those that were in the higher range pre-treatment increased disproportionately.

Cerebrospinal fluid studies   Results of assays of tryptophan levels in CSF have not been consistent. Oral doses of tryptophan, however, give a large increase in tryptophan and 5-HIAA levels, although one group of workers reported higher rises in tryptophan and lower rises in 5-HIAA than in controls. They postulated reduced accessibility of 5-HT neurons to tryptophan or diminished activity of tryptophan hydroxylase, but any 'accumulation of tryptophan' might more easily be attributed to changes in turnover of brain proteins. Their explanation could be partly correct, however, in that there is nothing to suggest that conversion of 5-hydroxytryptophan to 5-HT is altered in affective illness.

5-HIAA in lumbar CSF is derived from both the brain and the cord, the latter coming from descending tracts from the brain-stem. Of the 5-HIAA formed from degradation of 5-HT, perhaps 90 per cent finds its way to the blood stream, only the remaining 10 per cent being in CSF.

There is also a gradient of concentration down the cord which can be altered by sneezing, coughing, posture, etc. If added to this is the fact that 5-HIAA is that moeity of the 5-HT which is deaminated intracellularly, and is not a direct estimate of the physiologically active amine in the synapses, then interpretations of CSF data become difficult.

These uncertainties are reflected in the results. A number of studies have reported decreased levels of 5-HIAA, others no change or only slight falls in concentration. Most of the controls used, however, were non-depressed psychiatric patients or 'neurological' controls.

A more dynamic picture is obtained by treatment with probenecid between two lumbar taps. Probenecid blocks the passage of 5-HIAA from the CSF, and while it alters tryptophan metabolism by decreasing plasma binding of the amino acid, its results are probably more informative than 'basal levels'.

Not all the initial results were uniform though tending to indicate decreased turnover down the 5-HT–5-HIAA pathway. Later studies suggested decreased turnover in a proportion, about 40 per cent, of the total. Later a bimodal distribution in basal (i.e. non-probencid-treated patients) was found for 5-HIAA, perhaps thus accounting for discrepant earlier results. In patients with low 5-HIAA severity of depression was negatively correlated with levels; this did not hold in the patients with high basal 5-HIAA. These data have not been confirmed.

Post-mortem studies   Post-mortem studies of 5-HT are extremely difficult to do and interpret. One methodological error is that although losses of 5-HT are relatively small (10–20 per cent of the ante-mortem value in 48 hours in a body allowed to cool at the normal rate and then stored at 4 °C), losses once the skull is opened (and presumably exposed to oxygen) are extremely rapid. Similarly, if brains are stored for a long time in deep freeze, 5-HT tends to be converted to

5-HIAA. There is no need to stress the difficulty in getting accurate diagnosis frcm records retrospectively.

In one study in which no changes in 5-HT levels were observed, the control group were stored in deep freeze for significantly longer than the depressives, so this figure was in doubt.

Regional studies have shown 5-HT levels decreased in all areas studied, 5-HT lowered in the raphé nuclei, or no changes.

Endocrine studies in affective disorders

The studies of endocrine changes in affective disorder have reached a stage in development where there are many interlocking regions of ignorance, in an area where clearly abnormalities exist. In addition, an abnormality in one patient may not be seen in another, and even when a change has been recognized, its basis in terms of aminergic, other neuronal, peripheral or other processes is far from clear.

The hypothalamic–pituitary–adrenal axis

Of the neuroendocrine mechanisms studied to date in affective disorders, the hypothalamic–pituitary–adrenal axis has received most attention.

Corticotrophin-releasing factor liberates ACTH, which in turn stimulates the production of cortisol. One of the mechanisms of control is by feedback inhibition. There are cortisol and ACTH receptors in limbic areas which project to the hypothalamus, but feedback is only a minor part of the control exerted by the CNS. The main influence is by tonic inhibition of the hypothalamo–pituitary system, which is relaxed in accordance with the circadian secretory pattern. Normally ACTH is produced in 6–9 discrete secretory bursts between 5 A.M. and 2 P.M. with minimal activity at other times. Hypothalamo–pituitary adrenal activity is normally at its nadir between 11 P.M. and 3 A.M. and mechanisms which interrupt this pattern are most active when given during this period. The other controlling mechanism exerted directly by the response of the CNS to stress, apart from the 'release' process, is via binding of cortisol to proteins in plasma. Cortisol is bound to a protein (transcortin) in plasma, and in some illnesses and in surgery the binding protein can decrease in amount, which increases free cortisol levels without changes in total cortisol. It is the free cortisol level in plasma which determines the exposure of the tissues to cortisol.

The major changes in hypothalamo–pituitary function in depressive disorders is an increase in cortisol and corticosterone production. The pattern of diurnal variation is lost, so that production continues during the afternoon and night (*Figure 15.5*). Secretory bursts are more prolonged and more frequent, so that cortisol levels rise in plasma free cortisol (to $\times 2\frac{1}{2}$) and in CSF to double normal values (not confirmed in all studies), and urine free cortisol excretion levels are also increased. Binding capacity of transcortin is unchanged, and the sensitivity of the pituito-adrenal axis is normal.

Bipolar and unipolar patients are about the same in their cortisol levels, and in about 40 per cent urinary free cortisol excretion is in the range seen in Cushing's disease. Cortisol levels in CSF are raised in all newly admitted psychiatric patients, but are highest in depressives, especially in severe illness. Cerebrospinal fluid cortisol was weakly correlated with concentrations of 5-hydroxyindolacetic acid. Normally, cortisol production can be suppressed by the synthetic steroid dexamethasone, but many depressed patients, about a half, fail to suppress to 2 mg given at 12 midnight. 'Escape' from dexamethasone suppression correlates with severity and endogenous features, and there is a trend for the non-suppressors to have a poor response to drug treatment.

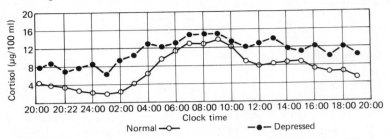

Figure 15.5 Plasma cortisol levels measured in 7 depressed patients over a 24 hour period were distinctly elevated in comparison with levels obtained from 54 normal individuals. In addition, cortisol levels in the depressives did not show pronounced circadian variation characteristics of normals, in whom cortisol secretion markedly decreased late at night and early morning

Patients still showing abnormal responses at discharge tend to relapse rapidly. Most patients have returned to a normal pattern on restoration of neutral mood.

There have been wide differences between centres, but about 46 per cent have abnormal dexamethasone tests as compared with 40 per cent showing abnormal urinary free cortisol levels. One author suggests that if there were 'late escapers' at a time perhaps when no observations were being made, the figure might be higher.

Since some of the results are in the Cushingoid range, why do depressives not show the physical stigmata of this disease? The answer usually given is that the time of exposure is too short, but if high cortisol levels persist in prolonged illness, this would not hold. These data are not available yet. However, in one series of brains from depressive suicides the sum of cortisol plus dehydrocortisols was lower than that of control brains, and in a second series cortisol plus corticosterone was reduced by 40 per cent in the depressives. These observations raise the question as to whether cortisol has normal access to brain in depression, and if so, whether this could apply to other tissues as well?

Raised cortisol levels are not seen in secondary depressives, or in mania (but *see* section on aldosterone, below). Changes similar to those seen in depressives have been observed in severely ill medical patients.

As one of the most consistent findings in affective disorder, suppression of cortisol to dexamethasone is coming to be considered as diagnostic in those for whom the test is positive. The test has stimulated considerable interest because of its practical and theoretical potential.

Corticotrophin-releasing factor is modulated by factors which include noradrenergic pathways (inhibitory), serotoninergic, muscarinic and nicotinic cholinergic pathways (both excitatory) and prostaglandins.

Dextroamphetamine and methylamphetamine suppressed cortisol in two groups of depressed patients, but the growth hormone response to the latter (presumably dopamine responsive) was unaltered. These findings suggested a central defect in alpha noradrenergic receptors, and this was supported by the finding that the

ACTH–corticosteroid effect was blocked by thymoxamine, a fairly specific alpha adrenergic antagonist, while that of growth hormone was unaltered. To the evidence of alpha noradrenergic receptor deficiency is added recent evidence of reduction in beta receptors after ECT and after chronic treatment with tricyclic antidepressants. The two findings are not 'mutually exclusive' (*see* section on antidepressants).

Schlesser, Winokur *et al.* have produced data showing that dexamethasone suppression occurs most frequently in the familial pure depressive group, in about half of their sporadic depressive disease individuals and rarely in those classified as depressive spectrum disease.

Growth hormone (GH)

Release of growth hormone is a complex matter. Dopaminergic stimulation and activation of adrenergic alpha receptors can release GH, while adrenergic beta receptors appear to be inhibitory. 5-HT also is involved, however, because release of GH in response to hypoglycaemia may be altered by, among other drugs, cyproheptidine and methysergide. In depression GH responses to hypoglycaemia but not to L-dopa are attenuated.

Prolactin

The release of prolactin is under tonic inhibition by the dopaminergic tuberoinfundibulum pathway. In general, prolactin levels are normal or near normal in depression and there is a normal prolactin response to thyrotrophin-releasing hormone, bromocriptine and L-dopa. It is likely but not certain that dopaminergic neurons function normally in depression.

Thyroid-stimulating hormone (TSH)

Thyroid function 'at rest' is normal in the great majority of depressed individuals. Abnormalities appear only when the releasing mechanism is stimulated. Thyrotrophin-releasing hormone (TRH) liberates both thyroid-stimulating hormone and growth hormone. When TRH is given to depressives, the response of TSH is often reduced. It may be that this is different in unipolar and bipolar patients, but confirmation is required.

In patients given TRH, growth hormone responses are not seen in manics or in patients with secondary depression. The bipolar patients, however, had an augmented TSH response, and the unipolar a blunted TSH response. Since both types of depression produce excess cortisol, this cannot be the explanation. It was pointed out that increased serotoninergic activity reduced the TSH response to TRH, and that there was an inverse relationship between CSF, 5-HIAA and TSH responses in unipolar illness. Conversely, increased noradrenergic activity enhanced the TRH responses. It should be noted, however, that the TRH/TSH response is reduced in Cushing's disease.

LH and FSH

Studies in this area are as yet at too early a stage for detailed report.

Renin–aldosterone system

A dysfunction of the renin–aldosterone system in bipolar patients has been reported with high renin levels, a reduced response of renin to posture and inappropriate secretion rates of aldosterone. A small group of manic-depressive patients received spironolactone for a year and five or six did well in an open trial.

Other studies have suggested abnormality in the form of high aldosterone levels in plasma in mania, usually without any change in cortisol. A small study used the technique of multiple sampling (every 20 minutes for 24 hours) in three patients in mania, and found levels of aldosterone to be higher than those of normal controls, with cortisol levels just above the normal range (but with some loss of diurnal variation). It was suggested that the latter might have been due to the abnormal sleeping pattern.

In drug-free bipolar patients CSF levels of arginine vasopressin (AVP) and plasma AVP responses to hypertonic saline were reduced during depression but not in 'mania'. Three out of four patients given L-desamino-8-D-arginine vasopressin (a synthetic analogue of vasopressin with a long half-life) had improved cognitive performance, as shown by recall of learnt material, with a dramatic improvement in one. Relapse tended to follow withdrawal. Two of the four improved also in mood.

Testing the amine hypothesis with amine precursors and drugs

Amines are of apparent importance in the treatment of affective disorders (most, if not all, of the active antidepressants alter amine metabolism, although this is not to prove that amines are of direct aetiological significance). This fact led naturally to the use of the amine acid precursors as possible methods of therapy.

5-Hydroxytryptophan (5-HTP)

This substance is difficult to give orally, because it causes nausea and vomiting. By giving a peripheral decarboxylase inhibitor, these side-effects can be prevented, but the substance has the disadvantage that it acts unphysiologically. It gets into 5-HT cells, but enters also into catecholaminergic neurons, when it is decarboxylated to 5-HT and may act as a false transmitter. Results of its use therapeutically have led to claims of success in depression (1) in those with reduced accumulation of 5-HIAA after probenecid, and (2) as a potentiator of dopamine. There is one report of a soluble ester of 5-HTP given intravenously with a peripheral decarboxylase inhibitor to normal individuals which gave consistent rises in mood lasting for up to 4 hours. On the whole, however, results with 5-HTP have not been consistent.

There has been a promising development, however, in which some of the problems with 5-HTP have been bypassed by use of a soluble ester intravenously or a coated capsule which did not disintegrate until the small intestine was reached (pH 8.6). Given with a peripheral decarboxylase inhibitor, this latter oral preparation was useful in 50 per cent of 99 treatment-resistant patients.

Tryptophan

The first use of tryptophan in this context was in an attempt to potentiate the antidepressant response to MAOIs, and a positive result was seen by a number of investigators. Tryptophan failed to potentiate tricyclic antidepressants in some early trials, including one using clomipramine (a drug with major effects on 5-HT neurons) and 0.1 g tryptophan per kg body weight (equivalent to 7 g in 70 kg persons). A similar trial with clomipramine using the same dose but using DL-tryptophan instead of L-tryptophan (equivalent to much smaller doses of L-tryptophan) gave a positive response—i.e. the smaller dose potentiated the antidepressant response to clomipramine. The result of the trials, including those giving tryptophan alone as a putative antidepressant, have been very confusing. It has been postulated, however, that most of the trials have been with a dosage above the upper range of the optimum and that there is a 'therapeutic window' above which increasing the dose is counterproductive.

The proponents of this idea gave nicotinamide with tryptophan or imipramine, or the three together, giving the amino acid in doses of initially 4 g then 6 g per kg. The effect of tryptophan in the tryptophan plus nicotinamide combination fell off as the dose was increased to 6 g in unipolar patients, but bipolar patients probably required more. They suggested that, given with nicotinamide, unipolar patients should have 4 g or less, bipolar patients 4 g or above, and half these amounts are appropriate if tryptophan is administered with imipramine.

Thus, while the action of tryptophan and MAOI has proved effective (with no obvious therapeutic window), the use of tryptophan with tricyclics and when given alone merits further investigation, and the presence of the 'therapeutic window' at low levels might explain the discordant findings.

Whatever the outcome, it must be realized that manipulation of the activity of 5-HT neurons—e.g. by tryptophan, or other aminergic neurons—does not occur in isolation, and giving L-tryptophan produces quite obvious changes in animals in noradrenergic and dopaminergic systems.

L-dopa

Results with L-dopa have not been consistent, whether it has been given with or without a peripheral decarboxylase inhibitor. One study shows a lessening of akinesia in depression but no change in depressed mood, and in another a proportion of bipolar depressed patients became hypomanic. In other studies the results have not been impressive, and L-dopa has not yet established a place for itself as an effective antidepressant.

Inhibitors of synthesis of biogenic amines: acute potentiation of aminergic activity

Imipramine is a tricyclic drug which, via its conversion to its desmethylated derivation, acts on both noradrenergic and serotoninergic drugs. There is a report from one centre only on giving imipramine to depressed patients who continued to get well when the synthesis of noradrenaline was blocked. As mentioned above, blocking the synthesis of 5-HT, however, resulted in deterioration, which suggests that the integrity of the 5-HT pathway was needed for the therapeutic action of imipramine.

Blocking the synthesis of noradrenaline in normal individuals with α-methylparatyrosine gave sedation, fatigue (and anxiety in a few), but nothing remotely resembling the depressive syndrome. Those sedated by the drugs had a pleasant feeling of alertness and also insomnia on withdrawal. The drug did not act consistently in mania, but three depressed patients became worse when given this substance.

Thus, there is very little to suggest a simple relationship between noradrenergic depletion and the depressive syndrome.

In comparable work using parachlorphenylalanine to inhibit synthesis of 5-HT, normal subjects experienced tiredness, restlessness, unease, anxiety, and at higher doses confusion and agitation. They did not become depressed, however, or have other symptoms resembling the depressive affective syndrome.

Acute depletion of all the amines with reserpine produces the classical 'neuroleptic syndrome', but in the short term no pattern of symptoms in the mode of depressive affective illness.

Some of the other 'therapeutic' experiments have been mentioned, and for a detailed discussion of tricyclics and MAOI drugs the chapter on neuropharmacology should be consulted. Other data include the possibility that patients with low 5-HIAA levels in CSF may be resistant to nortriptyline (which acts mostly on noradrenergic neurons) but respond to clomipramine (which acts powerfully on serotoninergic neurons). This points to differentiation between '5-HT abnormal' depressions and 'non-5-HT' depressions, but this is speculative.

Cocaine

Cocaine is a powerful potentiator of noradrenergic and dopaminergic neurons but is not antidepressant.

Receptor sensitivity

When the deficiencies in the simple amine hypothesis (decreased availability of amines ⟶ decreased aminergic function ⟶ depression) began to be apparent from data which were incompatible with it, two views were possible. One was that manipulation of aminergic systems was likely in therapeutic manoeuvres, but that the primary abnormality lay in another system in parallel or in series with aminergic pathways. The other was that aminergic systems were involved directly in the aetiological mechanisms but in a much more complex way than was hitherto thought. Aminergic pathways are controlled in a complex way by many regulatory mechanisms, and also interact with one another (particularly closely in the case of some dopaminergic and serotoninergic pathways).

The processes which have to be considered are availability of precursor amino acid in the plasma and its transport across the blood–brain barrier; activity of the amine-synthesizing enzymes, which can be controlled by product inhibition (via autoreceptors and also by feedback loops); intraneuronal binding and compartmentalization; activity of monoamine oxidase; the re-uptake mechanism across the presynaptic membrane; the sensitivity of the postsynaptic receptors at the time (i.e. probably their number); and the effect of modulators of the postsynaptic response (e.g. thyroxine at noradrenergic synapses). In addition, aminergic pathways 'in series' with another can modify its function. For instance, some 5-HT pathways are very dependent on conditions prevailing in related dopaminergic and GABAergic systems.

There followed a spate of papers mainly centred on some of these aspects, but with many directed to the properties of the postsynaptic neuron and its receptor.

It had been known for some time that denervation led to hypersensitivity of pathways, and the tachyphylaxis to drugs (the development of tolerance) in the central nervous system probably meant that a similar but reverse mechanism of hyposensitivity applied in the brain. The demonstration of hypersensitivity in the brain was first with dopaminergic and cholinergic mechanisms, and then for noradrenergic, serotoninergic and histaminic pathways. Originally, changes in receptor sensitivity were considered to be slow, but the process occurred in hours (although it may take 2–3 weeks to disappear). Changes in receptor sensitivity were studied by use of the measurement of the appropriate cyclic purine monophosphate where this was acting as '2nd messenger', from the assays of radioactively labelled receptor ligands to receptor sites, from the long-term changes in turnover of amines transmitter, and from behavioural responses to receptor agonists.

In general, hyposensitivity followed overstimulation of receptors; and hypersensitivity, understimulation. Some systems could be altered either way; other target systems only one way, as though they were already in maximal or minimal stimulation states, depending on the intensity of the 'natural' intensity of transmitter bombardment.

Data from the hypersensitivity to acetylcholine indicated that this might have been accompanied by the formation of new receptor sites, possibly outside the immediate area of the synapse.

Whereas in schizophrenia there is some direct evidence of changes in receptor sensitivity, no such evidence exists at present in affective disorder.

Tricyclic drugs depress noradrenergic and serotoninergic firing rates almost immediately, and the respective hydroxylases decline in activity in response to stimulation of autoreceptors and feedback loops from the postsynaptic pathways.

As far as postsynaptic effects of these drugs are concerned, the situation is complicated by two findings: (1) that the firing rates of 5-HT- and noradrenaline-sensitive neurons in the cortex show a biphasic response—potentiation by low doses of iontophoretically applied imipramine and desipramine and antagonism by higher doses; and (2) that the 5-HT receptor probably exists in one of two* alternative forms—an agonist form to which 5-$[H^3]$T binds and an antagonist configuration to which D-$[H^3]$LSD will bind. Amitriptyline and nortriptyline have been found to bind to some of the antagonist forms of the 5-HT receptors at levels which were insufficient to give significant re-uptake blockade at the presynaptic membrane. At these dose levels they blocked 5-HTP or D-LSD head twitches in rats. Some of these properties were shared by the new antidepressant mianserin.

These data make interpretation of treatment responses difficult to interpret in affective illness. However, observation from short-term effects of these drugs are of

*There is some evidence for more than two forms of 5-HT receptor.

less importance than those given at therapeutic doses (or near-therapeutic doses in animals) in prolonged experiments. Some of these in rat forebrain have shown that long-term treatments with tricyclic antidepressants (at the upper dose range) give an enhanced inhibitory response to forebrain neurons sensitive to 5-HT and a decreased formation of noradrenaline-sensitive cAMP in limbic forebrain after desmethylimipramine and iprindole. In lower doses hippocampal pyramidal cells were more responsive to 5-HT after iprindole given long term.

In general, however, hyposensitivity of postsynaptic aminergic receptors has been reported for tricyclic re-uptake inhibitors, monoamine oxidase inhibitors and, most interestingly, following spaced electrically or flurothyl-induced seizures.

The relative activities of tricyclic drugs for the alpha adrenoreceptors in rat brain correlated closely with their ability to cause sedation and hypotension, which suggests that these properties might well be related in therapy.

In contrast to these data and some of the evidence implicating changes in alpha adrenoreceptors in depression and effects of tricyclic drugs on these receptors, as mentioned above, a recent report has suggested that chronic treatment with tricyclic antidepressants reduced beta adrenoreceptor binding and that, unlike most other aminergic systems, beta receptor activity was reduced by ECT.

The situation is far from clear at the moment, but it seems likely that receptor sensitivity, turnover and release of amines via changes in firing rates and adaptive changes of other 'adjacent' systems may interact in the therapeutic effects of antidepressant treatments. Could it be that the very complexity of their actions, by combining advantageous and deleterious effects (as far as affective disorders are concerned) may delay their own therapeutic actions? (*See* section on psychopharmacology of modes of action of first- and second-generation tricyclics for a further discussion.)

The 'contraint hypothesis'

Attempts to put some of the foregoing data into a comprehensible pattern have resulted in what may be termed the 'contraint hypothesis'.

Accepting that the current views of the actions of tricyclic antidepressants are to block both presynaptic α_2-adrenergic sites and the uptake site, and to reduce postsynaptic β-receptor activity (a result of chronic treatment), the hypothesis begins with the α_2-receptor.

It is assumed that the system in noradrenergic cells becomes unstable and that the presynaptic α_2-adrenergic receptors, which block Ca^{2+}-dependent release of noradrenaline, become hypersensitive. This tends to reduce noradrenergic activity. The first action of a tricyclic drug is to block the α_2-receptor, which allows release of transmitter. Then the uptake back across the presynaptic membrane is blocked, which enhances noradrenergic function. At the same time the drug is reducing post-synaptic sensitivity presumably by decreasing the number of β-receptors.

This gives a push–pull situation. The instability of the system in this hypothesis, therefore, is prevented by blockade of the homeostatic and synaptic interacting mechanisms which are 'held' by the drug, preventing variations in levels of their function. In theory, 'holding the pathway steady' will allow recovery.

As with other hypotheses, the 'contraint hypothesis' is incomplete, as the mechanism initiating the original instability is unstated. It is an attractive view, however, made more so now by the possibility of linking it with 5-HT dysfunction.

Provided that there is an abnormality in the 5-HT system which has not become excessive, its behavioural manifestations depend on an 'intact' noradrenergic system, and the effects of these changes based on the serotoninergic system can be blocked by drugs which block re-uptake of noradrenaline at the presynaptic membrane.

With some minor modifications of the hypothesis, therefore, it is possible to account for pathology in either system.

Electrolyte and water studies in affective illness

The late 1950s and early 1960s witnessed a number of investigations of water and electrolytes in affective illness. These were stimulated partly by the appearance of suitable methods (mostly isotope dilution techniques) and partly by an increasing interest in the hypothesis that changes in the distribution of ions across neuronal membranes could alter excitability and induce changes in brain function. Unfortunately, good though the available techniques were, they were unable to carry the problem through to its logical conclusion, and the impetus to this line of enquiry has petered out at this barrier as far as whole body or brain studies are concerned. Studies of cells have taken over from these more 'global' tests.

Some of the initial investigations were of extracellular and intracellular fluid volumes. In general, both tended to be reduced in depressive illness, and also there was some evidence for some loss of extracellular volume in mania. The most striking change, however, was in the relative behaviour of two isotopes, ^{24}Na and ^{82}Br, which were used to measure the freely available pool of sodium in the body and the extracellular space, respectively. ^{82}Br was intended to mimic, as far as was possible, the measurement of the distribution of its 'cousin', the chloride ion. In general, it did so, but there were differences—notably in the stomach, where Br$^-$ and Cl$^-$ were handled differently. The main findings were that the 'sodium space' relative to the 'bromide space' was higher in depression than after recovery and, even more fascinating, the highest ratio of Na$^+$/Br$^-$ spaces was in the individuals suffering from mania. (This finding encouraged a view that the continuum was not mania–normality–depression, but normality–depression–mania.)

There were about four explanations for this 'greater penetrance of sodium' in the body in comparison with the lesser distribution of bromide in depression and mania. It was thought, but this may not be valid, that the first two had little heuristic value.

(1) In the pathological conditions existing during depression and mania, the bromide ion might be excluded from a sodium space which it normally occupies. The gastric mucosa was a likely candidate here, as this tissue normally concentrates bromide preferentially to chloride (the systematic difference mentioned above). If this process failed in affective illness, sodium would appear to have relatively greater or bromide relatively smaller distribution volumes.

(2) Some of the sodium in bone exchanges rapidly (within the time of the tests), another fraction exchanges slowly over 5–7 days, and some is relatively inaccessible to a circulating isotope of sodium. If part of the inaccessible pool became accessible, or if the slowly exchanging sodium became rapidly exchanging, this could account for the results. Data obtained earlier using ^{22}Na, an isotope of long half-life, did not support this possibility.

(3) The amount of sodium in cells had increased, thus altering the bioelectrical properties of the cell membranes. There were no data, however, to show whether the brain was similarly involved, even if this explanation of the finding were correct.
(4) There could have been an alteration in the ion-binding properties of the macromolecules in the extracellular space, so that the relative masses of sodium and chloride (and bromide) ions held in the tissues in association with these molecules had changed during affective illness.

If (3) and (4) were correct, even if the brain were not involved, these might produce significant changes in body function which could play a part in the aetiology of affective illness.

While, as already mentioned, it has not been technically possible to pursue whole-body studies of electrolyte distribution, or to locate the site of the observed changes, several other lines of investigation have pointed to peculiarities in electrolyte function in affective illness.

The rectal mucosa has a potential difference across it produced by a mechanism requiring active transport of sodium. This potential difference is increased by lithium and is low in depression.

Another group studied saliva and measured the sodium and bicarbonate 'activity' (using a microelectrode system) in the output of the parotid gland. The patients (bipolar and unipolar depressives) had higher 'sodium activity' and pH levels than did controls, which suggested decreased membrane transport. Manic patients tended to be similarly abnormal.

The system which has commanded most attention with regard to electrolytics is the erythrocyte. Early observations showed that the sodium content of the red cell tended to fall on recovery from both depression and mania, probably as a result of changes in transport of sodium. Later studies showed that the changes in active transport were secondary to an abnormality in $Na^+–K^+$ ATPase. In general, the results of various groups have been in the same direction, and in addition lithium has been shown to increase red blood cells (RBC) $Na^+–K^+$ ATPase activity in the red cells of patients suffering from affective illness, but not in those from normal subjects. This cannot be demonstrated *in vitro*. Two studies have suggested a link between increase in $Na^+–K^+$ ATPase activity during treatment with lithium and clinical response. This could be due to a change in the number of $Na^+–K^+$ ATPase molecules per cell or some alteration in activity of the individual ATPase molecules.

In investigations by Naylor's group, the data show decreased activity in $Na^+–K^+$ ATPase molecules in mania and depression and no alteration in the number of these molecules, the comparison here being between ill and recovered patients.

This is clearly an interesting area of study. One of the problems in this type of investigation is the life-long span of erythrocytes and the effect which previous drug treatments could have on them. These objections did not seem to apply to this investigation. Naylor's group have gone on to look for an external molecule in plasma which might decrease the activity of ATPase and have found a candidate in the form of vanadium. This is a naturally occurring trace element, normally present at a concentration in plasma near to that at which inhibition of the enzyme will occur. They have shown that lymphocytes incubated in plasma containing vanadium tend to increase the number of pump sites. In contrast, cells from patients with affective disorder do not have this recovery mechanism. A possible causative mechanism was suggested by the presence of higher concentrations of vanadium (statistically significant in mania but not in depressed or recovered groups). There were significant negative correlations between plasma vanadium concentrations and the ratio of Na^+-K^+ Mg ATPase and Mg ATPase in those with affective illness but none in normals. This suggests that the variation in Na^+-K^+ Mg ATPase and sodium pump activity is associated in the illness. Finally, clinical improvement was seen following lowering of the body burden of vanadium. This could be a promising line of research.

The effect of lithium has been followed both in RBCs and in other systems. Lithium increases the activity of Na^+-K^+ ATPase in red cells. In addition, some individuals have high RBC/plasma ratios (lithium index), while others have low ratios. These seem to be constant for the subject and dependent on a Na^+-dependent lithium counter-transport system, the characteristics of which are genetically determined.

A high ratio or an increasing ratio is said to indicate susceptibility to neurotoxicity to lithium, but carries no implications for response. Bipolar patients with high erythrocyte Na^+-K^+ ATPase and high levels of lithium in their red cells tend to do well. Attempts to identify a high lithium index with either bipolar or lithium responders remains controversial.

The other more general studies of the effect of lithium on electrolytes are difficult to interpret. The very early effects of lithium are likely to be irrelevant to antimanic activity, but the subacute changes (days to 1–2 weeks) may have some connection with therapeutic activity. When we come to long-term treatments, prophylactic therapy, the acute and subacute changes brought about by lithium may have nothing to do with changes in physiology/biochemistry which clinical observations suggest may be responsible for clinical benefit developing over 6 months or more.

However, looking at lithium from the point of view of electrolytes and the early effect on mania, the drug causes initial loss of Na^+, K^+ and water, and a transient increase in secretion of aldosterone. During mania patients are highly tolerant of lithium and retain more of the drug than they would if they were in normal mood (the half-life of lithium can be doubled in mania).

Later in time the body tends to lose sodium, and lithium may begin to replace some of the sodium and calcium in bone. An observed increase in sodium space is probably the result of mobilization of tissue sodium, including that from bone. Total body potassium decreases at about 2 weeks. Urinary losses and plasma levels of magnesium tend to rise.

Quite long-term readjustments in electrolyte balance—e.g. with potassium—take place over a period of months. It is undecided whether lithium has any chronic effects on the calcification of bones.

Recently, in a very small series which needs extension and replication, five out of six bipolar patients did well after a year's treatment with spironolactone, a drug which inhibits aldosterone.

The study of electrolytes, membrane energy mechanisms, cellular permeability, etc., remains an interesting and possibly promising field in which there appear to be a number of pieces of a jigsaw at least promising a useful picture at the end. However, the critics of this type of research claim that the findings are secondary phenomena.

Cyclic adenosine 3'5'-monophosphate (cAMP)

Cyclic adenosine 3'5'-monophosphate is formed inside cells in response to the triggering of that cell by a variety of hormones, and in neurons also by transmitter substances. This does not imply that all hormones or transmitter substances act via this mechanism.

The process involves interaction with a hormone or transmitter substance with a specific site on the cell membrane which is unique to its ligand and closely related molecules. This interaction activates the enzyme adenylate cyclase, which in the presence of Mg^{2+} catalyses the conversion of adenosine triphosphate (ATP) to cAMP and inorganic phosphate. This molecule goes on to initiate changes in cellular metabolism. Its levels are limited by 3'5'-cyclic nucleotide phosphodiesterases which convert cAMP to 5'-adenosine monophosphate (5'-AMP).

The discovery of this vital modulating process in cellular metabolism led to the search for an abnormality in affective illness. Initial studies suggested decreased urinary excretion of cAMP in depression and increased excretion in hypomania, with change towards normal on recovery. Comparisons were with euthymic patients, normal controls or patients with neurotic depression, or the patients themselves on recovery. Some alterations with mood change were observed in rapidly cycling manic depressive patients, but this was not confirmed in other investigations. In longitudinal studies the increase in cAMP excretion was greater in tricyclic-treated than in ECT-treated patients. Since urinary cAMP originates partly from the body but partly from the kidneys (about 50 per cent each), it is difficult to draw conclusions from these data, but cAMP was at normal levels in plasma CSF and platelets during depression.

The most likely explanation of the data is that there is a reversible abnormality of unknown origin in the renal excretion of cAMP in depressive illness. The changes (increase) in excretion of cAMP during treatment with tricyclic antidepressants could be due to some inhibition of hydrolysis of the compound by inhibition of the phosphodiesterases. Lithium inhibits the formation of cAMP in many tissues (and this is responsible for the polyuria refractory to antidiuretic hormone) but whether its interaction with the ATP–cAMP system is in any way related to its therapeutic actions is not known.

Cholinergic–adrenergic imbalance hypothesis

One of the relatively recent hypotheses for affective illness is that, in a way somewhat comparable with the situation in Parkinson's disease, alterations in mood may be the product of changes in the balance between opposing cholinergic –adrenergic (or serotoninergic) mechanisms. In this formulation, depressive affect and associated symptoms are the result of a predominance of cholinergic processes, and mania is the converse situation—relative overactivity in adrenergic (or serotoninergic) systems over cholinergic mechanisms.

Of course, such ideas are not entirely discordant with aminergic theories; because nobody could suggest that aminergic mechanisms exist in a neuronal vacuum, the search for simple changes in aminergic processes was much too unsophisticated an approach and aminergic networks are part of as yet incompletely described complex networks. Nevertheless, the cholinergic–adrenergic hypothesis is attractive in many ways and could provide an equal contender with other hypotheses for affective illness.

The arguments of the proponents of this hypothesis can be summarized as follows:

In peripheral vegetative systems in the body (heart rate, gastrointestinal activity, control of the pupil, etc.) adrenergic and cholinergic mechanisms have opposing effects, and there is some evidence for similar central balances—e.g. in arousal, and in the pathways mediating self-stimulation mechanisms. In addition, a psychostimulant drug, methylphenidate, which increases locomotor activity in animals by releasing noradrenaline and dopamine, is potentiated by physostigmine, an inhibitor of acetylcholine.

Anticholinergic agents which pass the blood–brain barrier increase locomotion, self-stimulation and behaviour activation in animals; and amphetamine and anticholinergic drugs are synergistic in increasing locomotor activity in mice.

The rate-limiting step in the synthesis of acetylcholine is choline acetylase, which is increased in animals after they have been given amphetamines or intravenous noradrenaline—presumably a compensatory readjustment. A mechanism of this type, a compensatory increase in cholinergic activity, in theory could account for the depression seen in amphetamine withdrawal.

In man the effects of methylphenidate are diminished by physostigmine, presumably by increasing cholinergic activity. The latter drug given initially produces an anergic syndrome reversed by methylphenidate.

A further argument is that reserpine, which induces depression in susceptible individuals, has cholinomimetic-like effects—salivation, increased gastric secretion, nausea, vomiting, asthma, bronchospasm, biliary colic, nasal congestion and diarrhoea.

Tricyclic antidepressants have anticholinergic side-effects and can give a confusional state comparable to atropine/scopolamine poisoning, which can be ameliorated with physostigmine.

Cholinesterase inhibitor, organophosphorous insecticides and nerve gases produce depression, lassitude, apathy, slowness and inefficiency of thinking, and a proportion of manic patients improved on intravenous physostigmine.

A disadvantage of the hypothesis is that neither acute blockade of noradrenergic synthesis with α-methylparatyrosine nor the effects of acute cholinomimetic drugs gives an accurate replication of the depressive syndrome.

Histamine receptors (H₁, H₂) in the brain and antidepressant drugs

The therapeutic actions of tricyclic antidepressants have usually been attributed to their ability to block re-uptake at the presynaptic membranes of noradrenergic and serotoninergic synapses in the brain. Yet they have other effects, some of which were outlined in the last section. These include the recent finding of blockade of the antagonist form of the 5-HT postsynaptic receptors in the cortex, antagonism of the muscarinic cholinergic receptors discussed in the section above, and blockade of H_1 receptors.

Histamine is a neurotransmitter in the central nervous system, and one such pathway passes up in the medial forebrain bundle to be distributed widely to the cortex. Histamine-sensitive adenylate cyclase has been found in the hippocampus and the cortex. Activation of H_2 receptors decreases the firing rate of some cortical cells, but the function of histaminergic neurons in the brain is not known.

It has been demonstrated recently that tricyclic antidepressants—particularly the tertiary amine drugs, iprindole, mianserin and also chlorpromazine, thioridazine, thiothixine and other neuroleptics—inhibited H_2 receptors in the brain at levels which would be expected from their usual therapeutic doses. The significance of this finding is not known.

Miscellaneous observations

REM sleep deprivation

Depressed patients tend to have decreased rapid eye movement (REM) sleep latency, higher REM frequency and abnormal distribution of REM throughout the night. These changes revert towards normal with recovery. Deprivation of sleep and of REM sleep have been tried with temporary improvement as treatments for depression.

Tendon reflexes

Hoffmann reflex recovery curves have been studied in psychiatric patients and facilitation of reaction time has been seen in patients with affective illness.

Treatment with phenylalanine and tyrosine

Both phenylalanine and tyrosine are catecholamine precursors and as such have been given in attempts to treat affective disorders. More details are required.

Augmentors and reducers: previous personality and affective disorder

There are a number of studies pointing to systematic differences between bipolar and unipolar patients. In evoked potential studies in bipolar individuals the signal tends to be enhanced, whereas the contrary tends to happen in unipolar individuals.

The subject can only be dealt with briefly here, but there seem to be systematic differences in premorbid personality—that of bipolar tends to be nearer the normal or cyclothymic, with only a few individuals of the obsessional type. Unipolar individuals differ in that some are orderly, conscientious, meticulous persons with a high value in achievement, conventional thinking and dependency in close relationships. They are often worrying individuals with obsessional tendencies.

It is not known whether personality and illness are manifestations of the same process, and what effect episodes have on personality (since the area is a difficult one to investigate and premorbid personality has been studied retrospectively).

Rhythms

One of the cardinal features of affective illness is in disturbance of rhythms. These include the well-known diurnal variation in mood (which often includes anxiety, appetite, energy, efficiency in thinking and other symptoms), sleep, hormones (e.g. cortisol, prolactin), and excretion of metabolites (e.g. 3-methoxy,4-hydroxyphenylglycol: MHPG) and temperature.

There are also longer-term rhythms. Some patients have a period of time when their illnesses recur regularly at one time of the year; patients with mania have a peak of admissions in June–July, decreasing as the summer goes on, and a 'trough' at mid-winter. Suicide rates reach a maximum in March–May and a minimum in December.

Conclusions

While there are many important approaches to the problem of affective illness, that concerned with its biological aspects and physical treatments is seeking aetiological mechanisms and improved therapies, respectively. The amount of information accruing may be pointing to further subdivisions in the types of affective illness while at the same time raising some most interesting and promising hypotheses.

Chapter 16

Schizophrenia

Introduction

Currently the problem of the aetiology of schizophrenia remains unsolved. The search for the causes of this illness or group of illnesses has covered many areas of enquiry (and we do not know how close we are to a fruitful approach). It is hoped that we may be entering an era in which our footholds on the problem are improving. When we have established beyond reasonable doubt that we are researching in the correct field, this indeed will be real progress.

With any condition of unknown aetiology, the first task is to define the condition clinically, and the history of the study of schizophrenia is one of unfortunate difficulties born of confusing differences in classification and the breadth of clinical syndromes included in the term 'schizophrenia'. In the USA in particular, the term 'schizophrenia' has included a much wider spectrum of conditions than is customary in Europe. The more limited boundaries of the term apply here.

Detailed descriptions of the phenomenology of schizophrenia are to be found in standard textbooks of psychiatry. A general outline of the basic clinical symptoms has been included here because the phenomenology of this illness is inseparable from the discussion of aetiological theories. This is because our starting points at one extreme are in the syndromes in humans with similar symptom patterns to those of schizophrenia and at the other are in animal models, some of the features of which mimic those seen in schizophrenia. The main groups of symptoms in this type of illness are as follows:

(1) *Hallucinations* In contrast to most other conditions accompanied by hallucinations, those in schizophrenia occur on a background of clear consciousness. Quite a variety of hallucinations are seen, but the characteristic ones tend to be auditory and to be structured and complex. Thus, patients may be quite absorbed in the messages and instructions they are 'receiving', or they may be involved in hallucinatory conversations. The content may include descriptions of actions or thoughts and may refer to the subject in the third person.

(2) *Delusions and perceptual disorders* Delusions in schizophrenia are varied and are elaborated with time to a varying degree. They may be persecutory or religiose or be beliefs interpreted in terms of paranormal or alien influences communicating with, influencing or controlling the patient. The patient may feel that thoughts are being put into their minds, that there is thought

broadcast, thought reading, thought echo, thought block or withdrawal. Delusions of reference or delusional misinterpretation are very common.

(3) *Affective change*   Affect in many schizophrenics appears to be non-existent or reduced—there is little of the normal affective response to the environment or emotional interplay with other people. In the absence of emotional interaction, it is difficult to feel rapport with the patient with schizophrenia who has the aura of coldness, aloofness or inexplicable strangeness. The impression engendered is that of emotional pallor. At other times or in other patients the affective response may be apparent but the emotional expression may be the opposite of what would be expected from a normal individual. The two types of affective change are referred to as 'flat' and 'inappropriate' affect.

(4) *General behaviour and motor activity*   Often schizophrenia is accompanied by extreme inertia, loss of any activity based on initiative and a marked depression of motor activity. The converse also occurs, so that the patient is in a state of frenetic excitement. Movements of the body may be abnormal, in that they are repetitive, or are unusual or awkward or may cease, with the body held in one position for long periods.

(5) *Thought*   The ability to experience thoughts in a logical, sequential stream may be reduced, in which case communication with the patient seems vague or oddly elusive. With increasing thought disorder, the point is reached at which speech becomes quite incomprehensible, which presumably indicates that the mental processes are governed in such individuals by the most remote associations or even are virtually random. Sometimes the thought processes come to an abrupt halt.

The main discernible clinical types of schizophrenia are:

(1) *Simple*   This type is characterized by lack of drive, initiative and sociability. Florid symptoms are few, and if they occur, do so usually in response to stressful situations.

(2) *Hebephrenic*   This type of illness is identified by the presence together of thought disorder, auditory hallucinations, delusions and inappropriate affect.

(3) *Catatonic*   Patients with this variety of schizophrenia tend to have predominance of disorders of movement such as stereotypy, stupor, overactivity, grimacing and the maintenance of seemingly uncomfortable postures for long periods.

(4) *Paranoid*   As the name implies, this condition is accompanied by persecutory and/or expansive delusions based on disturbing and often frightening hallucinations. The condition is characterized by hostility, suspicion, fearfulness and aggression, by a late onset in life and by the relative absence of other forms of schizophrenia; the personality is well preserved.

The existence of these various classifications of schizophrenia, with their related but in some respects diverse symptomatology, is one of the reasons why there is a question as to whether schizophrenia is one entity with a spectrum of varying manifestations or is a group of illnesses having the semblance of clinical similarities.

Hypotheses attempting to explain schizophrenia have tended to fall into one of four main categories of hereditary origin (with the assumption now that what is inherited is a susceptibility to illness with which stress, etc., interact to produce the condition):

(1) *Monogenic*   In this group of hypotheses a single mutant gene is responsible for

the appearance of the disorder and its main manifestations. The genetic abnormality would be in the form of a defective organizer or, more probably, dysfunctional enzyme, and in this way would determine susceptibility to illness and the appearances of the schizophrenic syndrome or syndromes.

(2) *Two interacting genes*

(3) *Polygenic* The polygenic theories are somewhat different, in that they imply a much wider distribution in the population of a minimum of three genes, none of which is essential to illness. The precipitation of illness in this hypothesis is by a threshold effect, environmental factors playing a major role in the various illness-precipitating processes.

(4) *Life experience only hypothesis* Here there is no inherited predisposition—all members of the population are equally at risk for developing schizophrenia. The agents producing illness are considered to be either positive (an excess of certain noxious influences) or negative (the absence of beneficial or protecting experiences or environmental circumstances). The illness is the psychological reaction to these abnormal environmental conditions. Many of the hypotheses of this type have devolved around mother–child relationships or parent–child communication.

The most important point of difference between these various groups of ideas puts (1), (2) and (3) together because they imply a genetic causative agent or agents, in contrast to (4), where genetic factors are not implicated at all. These do not exhaust the types of idea advanced to explain schizophrenic illness, which extend to infective and other noxious processes.

Research into the genetic basis of schizophrenia

According to several authorities, the genetic basis of schizophrenia can be regarded as a secure hypothesis. If this is accepted, then the life experience only hypothesis must be rejected. It is important to stress that this statement does not exclude life experiences from having a major role in the genesis of schizophrenia, because this would be patently untrue. It merely states that the prime mover or movers as regards vulnerability are inherited, and therefore have a biochemical basis.

Twin studies

Early studies of the hereditability of schizophrenia found that relatives of schizophrenics had the illness more frequently than would be expected from its incidence in the population at large.

The phenotypes of monozygotic twins (MZ) may differ slightly, but their genotypes are identical. In the first studies of such twins with one twin suffering from schizophrenia, the concordance rates (that is, the number of times illness was observed in the co-twin) was high, in the region of 69 per cent. In these studies the investigators relied on notes, but never or rarely saw the patients. The co-twins had passed through most of the period of their lives when they would be at risk. The subjects were also chronic schizophrenics of many years' standing and therefore a slightly 'skewed' population. Later studies gave somewhat lower levels of concordance for monozygotic twins, of 10–40 per cent. These were first admissions, more transiently ill and more fluctuant, and tended to get better. The co-twins had not passed through much of their period of risk. Less severely affected patients were included in these series. Increasing severity of illness in an individual increases the risk of illness in the relative, so that if less severely ill twins were accepted, a lower concordance rate would be expected in the co-twins.

Other relatives

Expectation of schizophrenia in other relatives is about 9 per cent for parents, 14 per cent for siblings and 16 per cent for children. The children of two schizophrenic individuals have about a 34 per cent chance of developing the illness.

Adoption studies

The proponents of the view that there is no hereditable factor in schizophrenia would suggest that schizophrenic parents evoke a schizophrenic environment in their families and thus give spurious evidence of a genetic endowment to the illness. Two strategies have been employed to study this. In one, Heston looked at the children of mothers suffering from schizophrenia where the children had been reared apart from their biological mothers from the first month of life onwards. Five of the adopted children of 47 schizophrenic mothers developed the illness, as compared with none of the adopted children of 50 non-schizophrenic mothers. In another investigation, the biological and adoptive parents of 10 adopted schizophrenic and 10 adopted normal persons were studied. It was found that the biological parents of the schizophrenic adoptees showed significantly raised psychopathology. The adoptive families of schizophrenics were indistinguishable from the adoptive and biological families of normal controls. On the other hand, there was significantly greater psychopathology in the biological relatives of the adopted schizophrenic individuals than among the adoptive relatives who lived with them. The conclusion that there is a significant genetic component in schizophrenia seems inescapable (with the proviso that a transmitted infective agent is still possible).

More detailed adoption studies by Rosenthal and his collaborators identified 5500 children who had been adopted outside their families. The incidence of schizophrenia in the adopted offspring of schizophrenic parents was compared with the control group from parents free from the disease. The diagnosis 'schizophrenia spectrum disease' was applied to those with acute or chronic illness, 'borderline state' or personality disorder—that is, a fairly wide view of the condition. Of the adopted offspring of schizophrenic parents, 31.6 per cent were given this diagnosis, as compared with 17.8 per cent of adopted offspring of normal individuals. None of the 67 controls had schizophrenia, whereas 3 of the index individuals had definite illness.

Kety and others assessed the biological and adoptive relatives of 33 of the schizophrenia group adoptees, and found 21 per cent and 5 per cent with schizophrenia spectrum disease, respectively. With the comparable control group (relatives of a control group of healthy adoptees) these figures were 11 per cent and 6 per cent, respectively.

From the previous section it can be seen that another concept has been introduced into the discussion on the genetics of schizophrenia. It has been felt for some time that the blood relatives of schizophrenics differ from the norm in their personality and behaviour, and this has led to the description of the 'schizoid' individual and schizophrenic spectrum disorder. By this was meant someone with many of the features and the bizarre characteristics of patients with schizophrenia but in attenuated form and without the overt psychotic manifestations.

Heston has suggested that a single autosomal gene could account equally for both schizophrenia and the schizoid state, and he has pointed out that the schizoid condition and schizophrenia occur with about equal frequency in monozygotic twins, and that the proportions of the two states in the relatives fit reasonably well with theoretical predictions. It is difficult to account for all the observations under this hypothesis—for instance, why increasing severity of illness in an index individual increases the probability of finding the disorder in a relative, why an increase in the proportion of schizophrenic relatives in a family increases the risk and why there are different forms of the illness.

Rosenthal studied the spouses of schizophrenics and showed that there had been some degree of assortative mating (i.e. schizophrenic individuals had tended to marry individuals with schizophrenic spectrum disorder). The prevalence of schizophrenic spectrum disorder was more than three times as common in the offspring where the co-spouse also had schizophrenic spectrum disorder.

Quite apart from these, there are other unanswered questions about the characteristics of this illness. We cannot yet understand why schizophrenia persists when the reproduction rate in schizophrenic illnesses is reduced and why such modifying effects as body build, intelligence and possibly body weight affect its manifestation.

A two-gene hypothesis proposed initially by Rüdin and Böök and co-workers suggests a dominant gene affecting monoamine oxidase activity and a recessive gene altering the properties of dopaminergic activity via an abnormal dopamine beta hydroxylase enzyme. Unfortunately, the evidence from post-mortem studies is that the latter enzyme is normal in the brain in schizophrenia.

An interesting genetic finding has been the observation that 14 of 22 twins (with an index individual with schizophrenia) were left-handed and in this left-handed group concordance rates were low and illness was not severe. Of the 8 right-handed individuals, 7 were concordant for schizophrenia. One possibility is that being a twin increases the chances of altered cerebral dominance and perhaps 'non-genetic' schizophrenia (so the twins would tend to discordance). There is no evidence of increased schizophrenia in twins, even though left-handedness is commoner in twins than in single births. The finding is of interest, however, in the light of the recent work of Jones on possible malfunction of the corpus callosum in schizophrenia.

Monoamine oxidase (MAO) is reduced in platelets in some schizophrenics. The presence of low MAO in platelets does not seem to be a specific marker for the illness—it occurs in other conditions and it has been proposed as an indicator of mental illness in general.

Biological studies in schizophrenia

The clinical classification of schizophrenia has been bedevilled by different criteria for its diagnosis, but the search for biochemical causes of the illness has run an even more erratic course. On the other hand, there are many formidable problems to solve in this type of investigation. The underlying abnormality in schizophrenia may be subtle—perhaps a change in a relatively small part of the brain or one caused by a substance of strong effect acting in micro-concentrations. The brain is partially isolated behind the blood–brain barrier, and it is asking a lot of biochemical techniques to expect them to detect minute quantities of, say, some abnormal central transmitter or modulator of neuronal activity from peripheral fluids at second hand (plasma) or even third hand (urine). Even the use of cerebrospinal fluid leaves much to be desired in this context.

If this fact is added to what might be termed the welter of biological noise—the considerable inter- and intra-individual variance produced by differences in age, sex, body mass and body activity; by differences in bacteriological, viral and nutritional environments; and by powerful neuroleptic drugs, the traces of which remain in the body for prodigous times—it is small wonder that biochemical studies in schizophrenia have been the graveyard of forlorn hopes.

Even if none of these problems existed, it might be impossible to replicate or control for the stress experienced by individuals in the height of a psychotic episode, and clearly this factor alone could generate a whole series of changes in the body which could be spuriously attributed to causative mechanisms. Yet, despite all these technical problems, there is sufficient circumstantial evidence to point to a biochemical aetiology of the illness and encourage research in this area. The genetic studies would be enough on their own to implicate a biological basis for schizophrenia, but other data have been used to support this view of the illness.

In 1952 Osmond and Smythies noted the similarity between noradrenaline and the hallucinogenic compound mescaline (*Figure 16.1*). They postulated an abnormality in schizophrenia which would result in production of a compound from noradrenaline, possibly 3,4-dimethoxyphenyl ethanolamine, which might have some of the properties of mescaline. This hypothesis assumed that the biochemical defect would become manifest during stress. The production of hallucinogenic compounds would itself be stressful, so that, once started, the condition would tend to be self-perpetuating.

The close similarity between other hallucinogens and possible hallucinogenic compounds and noradrenaline, 5-hydroxytryptamine (5-HT) and dopamine has been emphasized by many workers in this field (*Figure 16.2*).

As the subject developed, so strategies developed for testing the so-called 'transmethylation' hypothesis (*Figure 16.3*). It was argued that if transmethylation of amines to hallucinogens occurred in schizophrenia, increasing the supply of amines, the precursors of the hallucinogenic compounds, should exacerbate schizophrenia. This would also happen if the same end were achieved by preventing the destruction of amines—for instance, with monoamine oxidase inhibitors.

Similarly, the clinical state of schizophrenics should be worsened by increasing the methylating capacity of the brain and presumably also reduction in methylating capacity should give an improvement in symptoms.

A number of studies now have shown that sometimes detectable clinical changes may occur in experiments along these lines but not always in the direction predicted. Chronic schizophrenics given phenylalanine while receiving monoamine oxidase inhibitor (MAOI), in an attempt to increase the amounts of catecholamines in the brain, showed no change. There was some degree of euphoria, however, in patients given tryptophan as the additional treatment with MAOI, but neither treatment caused any significant worsening of their clinical state.

L-dopa has now been given with or without a peripheral decarboxylase inhibitor (to prevent transformation of dopa to dopamine in the body) to normal individuals

294

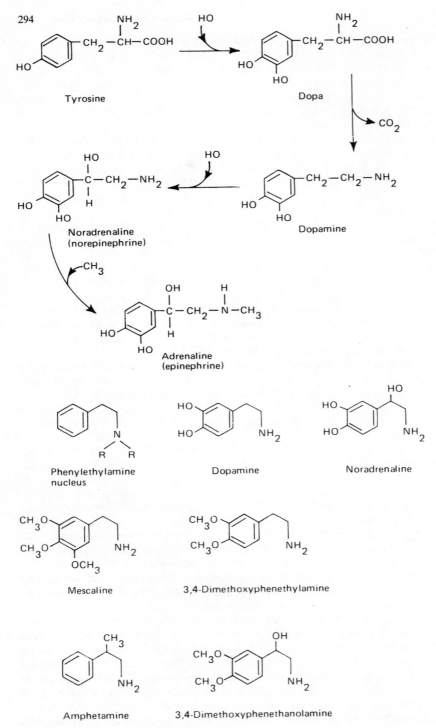

Figure 16.1 Catecholamines and mescaline

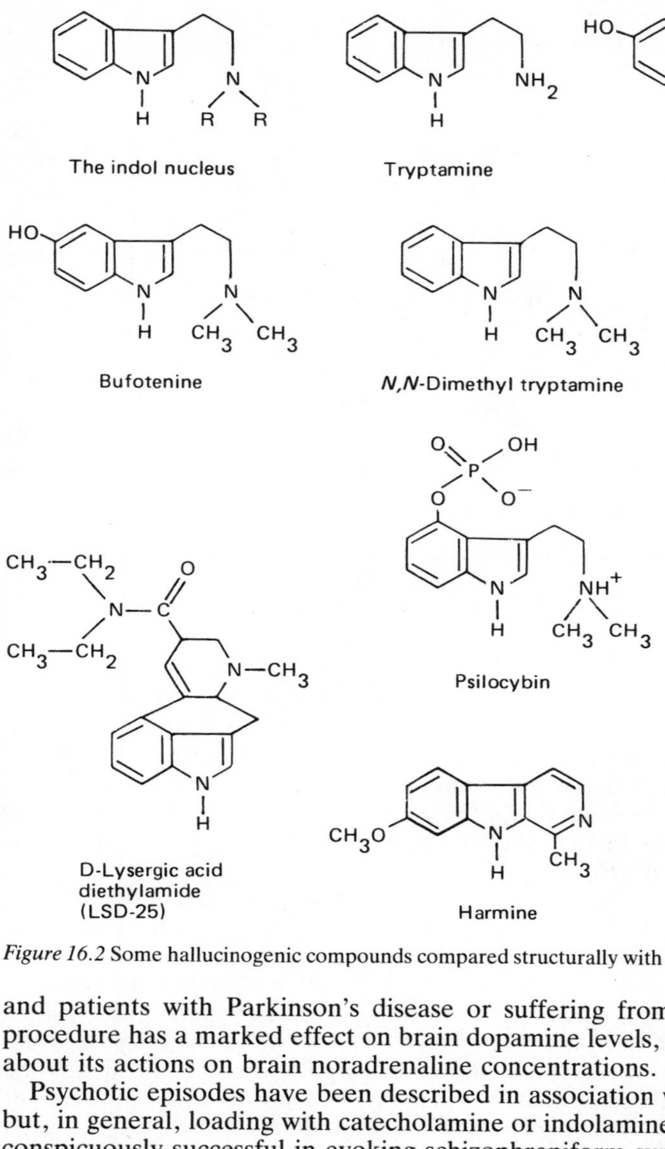

Figure 16.2 Some hallucinogenic compounds compared structurally with serotonin

and patients with Parkinson's disease or suffering from depressive illness. The procedure has a marked effect on brain dopamine levels, but there is less certainty about its actions on brain noradrenaline concentrations.

Psychotic episodes have been described in association with the giving of L-dopa but, in general, loading with catecholamine or indolamine precursors has not been conspicuously successful in evoking schizophreniform symptomatology.

The position with attempts to increase methylating capacity has produced more positive effects. Treating chronic schizophrenics with MAOI and adding methionine, a methyl donor, produces a quite clear-cut clinical deterioration in a significant proportion of schizophrenics, and this observation has been replicated by a number of groups. It could be argued that, at the dosage of methionine given, the side-effects might have been sufficient to activate a latent psychosis as a non-specific phenomenon. That was not the case. An alternative methyl donor, betaine, was given with MAOI to a group of chronic schizophrenics. The responses seen did not appear as rapidly as with methionine, but the substance increased the

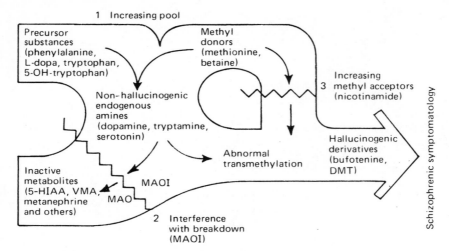

Figure 16.3 Strategies used to study the hypothesized abnormal transmethylation in schizophrenia. 1, Increasing available pool of substances thought necessary to process: precursor substances and/or methyl donors. 2, Interfering with normal enzymatic break-down by use of monoamine oxidase inhibitor. 3, Increasing available pool of methyl acceptors. From *Foundations of Biochemical Psychiatry*, 1976, by D.S. Segal, J. Yager and J.L. Sullivan, Butterworths

severity of schizophrenic symptomatology. Nicotinic acid and nicotinamide adenine dinucleotide, a methyl acceptor, have been given in large amounts to chronic schizophrenics to find out whether this would improve their symptoms. Claims for success by amelioration of the manifestations of schizophrenia have not been confirmed, and it has also been shown that nicotinic acid did not prevent the clinical deterioration produced by MAOI and methionine. Thus, attempts to promote demethylation in the brain had little, if any, effect.

There is, unfortunately, some doubt as to whether the compounds used do have any appreciable effect on the methylating potential of the body, so these investigations are somewhat inconclusive.

As can be seen from *Figure 16.2*, bufotenin, as the *N,N*-dimethyl derivative of 5-HT, was bound to come under close scrutiny as a potential 'endogenous' hallucinogen, particularly when it became known that there was an enzyme in the brain capable of synthesizing it. It was thought originally that bufotenin was the active principle in hallucinogenic snuff, but this was not found to be so. Subsequent attempts to demonstrate hallucinogenic activity with bufotenin have not produced an unequivocal answer. Undoubtedly, bufotenin provokes quite marked somatic symptoms, but that it is a hallucinogen now seems to be in some doubt.

Assuming that bufotenin was synthesized in the brain from serotonin only, very small quantities would be expected in the urine. Some writers have failed to detect any; others have identified substances in small amounts which, though thought to be bufotenin, turned out to be other substances (e.g. drug metabolites). Of the many studies performed, few have combined blind analysis with an exclusion of dietary and analytical artefacts. There is considerable doubt from the most carefully designed studies as to whether bufotenin occurs in urine in schizophrenia, even after the administration of MAOI.

The 'pink spot'

The 'pink spot' story began with the suggestion by Osmond and Smythies that noradrenaline might be converted to hallucinogenic phenylethylamines and with the report that 15 of 19 schizophrenics excreted dimethoxyphenethylamine (DMPEA; *Figure 16.1*). A similar number of control subjects were found not to excrete this substance, which was associated with the term 'pink spot' from its appearance on chromatograms stained with a modified Ehrlich's reagent. This sparked off a considerable research effort, designed to explore whether or not DMPEA was found in urine and, if it was found, whether it was present in larger amounts in schizophrenic individuals. Once again, general studies which have gone to the greatest possible lengths to exclude dietary and other artefacts have tended to be 'least positive', and to date there is no really reliable evidence to suggest that, as compared with controls, DMPEA is to be found in urine in greater amounts or in a larger number of schizophrenics. Support for the DMPEA hypothesis lessened even further when DMPEA failed to evoke schizophrenic symptoms, even when ingested, but before this negative was accepted finally, more would need to be known about its fate when taken orally.

'Malvaria'

Hoffer and his co-workers described the appearance of a mauve spot on the chromatograms of the urine of many schizophrenics and called the condition 'malvaria', from the colour of the spot. Unfortunately, this spot was found also in patients with other psychoses and other psychiatric states, and in some normal individuals. Since then, the mauve spot has been identified as 2,4-dimethyl-3-ethylpyrrole. This compound injected into rabbits produced sedation, and it is not thought to be a likely candidate for a schizophrenia-inducing compound.

Melatonin and harmine

In 1961 McIsaacs pointed out the very close similarity between melatonin and the hallucinogen harmine, suggesting that the pineal gland could be the source of an hallucinogenic compound of this type (*Figure 16.4*). This possibility has not been pursued further to date.

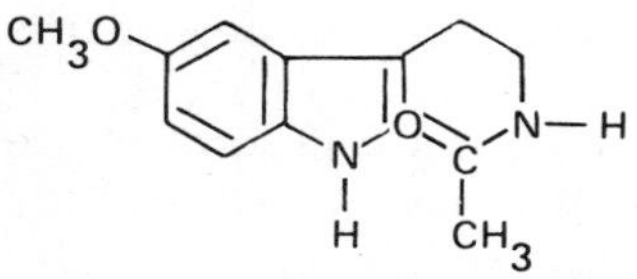

Melatonin

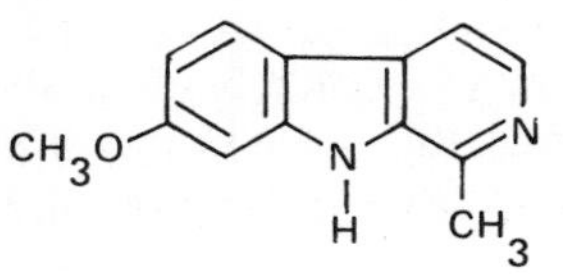

Harmine

Figure 16.4 Melatonin and harmine

Histamine

Just as the effects of MAOI combined with methionine or betaine have given consistent, tantalizingly positive results in schizophrenia, so also have some of the studies which have concerned themselves with histamine.

One observation is that patients with schizophrenia produce smaller skin wheals than do controls in response to intradermal injections of histamine and react less than non-schizophrenics to an injection of histamine, fall in blood pressure being used as a means of assessing histamine tolerance. There is even the suggestion that there may be two populations of schizophrenics, differentiated by high and low blood histamine concentrations. Methodological problems have made estimates of plasma and blood histamine levels difficult to interpret, but there is some evidence to suggest that there could be an abnormality in the metabolism of histamine. Various writers have suggested that allergic illness is relatively rare in schizophrenics and that asthma remits with the onset of schizophrenic episodes.

One of the difficulties in interpreting this type of study is that phenothiazines have some antihistamine activity and that schizophrenic episodes are very stressful and therefore may be expected to be associated with changes in catecholamines and cortisol output. Nevertheless, the position of histamine in schizophrenia may merit further studies.

Abnormal proteins in schizophrenia

There has been a whole series of hypotheses associating schizophrenia with the presence of abnormal proteins in blood.

One group has claimed that the plasma from schizophrenics contains a protein which alters the metabolism of chick red cells, producing in them a higher degree of anaerobic respiration, so that the ratio of their production of lactate to pyruvate was raised. Drug effects were not responsible for the observations, but subsequent studies have shown that chronic hospitalization could have been an important contaminating factor. Thus, there seems to be some doubt about the specificity of the finding to the illness.

Other groups have studied the effect of plasma or serum from schizophrenic patients on some form of learned or other response in animals. These investigations have included food-motivated bar pressing, avoidance learning, time taken to complete a learned precision task, the effect on evoked cortical responses, etc. The results, on the whole, have not been promising from the point of view of the replication of these findings.

One of the test systems studied was rope climbing by rats, which in some of the tests was more impaired after the injection of schizophrenic than it was after the injection of normal plasma. The active fraction was an α-2-globulin which also produced changes in evoked potentials in rabbits. One suggestion was that there was a small compound associated with the protein, possibly a phenylethylamine. Russian workers have postulated immunological abnormalities in schizophrenia, resulting in the production of an abnormal labile α-2-globulin and which could alter the properties of cell membranes. It has been suggested that the red cell factors, this protein and the one associated with changes in rope climbing may be one and the same substance.

A further claim has been made that plasma from schizophrenics alters the rate of entry of glutamic acid, tryptophan, 5-hydroxytryptophan and alanine into chick red cells, which, if operative in the brain, might increase the concentration of amine precursors of hallucinogens. Clearly, there is much in this area requiring clarification and further study.

Another group of hypotheses has centred around the suggestion that schizophrenics have abnormal electrical activity in the septal region of the brain, and that their plasma contains an abnormal protein 'Taraxein'. This serum protein has been claimed to produce schizophrenic symptoms when injected into normal non-schizophrenic individuals. It has also been claimed that when Taraxein was injected into monkeys, the abnormality in electrical activity seen in the septal region in schizophrenics was replicated. Attempts to repeat the induction of psychotic states using serum from schizophrenics under double blind conditions failed, but the serum had been kept for several days and the original group suggested that Taraxein, purported to be a subfraction of gamma G immunoglobulin, would be stable for only a few hours and would then become inactive. The work on monkeys has been replicated successfully by others but subsequent work has cast doubt on the specificity of the findings. These ideas have been developed further by the suggestion that schizophrenia is an autoimmune disease in which it is proposed that autoantibodies might be produced against proteins in the limbic system and might, therefore, interfere with brain activity, ultimately inducing a psychotic state. The latter part of the theory was based on immunofluorescence reported in schizophrenic brains in post-mortem studies, but other workers have been unable to find supporting evidence.

A significant proportion of acutely ill psychotic patients, including those suffering from schizophrenia, have demonstrable histological changes in muscle. In addition, this group of patients has raised levels of two muscle enzymes—creatine phosphokinase and aldolase in plasma. Liberation of creatine phosphokinase may occur as a result of the injection of phenothiazines, but it seems likely now that this can occur in the absence of the use of phenothiazines. The changes are associated with an acute psychosis and are not, therefore, specific to schizophrenia.

Model psychoses and schizophrenia

The experiences provoked by psychotomimetic drugs and by abuse of amphetamines have been considered as possible paradigms for the naturally occurring psychoses.

The hallucinogenic drugs, discussed above in connection with hypotheses for the aetiology of schizophrenia, have provoked interest by virtue of their evoking mental states characterized by changes in mood; distortion of perception, including that of the passage of time; depersonalization and derealization; disorders of thinking; and hallucinations, which are more often visual than auditory. There are considerable interindividual differences between the responses to these drugs and also differences in one individual on separate occasions. Within the usual dose, the condition occurs in clear consciousness.

It is difficult to know whether the similarities or dissimilarities between drug-produced and schizophrenic psychoses should be stressed. Certainly, schizophrenics given hallucinatory compounds recognize the difference between the naturally occurring illness and the drug-produced mental state. Such patients also seem to be more vulnerable to the effects of hallucinogenic drugs and to manifest more severe and more distressing changes than do normal individuals, who more frequently have a pleasant reaction to these substances. If we examine the symptoms usually associated with schizophrenic illness, the psychedelic condition does not mimic it closely in its affective, perceptual or hallucinatory experiences. Some authors have claimed, however, that the effects of hallucinatory drugs are not all that different from the mental states seen in the initial stages of schizophrenia.

No comparison should ignore the fact that drug-induced psychoses are acute phenomena occurring as isolated, explicable and self-limiting phenomena in the context of the security of previous normality and the expectation of subsequent normality. The established schizophrenic has no such secure base—his world has been turned upside-down by disruptive and bewildering catastrophes and, for all we know, earlier 'subthreshold' abnormal experiences.

The similarities between schizophrenic illness and the effects of drugs such as LSD and mescaline are striking enough for us to continue study in this area.

Amphetamine psychoses follow either an acute repeated administration of very large amounts of the drug or a more gradual escalation of the dosage over a longer period. The symptoms of this amphetamine-induced psychosis include persecutory delusions, ideas of reference, changes in body image, hyperactivity and stereotyped movements and behaviour. There is no loss of memory; on the contrary, if anything, recall of events (unlike delirious states—acute brain syndrome) is heightened. There is no disorientation and the condition occurs in clear consciousness.

There are both auditory and visual hallucinations in amphetamine psychoses, and the relative frequency of visual hallucinations—about 50 per cent in one series—has been taken by some to point to significant differences from the schizophrenic syndromes. However, one possible answer to this is the claim that visual hallucinosis is more a feature of the very acute high-dose amphetamine psychosis and is less evident in the syndrome seen following the more gradually induced disorder.

The production of compulsive repetitive movements in amphetamine psychoses is of considerable interest, because similar effects have been seen in animals and the symptoms have been compared with similar occurrences in schizophrenia. Of course, the expression of repetitive behaviour differs from species to species.

The euphoric actions of amphetamines are thought to be caused by the actions on catecholaminergic neurons (possibly in the lateral hypothalamus), and their actions in enhancing locomotor activity are similarly likely to be on this system.

Potentiation of dopaminergic neurons by amphetamines is probably responsible for the stereotyped behaviour, and its psychotogenic actions could also be via these pathways. Amphetamines exacerbate illness in schizophrenics, and the effects of amphetamines in both animals and man are antagonized by phenothiazines.

Antipsychotic drugs

Phenothiazines and other drugs with apparently specific antipsychotic actions in schizophrenia have become the starting point for research into this illness. The rationale parallels that used in the study of the mode of action of antidepressants— that an understanding of a specific antagonist for the symptoms could lead to a greater understanding of the illness.

The proponents of this research are only too aware of its possible main defect. The problem, as in work taking the action of antidepressant drugs as a starting point, is that although a specific antischizophrenic effect may be demonstrated very successfully, the point of action of that effect could be at a distance from the main aetiological change. The rapid advance of the subject might occur only if the drug acted directly on the pathological process. A drug might act on an effect of a pathological process which was several steps away from the central causative process. Antipsychotic drugs such as phenothiazines and butyrophenones interfere with an alarmingly large area of the body's chemistry, and the validity of selecting one of the pharmacological actions may be questionable. It has been suggested by a number of groups that schizophrenia could be due to an increase in activity at dopaminergic synapses and that the antipsychotic action of drugs lies in opposing these changes.

This is an attractive hypothesis, and there have been many other elegant experiments demonstrating that this class of drug blocks dopaminergic receptors. Some do this by antagonizing the effect of dopamine on dopamine-sensitive adenylcyclase at these receptors. This effect correlates well with the clinical efficacy, and the data fit better for dopaminergic than for noradrenergic systems. Further circumstantial evidence has accrued from the demonstration that the preferred molecular configuration of chlorpromazine and of similar drugs can be

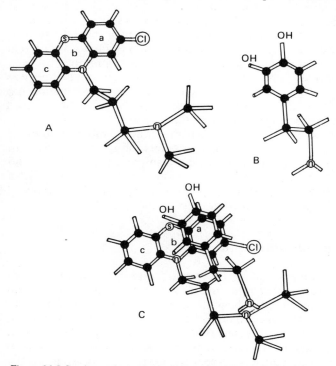

Figure 16.5 Conformations of chlorpromazine (A) and dopamine (B), and their superimposition (C), determined by X-ray crystallographic analysis. The a, b and c in (A) and (C) designate rings. (Reproduced from Horn and Snyder.) From *Foundations of Biochemical Psychiatry*, 1976, by D.S. Segal, J. Yager and J.L. Sullivan, Butterworths

superimposed on that of dopamine (*see Figure 16.5*). (It should be pointed out that chlorpromazine blocks 5-HT and noradrenergic receptors as well as those for dopamine.)

However, if this hypothesis were correct, then it might be expected that the antipsychotic actions of these drugs would correlate well with the Parkinsonian side-effects, because these symptoms are due to antagonism of dopaminergic neurons in the basal nuclei, allowing unopposed cholinergic function. This has not been found to be so—some drugs are notorious for this incidence of Parkinsonian side-effects, while others are virtually, but not completely, free of this activity. This discrepancy has been explained by the observation that the drugs with low Parkinsonian side-effects have their own built-in anticholinergic properties and may, therefore, have blocked their own Parkinsonian side-effects.

The question remains whether schizophrenia could be due to overactivity in dopaminergic neurons other than those in the nigrostriatal pathways. One of the other main dopaminergic pathways is a medial extension of the substantia nigra, whose efferent connections are to the nucleus accumbens, the olfactory tubercle, the interstitial nucleus, the stria terminalis and an area of frontal cortex. Certainly, with three neuroleptics accumulation of the breakdown product of dopamine in the nucleus accumbens is directly proportional to therapeutic potencies, which suggests that their antipsychotic activity could be here.

It seems at the present time that it is most likely that these drugs are acting at dopaminergic sites, but the dopaminergic hypothesis has some unanswered questions which it is not proposed invalidate what has become perhaps the most fruitful line of enquiry. For instance, there is no excess accumulation of homovanillic acid (HVA), the metabolite of dopamine in acute untreated schizophrenics; in fact, accumulation of this compound (when its removal from cerebrospinal fluid was blocked) was lower than normal. One group showed an inverse relationship between HVA accumulation and schizophrenic symptoms. Perhaps the affected neurons constitute too small a proportion of the total.

Prolactin release is inhibited by a dopaminergic pathway in the tuberoinfundibular region and prolactin is present in normal amounts of schizophrenics. In addition, dopaminergic activity is reduced in Parkinsonism, and schizophrenia and ideopathic Parkinsonism can co-exist. Thus, there seems to be little to support a generalized dopaminergic overactivity in schizophrenia. Assuming that the dopamine hypothesis is valid, the defect in function must be localized.

6-Hydroxydopamine and schizophrenia

Stein and Wise have taken a somewhat different tack in their hypothesis of the basis of schizophrenia. They have put forward the idea that the hallucinatory and delusional experiences are secondary phenomena in schizophrenia. The core symptoms, according to them, are loss of emotional reactivity, failure of activity in reward/pleasure centres and of goal directed thinking and activity. Thus, loss of ability to experience pleasure and all its consequences is, in their hypothesis, due to dysfunction in the noradrenergic pathways ascending from the brain-stem up the medial forebrain bundles to the frontal cortex, hypothalamus and limbic system.

An analogue of dopamine, 6-hydroxydopamine, if introduced into the brain, is taken into catecholaminergic neurons and damages or destroys them. Animals subjected to this treatment cease reward self-stimulation, and this effect of

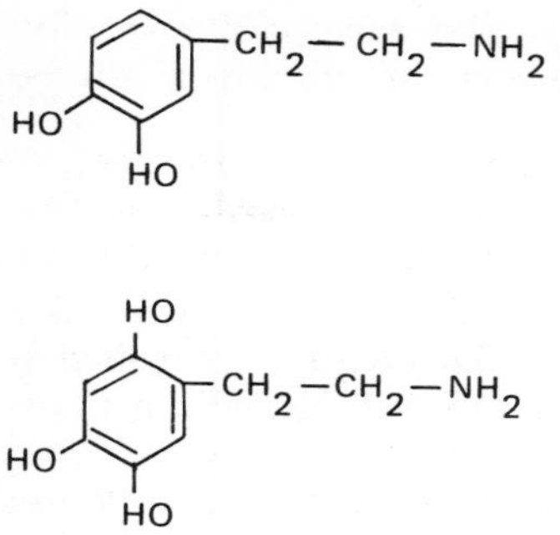

CH$_2$—CH$_2$—NH$_2$ Dopamine

CH$_2$—CH$_2$—NH$_2$ 6—Hydroxydopamine

Figure 16.6 6-Hydroxydopamine

6-hydroxydopamine is antagonized by chlorpromazine. The mode of action of chlorpromazine here is to prevent entry of the compound to the cells, so that 6-hydroxydopamine is unable to exert its noxious influence on these cells. The situation described here might occur in theory if dopamine-β-hydroxylase activity were reduced in schizophrenia. If this enzyme were relatively ineffective, dopamine could accumulate in noradrenergic cells and might be converted to 6-hydroxydopamine. This then is the hypothetical process whereby the noradrenergic reward system might be damaged or ultimately destroyed, according to this hypothesis.

Initial claims that dopamine-β-hydroxylase activity was reduced in schizophrenia have not been confirmed.

Environmental factors in schizophrenia

Environmental factors and the acute episode

LIFE EVENTS

Physiological measures in schizophrenia suggest a state of high arousal. It has now been amply demonstrated that 'independent' life events (events not triggered by the patient's behaviour, etc.) occur excessively frequently in the few weeks preceding an episode of schizophrenia. Drug therapy can offer some but not total protection from such life events, so that despite phenothiazine 'cover' an episode may break through if the trigger is of sufficient intensity. Perhaps schizophrenic patients are aware of this and this in part is responsible for a self-protective recluse-like life where the risk of life-events is reduced.

EMOTIONAL CONTACT WITH RELATIVES AND OTHERS

Patients living with their relatives have a poorer outlook on average than if they are living alone. The presence of a relative may be stressful to them by virtue of the degree of expressed emotion (positive or negative), excessive emotional involvement or a critical attitude. Patients living with relatives which have this 'high expressed emotion' can protect themselves with drugs and/or by keeping their contact to less than 35 hours per week in the same room. It is as though the overinvolvement or critical relation was a chronic stress (in distinction to the acute stress of a life event). There are several strategies employed by clinicians and social workers in this type of family to minimize contact and prevent relapse. Conversely, a warm but not overinvolved or critical relative, friend or employer can be protective in some ways and possibly raise the threshold to illness.

'Antecedent' environmental factors

The birth month of schizophrenics gives an excess in the winter months. This hints at something like a virus or other agent with a seasonal distribution which is acquired in pre-natal or early neonatal life. The seasonal effect is greater in patients with a low incidence of the disease in their family.

Although there is a high degree of concordance in monozygotic twins, why are some symptom-free? The ill twin tends to have the lower birth weight, higher incidence of cyanosis at birth, infantile colic, feeding problems and early illness, which suggests a less robust child which, it might be speculated, could have been exposed to a pathological agent *in utero*.

With monozygotic twins the risk of illness is roughly constant in the co-twin 6 months after the illness of the index twin. However, there is an excess of illness in the co-twin in the first 6 months which is confined to those who were living together—again in accord with the idea of an agent passed from one to the other.

Genetic vulnerability/viral infection theory

Could schizophrenia have some basis like polio or scrapie, which is influenced by genetic predisposition and involves immune/infective mechanisms, or could it be related to the slow virus illnesses with a predilection for neurological tissue? If so, one component would be transmitted genetically and this would be independent of expression of the illness. With regard to this view, it may be relevant that statistically the offspring of a schizophrenic twin have the same incidence of illness as do the offspring of the well monozygotic twin, where the twins are discordant for manifestation of the disease.

The idea of a genetic vulnerability and a viral infection remains an interesting theory, particularly in view of the proposed division by Crow of schizophrenia into Types I and II (*see* below).

Are there two distinct processes in schizophrenia?

It has been known for some time now that many schizophrenic patients suffer neurological loss. This takes the form of increase in the size of the ventricles, or widening of the Sylvian fissure, other fissures and the sulci. This loss of brain tissue is not correlated with age, length of illness, previous ECT treatment or hospitalization. As many as two-thirds of patients show some structural changes in the cerebral ventricles. The ventricular/brain ratio is correlated with deficits in neuropsychological performance. A further significant observation is that there is a poorer response with neuroleptics in patients with enlarged ventricles as compared with those with ventricles of normal size. Intellectual impairment is characteristic of patients who fail to respond to neuroleptics, and disorientation in time in the acute illness predicts a poor long-term outcome.

Negative symptoms correlate with intellectual impairment, with neurological signs, but none of these factors is related to positive symptoms.

About 30 per cent of a group of schizophrenics treated with chlorpromazine had evidence of antinuclear antibodies like the autoimmune disease lupus erythematosus. The EEGs of schizophrenics tend to have desynchronized low-voltage fast activity (possibly of limited importance), but assays of left hemispherical cortical blood flow have given values lower than controls.

Post-mortem findings in schizophrenia have varied between groups, but there are inconsistent reports of increases in dopamine and noradrenaline in the nucleus accumbens, the substantia nigra, the hypothalamus and the limbic system.

It seems to be reasonably well established that in some patients there is an increase in dopamine receptor activity in schizophrenics*. These and other data have led Crow to his Type I, Type II classification of schizophrenia—a scheme which, while posing more questions than answers, is a most attractive hypothesis.

The characteristics of Type I are the florid symptomatology as described by Schneider and others, with acute breakdown (sometimes in the setting of a deficit state) and good response to neuroleptics, and probably associated with dopaminergic supersensitivity and overactivity in one dopaminergic pathway. The Type II syndrome is accompanied by the negative symptoms of the condition (flat effect, poverty of speech, loss of volition), often intellectual impairment, chronic deterioration, poor response to neuroleptics and tissue loss from the brain.

Thus, under this classification there are two processes—one involving dopaminergic overactivity (Type I) and one involving cellular damage (Type II), with overlap between the two in some patients.

It might be speculated that Type II illness exists in simple schizophrenia *de novo*, and that late-onset paranoid illness and hebephenic illness of relatively good prognosis is predominantly Type I. Hebephenic schizophrenics might be a mixture of the two or pass from Type I to Type II.

Opiates and schizophrenia

The present position of endorphins and schizophrenia is unclear. Chronic naltrexone (long-acting opiate agonist) benefited two patients and was of no value in three. The two 'responding patients' were actively hallucinating, whereas the other three were not. Other studies have found endorphins to have apparent positive responses in some or no effect in others. One author has proposed the use of endorphins in acute as against chronic schizophrenia, and that neuroleptics may interfere with their action.

Cerebral laterality and schizophrenia

Several findings point to alterations in lateralization of function in schizophrenia, a subject which will be touched on only briefly here. For instance, 14 of 22 pairs of twins had at least one left-handed individual and the illness was less severe, and the concordance rate was lower than in 8 twins both of whom were right-handed. The importance of these findings has been underlined by the recent finding of Jones on abnormalities in evoked potentials (*see* reading list).

*Some of the patients had had neuroleptics, but in a small drug-free group enhanced binding by dopamine receptors ligands has been found.

Glossary

Drug	UK	USA	Canada	France	Australia	S. Africa	Sweden	Germany
Amitriptyline	Amizol Domical Lentizol Saroten Tryptizol	Elavil Endep	Deprex Elatrol Elavil Levate Mareline Novotriptyn	Elavil	Tryptanol Elavil	Tryptanol	Larozyl	
Clomipramine	Anafranil (Geigy)							
Nortriptyline	Aventyl Allegron	Aventyl		Psychostyl	Nortab	Nortrilin	Noritren Sensaval	Acetexa Nortrieen
Butriptyline	Evandyne							
Desipramine	Pertofran	Pertofrane Norpramin	Pertofrane Norpramin			Despramin Norpramin Quitaxon	Pertofrin	
Doxepin	Sinequan	Adaptin		Quitaxon	Quitaxon			Aponal Sinquan
Flupenthixol	Depixol Fluanxol							
Imipramine	Tofranil CoCaps Imipramine Norpramine Imipramine Berkomine Dimipressin Oppanyl Praminil	Imavate Janimine Presamine SK-pramine	Chemipramine Impranil Novopramine Impril		Censtim Imiprin Iramil Melipramine Prodepress Somipra	Panpramine Thymopramine		
Viloxazine	Vivalan							
Protriptyline	Concordin 5 Concordin 10	Vivactil	Triptil		Triptil			Maximed
Dibenzepin	Noveril							
Iprindol	Prondol							
Dothiepin	Prothiaden							
Trimipramine	Surmontil							Stangyl

Drug	UK	USA	Canada	France	Australia	S. Africa	Sweden	Germany
Opipramol	Insidon							
Maprotiline	Ludiomil						Ensidon	
Tranylcypromine	Parnate	Parnate		Tylciprine				
Phenelzine	Nardil	Nardil		Nardelzine				
Isocarboxazid	Marplan							
Nomifensine	Merital							
Mianserin	Bolvidon Norval							
Zimelidine	Zelmid							
Trazodone	Molipaxin							
Tryptophan	Optimax Pacitron							
Lithium **carbonate**	Camcolit Priadel Phasal Lisconum *Belgium:* Maniprex	Eskalith Lithonate Lithotabs Lithane	Carbolith Lithocarb Lithane	Lithium Oligosol Neurolithium [both gluconates]	Lithicarb	Lithionit (sulphate) Quinonum		Hypronex Lithium Duriles (sulphate) Quinonum
Benzodiazepines								
Bromazepam								
Chlordiazepoxide	Calmoden Librium Tropium *Poland:* Elenium	Libritabs	Chemidipoxide, Corax, C-Tran, Diapax Medilium Nack Novopoxide Protensin Relaxil Solium Trilium Via-Quil				Risolid	
Clorazepate	Tranxene						Tranxilen	Tranxilium
Diazepam	Atensine Tensium Valium Evacalm Sedapam *Poland:* Relanium		Paxel E-Pam Serenack Vivol				Apozepam Stesolid	

Drug	UK	USA	Canada	France	Australia	S. Africa	Sweden	Germany
Lorazepam	Ativan							
Medazepam	Nobrium							
Oxazepam	Serenid Forte *Finland and Norway:* Oxepam *Denmark:* Serepax *Austria:* Praxiten *Belgium, Netherlands and Switzerland:* Seresta	Serex	Serex	Seresta	Adumbran Serepax	Adumbran Serepax	Serepax Sobril	Adumbran Praxitin
Flurazepam	Dalmane					Dalmadorm		
Temazepam	Euhypnos Normison							
Triazolam	Halcion							
Nitrazepam	Mogadon Nitrados Remnos Somnused Surem					Mogadon		
Ketozolam	Anxon							
Clobazam	Frisium							
Clonazepam	Rivotril	Clonopin					Iktorivil	
Lormetazepam	Noctamid							
Phenothiazines								
Chlorpromazine	Amargyl Chloractil Largactil	Chlor-PZ Promachel Promapar Thoradex Thoradex Promachlor Vesprin	Chlor-Promanyl Elmarine Chlorprom-Ez -Ets Onazine Promosol Vesprin		Plegomazine Procalm Promacid Protran Serazone	Klorazin	Hibernal Klorpromex	Megaphen
Fluopromazine	*New Zealand:* Siquil *Italy:* Eliranol *Belgium, Netherlands and Switzerland:* Prazine			Psyquil	Psyquil			
Methotrimeprazine	Veractil	Levoprome	Nozinan	Nozinan	Neurocil	*Norway:* Protacty	Nozinan	Neurogil
Promazine	Sparine		Atarzin Intrazine Promanyl Promazettes Promerezine Pro-Tran		Protactyl		Protactyl	Protactyl
Propiomazine							Propavan	
Prothipendyl	Tolnate	Largon					Propavan	Dominal

Dimethylaminopropyl side-chain

Drug	UK	USA	Canada	France	Australia	S. Africa	Sweden	Germany
Piperidine side-chain								
Pericyazine	Neulactil		Neuleptil	Neuleptil				Aolept
Piperacetazine		Quide	Quide					
Thioridazine	Melleril	Mellaril	Mellaril Novoridazine Thoril				Mallorol	Melleretten
Piperazine side-chain								
Acetophenazine		Tintal					Tindala	
Butaperazine		Repoise						Randolectil
Carphenazine		Proketazine						
Fluphenazine	Modecate Moditen Motipress	Permitil Prolixin			Anatensol Sevinol		Pacinol Siqualone	Dapotum Lyogen Omca
Perphenazine	Fentazin	Trilafon	Trilafon	Trilifan	Trilafon	Trilafon	Trilafon	Decentan
Pipothiazine	Piportil-L4							
Prochlorperazine	Stemetil							
Thiethylperazine	Torecan							
Thioproperazine	Majeptil							Majeptil Jatoneural
Trifluoperazine	Amylozine spansule *Stelazine		Chemflurazine Clinazine Fluazine Novoflurazine Pentazine Solazine Trifluoper-Ez-Ets Triflurin Terfluzine	Terfluzin	Calmazine Terfluzin		Terfluzin	
Thioxanthenes								
Chlorprothixene	Taractan *Denmark:* Truxal		Tarasan		Truxal	Truxal	Truxal	Truxal Truxaletten
Flupenthixol	Depixol Fluanxol		Fluanxol Depot	Emergil Fluanxol Retard		Fluanxol Depot	Fluanxol Depot	Fluanxol Depot
Thiothixene	Narvane							Orbinamon
Clopenthixol	Clopixol						Cisordinol Depot	Ciatyl Depot
Butyrophenones and related compounds								
Benperidol	Anquil			Frénactil				Glianimon
Droperidol	Droleptan	Inapsine	Inapsine			Inapsin	Dridol	
Fluspiriline	Redeptin *Belgium:* Imap							Imap

Drug	UK	USA	Canada	France	Australia	S. Africa	Sweden	Germany
Haloperidol	Haldol Serenace							
Penfluridol	*Belgium*: Semap			Opiran				
Pimozide	Orap							
Trifluperidol	Triperidol							

Reading list

ADOLFSON, R., GOTTFRIES, C.G., ROOS, E.E. and WINBLAD, B. (1979). Changes in the brain catecholamines in patients with dementia of Alzheimer type. *Brit. J. Psychiat.*, **135**, 216–223

AIDLEY, D.J. (1978). *The Physiology of Excitable Cells*. Cambridge University Press, Cambridge

BADAWY, A.A.B. (1978). The Metabolism of Alcohol, In: *Clinics in Endocrinology and Metabolism*, 7(2), 247–267

BARCHAS, J.D., BERGER, P.A., CIARANELLO, R.D. and ELLIOTT, G.R. (Eds) (1977). *Psychopharmacology*. Oxford University Press, New York

BARR, M. (1979). *The Human Nervous System*. Harper and Row, Hagerstown

BERTELSEN, A., HARVALD, B. and HUAGE, M. (1977). A Danish twin study of manic depressive disorders. *Brit. J. Psychiat.*, **130**, 330–351

BEUMONT, P.J.V. (1979). The endocrinology of psychiatry, In: *Recent Advances in Clinical Psychiatry*, Vol. 3, pp. 185–224. Ed. K. Granville-Grossman. Churchill Livingstone, Edinburgh, London and New York

BIRLEY, J.L.T. and BROWN, G.W. (1970). Crisis and life changes preceding the onset or relapse of acute schizophrenia: clinical aspects. *Brit. J. Psychiat.*, **116**, 327–333

BRIERLEY, J.B. (1977). Neuropathology of amnesic states. In: *Amnesia*: Clinical Psychological and Medicological Aspects, 2nd edn, pp. 199–223. Eds C.W.M. Whitty and O.L. Zangwill. Butterworths, London

CHECKLEY, S.A. (1980). Neuroendocrine tests of monoamine function in man: a review of basic theory and its application to the study of depressive illness. *Psychol. Med.*, **10**, 35–73

COOPER, J.R., BLOOM, F.E. and ROTH, R.H. (1978). *Biochemical Basis of Neuropharmacology*. Oxford University Press, Oxford

CORNWALL, G.C. and WESTERMARK, P. (1980). Senile amyeloidosis, In: A protean manifestation of the ageing process. *J. Clinical Pathology*, **33**, 1146–1152

CRAMMER, J., BARRACLOUGH, B. and HEINE, B. (Eds) (1978). *The Use of Drugs in Psychiatry*. Gaskell Books, Headley Bros Ltd., Ashford, Kent

CROWE, T.J. (1980). Molecular Pathology of Schizophrenia, more than one disease process? *Brit. Med. J.*, **280**, 66–68

CROWE, T.J., JOHNSTONE, E.C. and OWEN, F. (1979). Research into schizophrenia, In: *Recent Advances in Clinical Psychiatry*, Vol. 3, pp. 1–36. Ed. K. Granville Grossman. Churchill Livingstone, Edinburgh, London and New York

FOTTRELL, E. (1981). Violent behaviour by psychiatric patients. *B.J. Hosp. Med.*, **25**, 28–37

GAZZANIGA, M.S. (1974). Cerebral dominance viewed as a decision system. In: *Hemisphere Function in the Human Brain*, pp. 367–380. Eds S. Dimond and J.G. Beaumont. Elek Science, London

GOODMAN, L.S. and GILMAN, A. (Eds) (1900). *The Pharmacological Basis of Therapeutics*, 5th edn. Macmillan, New York (Baillière Tindall, London)

GOTTFRIES, C.G. (1980). Biochemistry of dementia and normal ageing. *T.I.N.S.*, **3**, 55–57

GRAY, J.A. (1979). Anxiety and the brain. Not by neurochemistry alone. *Psychol. Med.*, **9**, 605–609

HEMMINGS, G. (Ed.) (1980). *Biochemistry of Schizophrenia and Addiction*. M.P.P. Press, London

HESTON, L.L. (1970). The genetics of schizophrenia and schizoid disease. *Science, N.Y.*, **167**, 249–256

JACQUET, Y.F. (1979). β-Endorphin and ACTH-opioid peptides with coordinated roles in the regulation of behaviour. *T.I.N.S.*, **2**, 140–143

JENNETT, B. (1980). Research in brain trauma. *T.I.N.S.*, **3**(10), I–IV

KANDEL, E.R. and SCHWARTZ, J.H. (Eds.) (1981). *Principles of Neural Science*. Edward Arnold, London

KATZ, B. (1966). *Nerve Muscle and Synapse*. McGraw-Hill, New York

KAY, D.W.K. (1978). Assessment of familial risks in the functional psychoses and their application in geriatric counselling. *Brit. J. Psychiat.*, **133**, 385–403

KILOH, L.G., McCOMAS, A.J., OSSELTON, J.W. and UPTON, A.R.M. (1981). *Clinical Electroencephalography*, 4th Edn. Butterworths, London

KOLATA, G.R. (1981). Clues to the cause of senile dementia. *Science, N.Y.*, **4**, 1032–1033

KUHAR, M.J. (1981). Radiographic localisation of drug and neurotransmitter receptors in the brain. *T.I.N.S.*, **4**, 60–63

LADER, M.H. (Ed.) (1970). *Studies of Anxiety*. W.P.A. and R.M.P.A. Publications, Headley Bros Ltd., Ashford, Kent

LADER, M.H. (1975). *The Psychophysiology of Mental Illness*. Routledge and Kegan Paul, London and Boston

LEONARD, B.E. (1981a). Speculation on the biochemical basis of depression. *Royal Society of Medicine. International Congress and Symposium Series*, No. 46, pp. 3–16

LEONARD, B.E. (1981b). Pharmacological properties of some second generation antidepressants. *Neuropharmacol.*, **19**, 1175–1184

MANN, D.M.A., LINCOLN, J., YATES, P.O., STAMP, J.E. and TOPER, S. (1980). Changes in the monoamine containing neurons of the human CNS in senile dementia. *Brit. J. Psychiat.*, **136**, 533–541

PAYKEL, E.S. (1979). Causal relationships between clinical depression and life events; In: *Stress and Mental Disorder*, pp. 71–86. Ed. J.E. Barrett. Raven Press, New York

PAYKEL, E.S. and COPPEN, A. (Eds) (1979). *Psychopharmacology of Affective Disorders*. British Association for Psychopharmacology Monograph. Oxford University Press, Oxford

PAYKEL, E.S. (Ed.) (1982). *Handbook of Affective Disorders*. Churchill Livingstone, Edinburgh, London and New York

PRIBAM, K.H. (1971). *Languages of the Brain: Experimental Paradoxes and Principles in Neuropsychology*. Prentice-Hall, Englewood Cliffs, N.J.

REVELEY, A. and MURRAY, R.M. (1980). The genetic contribution to the functional psychoses. *Brit. J. Hosp. Med.*, **24**, 166–170

RICHTER, D. (Ed.) (1980). *Addiction and Brain Damage*, Chapters 10–11. Croom Helm, London

ROSENTHAL, D. *et al.* (1971). The adopted-away offspring of schizophrenics. *Am. J. Psychiat.*, **128**, 307–311

SCHOU, M. and AMDISEN, A. (1971). The practical management of lithium treatment. *Brit. J. Hosp. Med.*, **6**, 53–60

SEARLE, A. (1977). A review of right hemisphere linguistic capabilities. *Psychol. Bull.*, **84**(3), 503–528

SHAW, D.M. (1977). The practical management of affective disorders. *Brit. J. Psychiat.*, **130**, 432–451

SHAW, S.H., MARJOT, D.H., PUXON, M. and ELLIOTT, F.A. (1982). Special Report: Violence. *Practitioner*, **226**, 281–304

SHIELDS, J. (Ed.) (1977). High risk for schizophrenia: genetic considerations. *Psychol. Med.*, **7**, 7–10

SHIELDS, J. and SLATER, E. (1975). Genetic aspects of schizophrenia, In: *Contemporary Psychiatry*. Eds T. Silverstone and B. Barraclough. Headley Bros Ltd., Ashford, Kent

SILVERSIDE, T. and TURNER, P. (1974). *Drug Treatment in Psychiatry*. Routledge and Kegan Paul, London and Boston

SLATER, P.J.B. (1980). Ethological approach to aggression. *Psychol. Med.*, **10**, 607–609

SPOKES, E.G.S. (1980). Neurochemistry of Huntingdon's Chorea. *T.I.N.S.*, **3**, 115–118

STORR, A. (1970). *Human Aggression*. Penguin Books, Harmondsworth

TENNENT, T.G. (1971). The dangerous offender. *Brit. J. Hosp. Med.*, **6**, 269–274

TYRER, P. (1976). *The Role of Bodily Feelings in Anxiety*. Institute of Psychiatry Maudsley Monograph. Oxford University Press, Oxford

TYRER, P. (1979). Anxiety states. In: *Recent Advances in Clinical Psychiatry*, Vol. 3, pp. 161–184. Ed. K. Granville-Grossman. Churchill Livingstone, Edinburgh, London and New York

TYRRELL, D.A.J. (1981). Schizophrenia and virus infection. *T.I.N.S.*, **4**(4), VII–IX

VAUGHAN, C.E. and LEFF, J.P. (1979). The influence of family and social factors on the course of schizophrenia, In: *Current Themes in Psychiatry*, Vol. 2, pp. 257–270. Eds R.N. Gaind and B.L. Hudson. Macmillan Press Ltd., London

VINGOE, F.J. (1981). *Clinical Psychology and Medicine: An Interdisciplinary Approach*. Oxford University Press, Oxford

WISINIEWSKI, H.M. and IQBAL, K. (1980). Ageing of the brain and dementia. *T.I.N.S.*, **3**, 226–228

Index